Lippincott's Primary Care

Rheumatology

EDITORS

Dennis W. Boulware, MD
Professor of Medicine
University of Alabama at Birmingham
Chief of Rheumatology
Hawaii Permanente Medical Group
Honolulu, HI

Gustavo R. Heudebert, MD
Division of General Internal Medicine
The University of Alabama at Birmingham
Birmingham, AL

 Wolters Kluwer | Lippincott Williams & Wilkins
Health

Philadelphia • Baltimore • New York • London
Buenos Aires • Hong Kong • Sydney • Tokyo

Acquisitions Editor: Sonya Seigafuse
Product Manager: Kerry Barrett
Production Manager: Alicia Jackson
Senior Manufacturing Manager: Benjamin Rivera
Marketing Manager: Kim Schonberger
Design Coordinator: Doug Smock
Production Service: Aptara, Inc.

© 2012 by LIPPINCOTT WILLIAMS & WILKINS, a WOLTERS KLUWER business
Two Commerce Square
2001 Market Street
Philadelphia, PA 19103 USA
LWW.com

Printed in China

ISBN-13: 978-1-60913-808-0
ISBN-10: 1-60913-808-2
Library of Congress Cataloging-in-Publication Data
available upon request

Care has been taken to confirm the accuracy of the information presented and to describe generally accepted practices. However, the authors, editors, and publisher are not responsible for errors or omissions or for any consequences from application of the information in this book and make no warranty, expressed or implied, with respect to the currency, completeness, or accuracy of the contents of the publication. Application of the information in a particular situation remains the professional responsibility of the practitioner.

The authors, editors, and publisher have exerted every effort to ensure that drug selection and dosage set forth in this text are in accordance with current recommendations and practice at the time of publication. However, in view of ongoing research, changes in government regulations, and the constant flow of information relating to drug therapy and drug reactions, the reader is urged to check the package insert for each drug for any change in indications and dosage and for added warnings and precautions. This is particularly important when the recommended agent is a new or infrequently employed drug.

Some drugs and medical devices presented in the publication have Food and Drug Administration (FDA) clearance for limited use in restricted research settings. It is the responsibility of the health care providers to ascertain the FDA status of each drug or device planned for use in their clinical practice.

To purchase additional copies of this book, call our customer service department at (800) 638-3030 or fax orders to (301) 223-2320. International customers should call (301) 223-2300.

Visit Lippincott Williams & Wilkins on the Internet: at LWW.com. Lippincott Williams & Wilkins customer service representatives are available from 8:30 am to 6 pm, EST.

10 9 8 7 6 5 4 3 2 1

Dedication

Where would we be without our beloved wives, Diane Boulware and Carmen Heudebert, and our families? For their endless love, support, patience, understanding, and tolerance of us and our absences as we developed this book and our careers, this book is dedicated to all of them.

Contributors

Graciela S. Alarcón, MD
Jane Knight Lowe Chair of Medicine in
  Rheumatology, Emeritus
Division of Clinical Immunology and
  Rheumatology
The University of Alabama at Birmingham
Birmingham, AL

Seth M. Berney, MD
Department of Rheumatology
Louisiana State University
Shreveport, LA

Dennis W. Boulware, MD
Professor of Medicine
University of Alabama at Birmingham
Chief of Rheumatology
Hawaii Permanente Medical Group
Honolulu, HI

S. Louis Bridges Jr, MD, PhD
Marguerite Jones Harbert-Gene V. Ball, MD,
  Professor of Medicine
University of Alabama at Birmingham
Birmingham, AL

Amy C. Cannella, MD
Section of Rheumatology
University of Nebraska Medical Center
Omaha, NE

W. Winn Chatham, MD
Division of Clinical Immunology and
  Rheumatology
The University of Alabama at Birmingham
Birmingham, AL

Gregory A. Clines, MD, PhD
Assistant Professor of Medicine and Cell Biology
The University of Alabama at Birmingham
Endocrinology Section, Birmingham VA Medical
  Center
Birmingham, AL

Carol Croft, MD
Professor of Medicine
Division of General Internal Medicine
University of Texas-Southwestern
Dallas, TX

Carlos A. Estrada, MD, MS
Professor of Medicine
Director, Division of General Internal Medicine
University of Alabama at Birmingham
Fellowship Director, Birmingham VA National
  Quality Scholars Program
Birmingham, AL

Barri Fessler, MD, MSPH
Associate Professor of Medicine
Division of Clinical Immunology and
  Rheumatology
University of Alabama at Birmingham
Birmingham, AL

Angelo Gaffo, MD, MSPH
Division of Clinical Immunology and
  Rheumatology
The University of Alabama at Birmingham
Birmingham, AL

Gustavo R. Heudebert, MD
Division of General Internal Medicine
The University of Alabama at Birmingham
Birmingham, AL

Katherine Holman, MD
Fellow
Division of Infectious Diseases
Department of Medicine
University of Alabama at Birmingham
Birmingham, AL

Laura B. Hughes, MD, MSPH
Division of Clinical Immunology and
  Rheumatology
The University of Alabama at Birmingham
Birmingham, AL

Bao Quynh N. Huynh, MD
Second Year Fellow in the Division of
  Rheumatology and Clinical Immunology
University of Alabama at Birmingham
Birmingham, AL

Kristin M. Ingraham, DO, MBA
Lehigh Valley Health Network
Allentown, PA

William F. Iobst, MD
Vice President, Academic Affairs
American Board of Internal Medicine
Philadelphia, PA

Arthur Kavanaugh, MD
Professor of Medicine
Director, Center for Innovative Therapy
Division of Rheumatology, Allergy, and
    Immunology
Department of Medicine
The University of California at San Diego
San Diego, CA

Michael Lockshin, MD
Professor of Medicine and Obstetrics/Gynecology,
    Weill Cornell Medical College
Director, Barbara Volcker Center for Women and
    Rheumatic Disease and Co-Director, Mary
    Kirkland Center for Lupus Research
Hospital for Special Surgery-Cornell
New York, NY

Carlos J. Lozada, MD
Professor of Clinical Medicine
Director, Rheumatology Fellowship Program
University of Miami Miller School of Medicine
Miami, FL

Leann Maska, MD
Rheumatology Fellow
Division of Rheumatology and Immunology
University of Nebraska Medical Center
Omaha, NE

Ted R. Mikuls, MD
Division of Rheumatology
University of Nebraska Medical Center
Omaha, NE

Frederick W. Miller, MD, PhD
Chief, Environmental Autoimmunity Group
Office of Clinical Research
NIEHS/NIH
Bethesda, MD

Sarah L. Morgan, MD, RD, FADA, FACP, CCD
Professor of Nutrition Sciences and Medicine
Medical Director, UAB Osteoporosis Prevention and
    Treatment Clinic
The University of Alabama at Birmingham
Birmingham, AL

Iris Navarro-Millán, MD
Rheumatology Fellow
Division of Clinical Immunology and
    Rheumatology
The University of Alabama at Birmingham
Birmingham, AL

James R. O'Dell, MD
Division of Rheumatology & Immunology
Department of Internal Medicine
University of Nebraska Medical Center
Omaha, NE

Maika Onishi, MD
Medical Student
University of California, San Diego School of Medicine
San Diego, CA

Michelle A. Petri, MD
Division of Rheumatology
Johns Hopkins Hospital
Baltimore, MD

Zachary M. Pruhs, MD
Division of Rheumatology & Immunology
Department of Internal Medicine
University of Nebraska Medical Center
Omaha, NE

Martin Rodriguez, MD
Assistant Professor of Medicine
Division of Infectious Diseases
The University of Alabama at Birmingham
Birmingham, AL

Kenneth G. Saag, MD, MSc
Jane Knight Lowe Professor of Medicine
Director, Center for Outcomes Effectiveness
    Research and Education (COERE) and Center for
    Education and Research on Therapeutics (CERTs)
    of Musculoskeletal Disorders
Division of Clinical Immunology and
    Rheumatology
The University of Alabama at Birmingham
Birmingham, AL

Terry Shaneyfelt, MD, MPH
Chief, General Medicine
Birmingham VA Medical Center
Associate Professor of Medicine
UAB Department of Medicine
Birmingham, AL

Jerome Van Ruiswyk, MD, MS
Division of General Internal Medicine
Professor of Medicine
Medical College of Wisconsin
Zablocki VA Medical Center
Milwaukee, WI

Mary S. Walton, MD
Fellow, Division of Rheumatology and Immunology
Center of Excellence for Arthritis and
    Rheumatology
Louisiana State University Health Sciences Center
School of Medicine
Shreveport, LA

Irene Z. Whitt, MD
Staff Clinician
NIH | NIEHS | EAG
Bethesda, MD

Lisa L. Willett, MD
Division of General Internal Medicine
Associate Professor of Medicine
The University of Alabama at Birmingham
Birmingham, AL

Introduction to Lippincott's Primary Care Series

Welcome to Lippincott's Primary Care Series. The intended goal of this series is to help assist you in all of the use-case scenarios that you might encounter each day.

In this product, <u>Primary Care Rheumatology</u>, you will find:

1. **Book:** The book contains both bulleted points for quick look-up access when you need an answer right away, as well as longer text for the occasions when you need a little more information.

   Additionally we have included pedagogy to highlight certain aspects of the text. These elements include:

 Patient Assessment—Quick reference for the physical examination

 Not to Be Missed—Things to watch out for or possible diagnoses to keep in mind during the examination

 When to Refer—When to suggest further options to your patient

 Patient Education Information Available Online

2. **Website** that includes:
   - Fully searchable text of the book
   - Image bank that can be downloadable into PowerPoint for presentations
   - PDF downloadable Patient Information Sheets

3. **Anatomical Chart for Your Office**

We certainly hope this product is useful and meets your needs.

Please look for other titles in the Lippincott's Primary Care Series.

Preface

Current clinic life for a primary care clinician is fast paced and multidimensional requiring the clinician to manage a host of clinical problems quickly, effectively, and efficiently. The prevalence and scope of arthritis and musculoskeletal problems are large and expected to increase in the future as the world's population ages and life expectancy lengthens. Today's primary care clinicians are expected to manage more clinical problems for more people and with improved outcomes in the future making reliable, factual, practical, and easily accessible resources a key tool for their clinics.

To meet the anticipated needs of the busy primary care clinician, this book is formatted to allow the clinician quick and easy access to reliable and practical information. The opening chapter focuses on the usefulness and pitfalls of the clinical presentation and physical examination; it describes a systematic yet efficient approach leading to the correct diagnoses of musculoskeletal disorders. The following chapters are organized by common clinical complaints of undiagnosed clinical problems like the painful knee, painful feet, and neck or low back pain as well as common musculoskeletal diagnoses like osteoarthritis, gout, or rheumatoid arthritis. The final chapters address special diagnostic and therapeutic considerations such as use of the laboratory, monitoring patients on disease modifying antirheumatic drugs, and arthrocentesis and injection.

Each chapter is formatted on a common template such that the reader can consistently find information on clinical presentation, the physical examination, diagnostic studies, treatment options, and the clinical course or outcome in a common location within each chapter. Tables and illustrations are used liberally to make information retrieval quicker and easier. All chapters were written and edited by a team comprising experienced clinical rheumatologists and primary care physicians.

We appreciate immensely the time and efforts of our many authors who contributed toward this new textbook and provided the expertise, knowledge, skills, and clinical judgment for the benefit of all patients.

Dennis W. Boulware, MD
Gustavo R. Heudebert, MD

Acknowledgments

This book is the outcome of a collaborative effort from many people. Our deepest appreciation is extended to Lisa Consoli, Developmental Editor, for her guidance and ability to keep us working at a productive pace through the gestational period of this book. The "heat and pressure" was maintained at an optimal balance to prevent burn out or worse yet, failure to produce. We also want to recognize and extend our appreciation to Sonya Seigafuse, Senior Acquisitions Editor, and to Kerry Barrett, Senior Product Manager, for extending this opportunity to us and assisting us in creating this textbook. Finally, we are indebted to our many contributing authors for their contribution of their expertise, time, and efforts in writing this book.

Contents

Contributors   v

Preface   xi

Acknowledgments   xiii

Section 1   Introduction to the Rheumatic Diseases   1

CHAPTER 1:   **Evaluation of Patients with Rheumatic Diseases**   3
Carlos A. Estrada and Gustavo R. Heudebert

Section 2   Sport-Related, Occupational, and Other Regional Pain Syndromes   9

CHAPTER 2:   **Neck Pain**   11
Jerome Van Ruiswyk

CHAPTER 3:   **Low Back Pain and Lumbar Stenosis**   23
Lisa L. Willett

CHAPTER 4:   **Shoulder Pain**   30
Dennis W. Boulware

CHAPTER 5:   **Painful Feet**   37
Dennis W. Boulware and Gustavo R. Heudebert

CHAPTER 6:   **Mechanical Disorders of the Knee**   48
Dennis W. Boulware

CHAPTER 7:   **Hip Pain**   55
Carol Croft

CHAPTER 8:   **Sports-Related Conditions and Injuries**   66
Lisa L. Willett

Section 3   Specific Rheumatic Diseases: Diagnosis and Treatment   75

CHAPTER 9:   **Rheumatoid Arthritis, Including Sjögren's Syndrome**   77
Zachary M. Pruhs, James R. O'Dell, and Ted R. Mikuls

CHAPTER 10:   **The Seronegative Spondyloarthropathies   95**
Dennis W. Boulware

CHAPTER 11:   **Systemic Lupus Erythematosus   103**
Michelle A. Petri

CHAPTER 12:   **Raynaud's Phenomenon and Systemic Sclerosis   111**
Laura B. Hughes and Barri Fessler

CHAPTER 13:   **Inflammatory Myopathies: Polymyositis, Dermatomyositis, and Related Conditions   118**
Irene Z. Whitt and Frederick W. Miller

CHAPTER 14:   **Vasculitis   132**
Bao Quynh N. Huynh and S. Louis Bridges, Jr

CHAPTER 15:   **Giant Cell Arteritis and Polymyalgia Rheumatica   140**
Angelo Gaffo

CHAPTER 16:   **Overlap Syndromes and Unclassified or Undifferentiated Connective Tissue Disease   150**
Iris Navarro-Millán and Graciela S. Alarcón

CHAPTER 17:   **Fibromyalgia   158**
Graciela S. Alarcón

CHAPTER 18:   **Pregnancy and Rheumatic Diseases   167**
Michael Lockshin

Section 4   Osteoarthritis and Metabolic Bone and Joint Disease   171

CHAPTER 19:   **Osteoarthritis   173**
Mary S. Walton, Carlos J. Lozada, and Seth M. Berney

CHAPTER 20:   **Gout and Crystal-Induced Arthropathies   183**
Angelo Gaffo

CHAPTER 21:   **Osteopenic Bone Diseases and Osteonecrosis   199**
Kenneth G. Saag, Gregory A. Clines, and Sarah L. Morgan

CHAPTER 22: **Arthropathies Associated with Systemic Diseases 223**
Leann Maska and Amy C. Cannella

Section 5 Infectious Arthritis 237

CHAPTER 23: **Bacterial Arthritis 239**
Arthur Kavanaugh and Maika Onishi

CHAPTER 24: **Lyme Disease 247**
William F. Iobst and Kristin M. Ingraham

CHAPTER 25: **Viral Arthritis 257**
Katherine Holman and Martin Rodriguez

Section 6 Special Diagnostic and Therapeutic Conditions 267

CHAPTER 26: **Use of the Laboratory in Diagnosing Rheumatic Disorders 269**
Terry Shaneyfelt and Gustavo R. Heudebert

CHAPTER 27: **Techniques of Arthrocentesis 274**
Dennis W. Boulware

CHAPTER 28: **Monitoring of Patients on Antirheumatic Therapy 280**
W. Winn Chatham

INDEX 297

Introduction to the Rheumatic Diseases

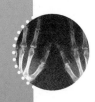

Chapter 1

Evaluation of Patients with Rheumatic Diseases

Carlos A. Estrada and
Gustavo R. Heudebert

Evaluation of Patients with Rheumatic Diseases

Carlos A. Estrada and Gustavo R. Heudebert

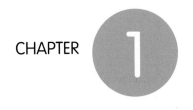

A 24-year-old female comes to the Emergency Department with a 3-day history of pain in the right knee that resolved in 48 hours, followed by pain in her left wrist (migratory arthritis). She has also noticed difficulty holding to flatware on her right hand (tenosynovitis). She noticed onset of symptoms shortly after her menses (seen in disseminated gonococcal infection). Physical examination reveals pain with motion of the left wrist with a thickened synovium; flexion of digits is tender at the right hand (tenosynovitis), however, wrist flexion is not painful. There are a few pustules noted in the left forearm and right foot (arthritis–dermatitis syndrome).

Approach to the Patient with Articular Complaints

CLINICAL PRESENTATION

The clinical presentation of rheumatic diseases is framed on the unique patient's background including age, gender, ethnicity, associated conditions, family history, and habits. Such characteristics can provide useful clues for patients presenting with signs or symptoms consistent with a rheumatic disease. We will consider these characteristics separately, consider mostly adult patients, organize on the basis of etiologic causes, and provide examples. We recognize that typical patterns occur in a few instances; however, we present a framework to efficiently recognize disease patterns. Table 1.1 summarizes the patient's background and common clinical entities.

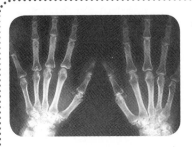

PATIENT ASSESSMENT

- Determine the pattern of joint involvement:
  - Number of joints involved: monoarticular, oligoarticular, polyarticular (>3 joints)
  - Evolution of involvement: additive, migratory
  - Anatomic location: axial, peripheral
  - Symmetry: symmetric, asymmetric
- Determine presence of inflammation:
  - Joints, tendon insertion, synovium

(Continued)

Patient's Background

Age

Crystal-induced arthropathies (gout and pseudogout) can present at any age; although, pseudogout usually presents in the fifth or sixth decade of life. Gout diagnosed in the twenties should raise the suspicion of lead exposure (saturnine gout), increased endogenous production of uric acid (e.g., lymphoproliferative disorder), or an inherent defect of production or excretion of uric acid.

Osteoarthritis (OA) usually presents in individuals older than 50 years of age. OA can be diagnosed in younger patients with past trauma (e.g., gymnasts) or in the familial form of the disease.

The infectious etiology of arthritis varies based on age. *H. influenza* arthritis presents almost exclusively in children, whereas gonococcal arthritis is diagnosed almost exclusively in sexually active individuals <40 years of age. Older patients are more likely to have comorbidities or underlying articular diseases such as OA or joint replacement. The affected joints are more vulnerable to synovial invasion, especially in the presence of bacteremia.

Ankylosing spondylitis, psoriatic arthritis, Reiter's syndrome, and reactive arthritis (seronegative spondyloarthropathies) are more commonly seen in

PATIENT ASSESSMENT (*Continued*)

- Determine pattern of muscle involvement:
  - Proximal versus distal
  - Painful versus painless
- Careful neurological examination for patients with muscular complaints
- Careful assessment of the skin, eyes, and mucous membranes

Table 1.1 Patient's Background and Diagnosis of Patients Presenting with Articular Complaints

	FEMALE	MALE	AFRICAN–AMERICAN	WHITES
Age ≤40 y	Takayasu's arteritis, SLE, SS	Reiter's syndrome, AS	Sarcoidosis	Reiter's syndrome, AS
Age ≥50 y	RA, OA, GCA	Gout, pseudogout		OA, GCA

AS, ankylosing spondylitis; GCA, giant cell arteritis; OA, osteoarthritis; RA, rheumatoid arthritis; SLE, systemic lupus erythematosus; SS, systemic sclerosis.

young adults. Systemic sclerosis presents in the third and fourth decades of life. Systemic lupus erythematosus (SLE) mostly affects women during their reproductive years. Rheumatoid arthritis (RA) presents in the fourth and fifth decades of life.

Systemic vasculitis exhibits a wide range of age distribution. For example, Henoch-Schönlein purpura is seen mostly in children (some present in their twenties), Takayasu's arteritis presents in young females, giant cell arteritis mostly occurs in the elderly, and polymyalgia rheumatica is seldom seen in individuals <50 years of age.

Gender

The best known rheumatic diseases with female predilection are SLE and systemic sclerosis. Other conditions with female predominance include Takayasu's arteritis, giant cell arteritis, Sjögren syndrome, and rheumatoid arthritis. However, the gender difference in RA is less prominent among older patients. Rheumatic conditions with male predominance include gout, Reiter's syndrome, and ankylosing spondylitis. Most of the systemic vasculitides exhibit a small male preponderance.

Ethnicity

A clear ethnic predilection is seen in few rheumatic disorders. More common in whites are the HLA-B27-positive seronegative spondyloarthropathies (Reiter's syndrome and ankylosing spondylitis), giant cell arteritis, and OA. Sarcoidosis is more common in young blacks, at least in the United States. For example, sarcoidosis should be considered in a young black patient presenting with ankle arthralgias. Takayasu's arteritis tends to be present in women of Asian descent. Behçet's disease is more common in the Mediterranean basin, especially among Turkish people. Familial Mediterranean fever is seen more commonly in individuals from the Middle East.

Patients with rheumatic conditions can present with a myriad of complaints. Symptoms can be localized and specific for a certain diagnosis; however, symptoms can be ill-defined and physical findings subtle on many occasions. Rheumatic diseases lend themselves well to a systematic approach of assessment and diagnosis. The patient's background, as previously mentioned, can provide useful clues. The pattern of joint involvement, the presence of inflammation (see physical findings below), and signs and symptoms in other organs can also guide the differential diagnosis.

Symptomatology
Pattern of Joint Involvement

A summary of typical patterns of joint involvement and certain diagnosis is included in Table 1.2. The number of joints involved, evolution of joint involvement, anatomic location of joints, and symmetry are important features in the history and physical examination of patients with joint complaints.

Table 1.2 Pattern of Joint Involvement and Diagnosis

	AXIAL	PERIPHERAL	ADDITIVE	MIGRATORY	SYMMETRIC	ASYMMETRIC
Mono-	OA	Gout, OA				
Oligo-	Reiter's Syndrome. AS		Gonococci, rheumatic fever	Gonococci, viral		Reiter's syndrome, AS
Poly-		SLE, RA, SS, psoriatic	RA, rheumatic fever	Gonococci, viral	SLE, RA, SS, psoriatic	Reiter's syndrome, AS

AS, ankylosing spondylitis; OA, osteoarthritis; RA, rheumatoid arthritis; SLE, systemic lupus erythematosus; SS, systemic sclerosis.

Joint involvement can be monoarticular (one joint), oligoarticular or pauci-articular (two to three joints), or polyarticular (>3 joints). In general, monoarticular involvement is characteristic of bacterial infections, crystal-induced disease, and trauma. Oligoarticular involvement is seen in patients with seronegative spondyloarthropathies and juvenile RA. Finally, polyarthritis is typical in patients with adult onset RA and frequently seen in patients with SLE and systemic sclerosis.

The evolution of joint involvement can be additive or migratory. Additive refers when a second joint becomes affected while the first one is still involved—characteristic of RA and Reiter's syndrome. Migratory refers when another joint becomes affected after resolution of the last one—characteristic of gonococcal and viral arthritis.

The anatomic location of joints can be broadly divided as axial or peripheral. The joints of the axial skeleton include the spine, sacroiliac, sternoclavicular, acromioclavicular, shoulder, and hip joints. Seronegative spondyloarthropathies and osteonecrosis typically involve the axial skeleton. The joints of the peripheral skeleton include the joints distal to the elbows and knees—characteristic of RA and many of the connective-tissue diseases. Furthermore, distinct joints can help in the differential diagnosis. For example, bilateral hand involvement of the metacarpophalangeal (MCP) and proximal interphalangeal (PIP) joints is characteristic of RA, whereas involvement of the distal interphalangeal (DIP) joints is more common in OA and psoriatic arthritis. The combination of an enthesitis (e.g., Achilles tendonitis, plantar fasciitis) with sacroiliitis should raise the suspicion of Reiter's syndrome.

Joints affected can be symmetric or asymmetric. Monoarticular and oligoarticular diseases are by definition asymmetric. Bilateral involvement, symmetric, of the DIP joints is seen in psoriatic arthritis and in occasional patients with polyarticular gout. Of the polyarticular entities, RA and the connective-tissue diseases are more likely to present in a symmetric fashion.

Presence of Inflammation

Determining the presence of inflammatory changes is one of the most important aspects in the evaluation of patients with joint complaints. The history is helpful, as patients can accurately describe if a joint has been or is currently warm, red, swollen, or simply painful.

Crystal deposition disease usually presents with inflammation. Gout tends to be an acute monoarthritis typically affecting the first metatarsal joint (podagra), followed by the knee (gonagra), or the wrist (chinagra). Occasionally, gout can mimic RA with polyarticular involvement. Usually, patients with gout have tophi elsewhere. Pseudogout can mimic gout in terms of acuteness and degree of inflammation; the joints most commonly affected in pseudogout are the knee, shoulder, and wrist.

Determining the duration of morning stiffness is also very helpful. Characteristically, patients with RA and other inflammatory arthropathies experience stiffness for more than an hour after awakening, for weeks or months. Conversely, patients with OA usually feel loosening of their joints before the hour has elapsed.

Patients with systemic vasculitis commonly complain of diffuse, symmetric arthralgias with little inflammation. For example, significant arthralgias is commonly seen in patients with Henoch-Schönlein purpura and cryoglobulinemia.

In summary, no single particular sign or symptom is likely to have enough discriminatory quality to diagnose a rheumatologic condition. A detailed history, a complete or relevant review of systems, and a systematic approach provide the necessary framework for an initial differential diagnosis.

Signs and Symptoms in Other Organs

The presence of signs or symptoms in other organs can guide the differential diagnosis. For example, the presence of subcutaneous nodules in extensor surfaces raises the possibility of tophaceous gout or RA nodules. Although eye findings such as conjunctivitis, iritis, and episcleritis are nonspecific, they can occur in many rheumatic conditions. The recent history of diarrhea or sexually transmitted disease should alert the possibility of reactive arthritis. The presence of hilar adenopathy in the setting of symmetric additive polyarthritis of the ankles and knees and erythema nodosum characterizes Lofgren syndrome (sarcoidosis). Purpura, arthralgias, and proteinuria are characteristic of cryoglobulinemia in patients with chronic hepatitis C infection.

Comorbidities and Associated Conditions

Comorbidities and associated conditions are also important in framing the clinical problem. For example, conditions associated with diabetes mellitus include diffuse idiopathic skeletal hyperostosis (DISH), adhesive capsulitis, trigger finger, stiff-hand syndrome, scleredema, Dupuytren's contracture, carpal tunnel syndrome, and reflex sympathetic syndrome among others. Occasionally, patients present with unusual patterns of articular involvement that might be highly characteristic of certain clinical entities. For example, patients with hemochromatosis present with arthralgias of the MCP joints and sparing of the DIP and PIP joints.

PHYSICAL FINDINGS

An important first step in patients presenting with complaints related to the joints is to determine if the problem is articular, periarticular, or nonarticular. Careful examination of periarticular ligamentous structures, pain at the site of tendon insertion (i.e., enthesitis), or pain around the joint itself (periarthritis) is important to determine the likely etiology of the patient's "articular" complaint. Also, during the physical examination, the clinician may confirm or refute the presence of inflammation and pattern joint involvement obtained in the history. The reader is referred to standard books on physical examination for a detailed review.

The physical examination is very helpful in determining the presence of inflammation. For example, the elbow and knee are normally colder than the rest of the body—even a slightly warm temperature in these locations suggests inflammation. Arthralgias alone do not support inflammation.

Bacterial causes of infectious arthritis are likely to present with obvious inflammatory changes; the most common clinical pattern is that of an acute monoarthritis. Inflammatory changes might not be present in patients on steroids or those with severe neutropenia. Another special case of infectious arthritis without or with minimal inflammation is that of bacterial infections in prosthetic devices. Fungal and mycobacterial infections can present with little or no inflammatory changes. Viral infections present clinically more like

CLINICAL POINTS: PHYSICAL EXAMINATION

- Not all joint pain is truly articular; point at tendon insertion and along tendons are helpful in differentiating rheumatologic conditions

- Joint pain might not be associated with inflammatory changes

- Pattern of joint involvement is helpful in the differential diagnoses

arthralgias than arthritis; parvovirus B19 infections usually present as a very acute and disabling polyarthralgia.

Rheumatoid arthritis almost universally presents with inflammatory changes in the affected joints. Patients with "burnout" rheumatoid joints present with severe deformities associated with little or no appreciable inflammatory changes. Over time patients with advance OA exhibit deforming changes of the affected joints with little or no inflammatory changes. The main difference between advanced RA and OA with deformities resides in the joints being affected (i.e., large joints in OA like the knee vs. small joints in RA like MCP or PIP). The presence of a new inflamed-appearing joint in a patient with OA should alert the clinician to the possibility of an infectious or crystal-induced etiology.

Patients with connective-tissue diseases can present with either arthralgias or arthritis. Characteristically, the joint involvement in SLE tends to be more of a polyarthralgia than polyarthritis. Patients with systemic sclerosis present with diffuse arthralgias; the changes observed in the digits (sausage-like changes) are due to infiltration of the skin and not due to that of the synovial space.

Patients with seronegative spondyloarthropathies can manifest joint involvement in various ways: those with psoriatic arthritis can have asymmetric polyarthritis indistinguishable from that in patients with RA; the most severe form of psoriatic arthritis produces a classic destruction of the distal phalanx known as arthritis mutilans. Patients with ankylosing spondylitis usually present with little or no evidence of a peripheral arthritis; these individuals have predominant involvement of the axial skeleton. Individuals with inflammatory bowel disease can present with either oligoarthritis or, more commonly, oligoarthralgias.

Approach to Patients with Muscle Disorders

CLINICAL PRESENTATION

Certain demographic characteristics can be linked to specific inflammatory muscle disorders. For example, inclusion body myositis is characteristically seen in elderly men; polymyositis/dermatomyositis (PM/DM) occur more commonly in females. Age is an important criterion for differentiation between inflammatory and noninflammatory myopathies. Adult patients with polymyositis and dermatomyositis are usually diagnosed in the fifth decade of life; patients with paraneoplastic PM present at around 60 years of age. The noninflammatory myopathies of glycogen or lipid storage diseases present in childhood or in early adulthood; the myopathies associated with connective-tissue disease usually present in the second or third decade of life.

The patient with myopathy may present with: (a) painless weakness that is diffuse (such as in polymyositis) or localized (distal, such as inclusion body myositis); (b) painful weakness (such as in polymyalgia rheumatica); and (c) pain without weakness that can be generalized (influenza, systemic infections) or localized (fibromyalgia).

PHYSICAL FINDINGS

Distinguishing muscle weakness of a neuropathic versus myopathic etiology can be difficult. Weakness due to upper motor neuron disease typically present with asymmetric weakness (such as hemiparesis), hyperreflexia, positive Babinski's sign, and ultimately, spasticity. Patients with lower motor neuron disease might be more challenging to differentiate from patients with a primary myopathic process; they present with distal weakness, fasciculations, hyporeflexia, and ultimately, decreased muscle tone. Patients with disorders affecting the neuromuscular junction are challenging to differentiate from

NOT TO BE MISSED

- Septic arthritis
- Inflammatory arthropathies

CLINICAL POINTS: PHYSICAL FINDINGS

- Likelihood of certain diagnoses is associated with age and gender.
- Pattern of involvement (proximal vs. distal) is important for the differential diagnoses.
- Consider metabolic and neurological conditions carefully when assessing patients with muscle complaints.

Table 1.3 Demographic and Clinical Characteristics of Patients Presenting with Muscular Complaints

	MALE	FEMALE	PROXIMAL	DISTAL
Age <50 y		CTD	Endocrine, CTD	LMN (?)
Age >50 y	Inclusion body myositis	PM/DM	PM/DM endocrine	Inclusion body myositis

CTD, connective-tissue disorder; DM, dermatomyositis; LMN, lower motor neuron disease; PM, polymyositis.

patients with myopathic processes, as they share similar characteristics (proximal distribution, normal reflexes, no Babinski's sign, and normal muscle tone). Not uncommonly, clinicians resort to electromyographic studies (EMG/NCV) and muscle biopsies to distinguish between these latter two groups of patients. Table 1.3 summarizes the patient's demographics and common muscular disorders.

The pattern of muscle involvement can be helpful in the differential diagnosis of patients with weakness. Proximal muscle weakness of insidious onset is more characteristic of polymyositis. Individuals with inclusion body myositis tend to have both proximal and distal muscle weakness. Proximal weakness is characteristic of the metabolic myopathies (hypokalemia, hypercalcemia) and the myopathies associated with endocrine disorders (thyroid disorders, hypercalcemia). Patients with periodic hypokalemic paralysis can present with profound generalized weakness of rather acute onset; a search for hyperthyroidism is warranted in such patients, especially if they are of Asian descent.

Individuals presenting with regional pain and/or weakness need to be approached in a different manner. Patients with clear regional muscle pain should be carefully questioned for a history of trauma. Occasionally, infections might be responsible for the regional nature of the pain. Pyomyositis, a relatively unusual disorder outside of the tropics, should be suspected in patients with known human immunodeficiency virus who present with fever and localized muscle pain. On occasion these patients might also have associated weakness. The presence of gluteal muscle weakness and atrophy among diabetics should alert the clinician to the possibility of diabetic amyotrophy. Diabetics with long-standing, poorly controlled diabetes can present with localized pain and weakness due to diabetes myonecrosis. More common, however, is the patient with fibromyalgia who presents to the clinician with complaints of profound generalized fatigue and diffuse muscle pains. Differentiating fatigue from weakness can be challenging. In these patients documentation of normal muscle strength and tone is of great importance. Elicitation of painful trigger points might help the clinician to make this diagnosis.

Additional Reading

1. Bowen JL. Educational strategies to promote clinical diagnostic reasoning. *N Engl J Med* 2006;355: 2217–2225.
2. Chew FS. Radiologic manifestations in the musculoskeletal system of miscellaneous endocrine disorders. *Radiol Clin North Am* 1991;29:135–147.
3. DeGowin RL. *DeGowin & DeGowin's Diagnostic Examination.* New York: McGraw-Hill, Inc, 1994.
4. McCluskey P, Richard J, Powell RJ. The eye in systemic inflammatory diseases. *Lancet* 2004;364:2125–2133.
5. Naschitz JE, Rosner I, Rozenbaum M, et al. Rheumatic syndromes: clues to occult neoplasia. *Semin Arthritis Rheum* 1999;29:43–55.
6. Sapira JD. *The art and science of bedside diagnosis.* Baltimore–Munich: Urban & Schwarzenberg, 1990.

Sport-Related, Occupational, and Other Regional Pain Syndromes

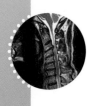

Chapter 2 **Neck Pain**

Jerome Van Ruiswyk

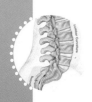

Chapter 3 **Low Back Pain and Lumbar Stenosis**

Lisa L. Willett

Chapter 4 **Shoulder Pain**

Dennis W. Boulware

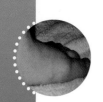

Chapter 5 **Painful Feet**

Dennis W. Boulware and Gustavo R. Heudebert

Chapter 6   **Mechanical Disorders of the Knee**

Dennis W. Boulware

Chapter 7   **Hip Pain**

Carol Croft

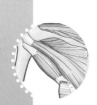

Chapter 8   **Sports-Related Conditions and Injuries**

Lisa L. Willett

2 Neck Pain

Jerome Van Ruiswyk

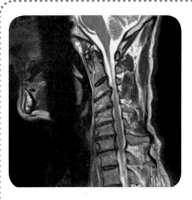

A 62-year-old man presents with chronic neck and left arm pain that have been getting progressively worse over the last 2 years. The pain radiates down to the left forearm and up into the head; he does admit some associated numbness in the left hand and occasionally in the right hand. He denies bowel or bladder incontinence but feels that his sense of balance has been off for years. He has a history of prior lumbar decompression for lumbar spinal stenosis and radiculopathy.

On examination, he has diminished light touch sensation on the dorsum of the left forearm and hand. Strength in the arms is 5/5 in the deltoids, biceps, triceps, and handgrip. Deep tendon reflexes in the arms and legs are normal except the left biceps is 3+. Hoffman's reflex is negative. There is no ankle clonus.

A magnetic resonance imaging of the cervical spine shows severe multilevel degenerative disc disease with broad-based disc protrusion at C3-C4 resulting in spinal cord deformity (see image), severe foraminal narrowing at bilateral C5, left C7, and bilateral C8 nerve roots. Electromyogram shows a chronic neurogenic lesion affecting the left C7 nerve root.

He is initially managed conservatively. However, 3 months later he presents with a worsening of symptoms with numbness and tingling in both arms and hands that is exacerbated by movement of his neck. He continues to deny bowel or bladder incontinence. His neurologic examination is unchanged except that he now has a positive Hoffman's reflex in the right arm.

Because of progression of symptoms and subtle signs of myelopathy, he undergoes posterior cervical decompression and fusion. Postoperatively, his neurologic symptoms abate, but his pain continues, and his neurologic examination continues to show diminished light touch sensation on the dorsum of the left hand and 5/5 motor strength in both arms except for 4+/5 motor strength in the left wrist extensors and triceps.

Clinical Presentation

Neck pain is a common presenting complaint in primary care settings. Studies suggest that up to two thirds of individuals experience neck pain at least once during their lifetime. The prevalence of neck pain increases with age and is more common in women than in men. Although up to 10% of the adult population has neck pain at any one time, most neck pain is self-limited. Consequently, patients seeking care for neck pain tend to have more severe pain, other associated symptoms, or chronic symptoms that have not responded to rest or over-the-counter analgesics; or they report neck pain as a secondary symptom of a more generalized condition. Those patients seeking care with neck pain as a primary complaint tend to have symptoms bothersome enough to cause functional limitations. Functional classification systems such as the World Health Organization's International Classification of Functioning, Disability, and Health (ICF) can be used to more fully describe patient impairments.

Multiple-risk factors for neck pain have been identified (1) including increasing age, obesity, smoking, unusual postures, and heavy lifting or other heavy work. However, an even greater number of psychosocial factors have been associated with neck pain including depression, drug abuse, low job satisfaction, monotonous or dissatisfying work, lack of coworker support, and lack of control over the work situation. Psychosocial and cultural factors can also impact the prevalence and natural history of neck pain. For example, in Australia, after legislation removed financial compensation for pain and suffering from whiplash injuries, subsequent whiplash patients reported lower pain scores and better functional outcomes compared with historical controls (2). Interestingly, in Lithuania where there is no legal tort system, late whiplash syndrome does not exist (3).

When evaluating neck pain, the history should include the elements of all basic pain histories including location, severity, quality, onset, duration, aggravating and alleviating factors, radiation, history of injury or overuse, any associated symptoms especially neurologic or constitutional symptoms, chronic and prior conditions especially infections or malignancy, common work or leisure activities and any recent unusual activities, and response to prior interventions or treatments.

In clinical practice, patients present much more commonly with posterior neck pain than with anterior neck pain. The most common ICD-10 codes specifically associated with neck pain include cervicalgia (M54.2), sprain and strain of cervical spine (S13.4), spondylosis with radiculopathy (M47.2), cervical disc disorder with radiculopathy (M50.1), and cervicocranial syndrome (M53.0).

The neck is the most flexible part of the spinal column. The less rigid bony structure that allows this flexibility, particularly the unique structure of C1 and C2, means that the neck must rely more heavily on soft tissue structures for support which contributes to the pathophysiology of some important cervical spine conditions. The atlas (C1) is a ring without any vertebral body (Fig. 2.1A). The superior lateral bodies of the atlas articulate with the occipital condyles to form the atlanto-occipital joint, which is responsible for about 50% of the flexion and extension in the neck. The axis (C2) more closely resembles the remainder of the vertebrae with a vertebral body, ring, and prominent spinous process (especially noticeable on lateral cervical spine x-rays), but it also has an odontoid process or dens projecting superiorly off its vertebral body (Fig. 2.1B). A transverse ligament holds the dens to the anterior arch of the atlas; this functional peg-in-hole joint provides about 50% of the rotation of the neck. Inflammation of the synovial joint that articulates the axis to the atlas, from conditions such as rheumatoid arthritis, can damage this ligament leading to subluxation of the C1-C2 joint. Radiologic evidence of C1-C2 subluxation can be seen on flexion–extension views of 20% patients with rheumatoid arthritis. Therefore, screening lateral flexion–extension x-rays should be obtained during preoperative evaluation of patients with rheumatoid arthritis who will be undergoing endotracheal intubation.

The remainder of the cervical vertebrae have standard vertebral anatomy with a body, a posterior arch that provides bony protection for the spinal cord and with intervertebral discs between the vertebral bodies of all the remaining cervical vertebrae (Fig. 2.1C). The intervertebral disc has an outer annulus fibrosis and an inner nucleus pulposus with superior and inferior end plates. The gelatinous nucleus pulposus acts as a shock absorber for compressive forces, whereas the annulus fibrosis acts as a fibrous sheath restraining the nucleus pulposus. When rents occur in the annulus fibrosis, the inner nucleus pulposus may protrude or be partially extruded; when the resulting bulge occurs in a posterolateral location it may compress a nerve root, and when it occurs in a posterior midline location it may compress the anterior spinal cord. Anterior and posterior longitudinal ligaments run along the vertebral body front and back, respectively. The posterior longitudinal ligament can become calcified in conditions such as diffuse idiopathic skeletal hyperostosis. In patients with either acquired or congenital stenosis of the spinal column, this calcified ligament

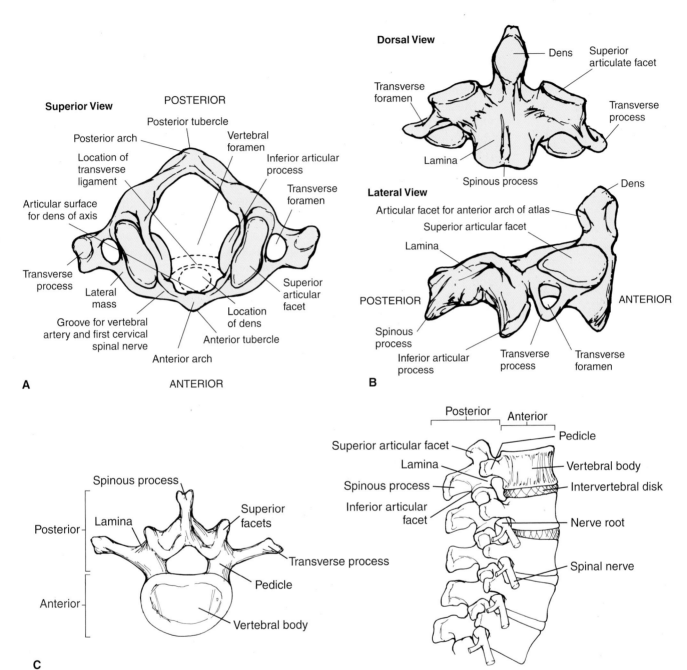

Figure 2.1 **(A)** Anatomy of atlas; **(B)** anatomy of axis; and **(C)** anatomy of typical vertebra. All illustrations from Oatis CA. *Kinesiology. The Mechanics and Pathomechanics of Human Movement.* Baltimore: Lippincott Williams & Wilkins; 2003.

may compress the anterior spinal cord, especially with neck flexion which causes a 3-mm reduction in spinal canal diameter.

The posterior arch of each vertebra is formed by pedicles, lateral bodies, and laminae. The lateral body is formed on each side where the pedicle meets the lamina. There are five articulations between each of the typical vertebra: the intervertebral disk, along with uncovertebral joints (joints of Luchska), and facet (zygapophyseal) joints along each side of the vertebra. The uncinate process is a vertical projection from the posterolateral vertebral body that contacts the adjoining vertebral body to form the uncovertebral joint. The uncovertebral joint is not a true synovial joint but it is a frequent site of osteophytes. Two articular projections arise from each lateral body—a superior articular projection that faces posteriorly and an inferior articular projection that faces anteriorly. Each projection forms a true synovial joint with its neighboring vertebra, and notches anterior to these projections coapt with complementary notches on adjacent vertebrae to form the intervertebral foramina. The facet joints formed by the articulation of these projections with neighboring vertebra are subject to degeneration or can be affected by inflammatory arthritis. Pain arising from arthritis in these joints typically is exacerbated by extension of the neck. For patients with focal posterior neck pain, injection of local anesthetic into the facet joint is sometimes used to confirm the joint as the generator of pain symptoms. Osteophytes arising from uncovertebral joints can cause anterior narrowing of the intervertebral foramina and osteophytes arising from the facet joints can cause posterior narrowing of the intervertebral foramina, which in either case can contribute to cervical spinal nerve compression causing radicular symptoms. The ligamentum flavum joins adjacent laminae; thickening of this ligament by degenerative processes can contribute to spinal stenosis and to spinal cord injuries in patients with spondylosis who suffer a hyperextension injury of the neck.

A transverse process off the side of the arch in the area of each lateral body and a midline posterior spinous process serve as anchor levers for musculature and ligaments. An intraspinous ligament joins adjacent spinous processes and helps prevent hyperflexion of the neck. The transverse process from C1 to C6 also has a transverse foramen where the vertebral artery courses until it enters the skull; in some patients extreme extension of the neck has been shown to lead to occlusion of the vertebral artery.

There are eight cervical spinal nerves with each cervical nerve root exiting through the intervertebral foramina above its corresponding vertebra except C8 which exits between C7 and T1. Each cervical spinal nerve is formed from an anterior root arising from motor neurons in the ventral horn of the spinal cord and a posterior root that carries afferent sensory fibers from the dorsal root ganglion. After exiting through the intervertebral foramina, the spinal nerves split into anterior and posterior rami. The anterior rami form the brachial plexus and provide motor innervation to the prevertebral and paravertebral muscles, whereas the posterior rami provide motor and sensory function of the posterior neck muscles, bones, and skin. Temporary and permanent blocks of the medial branch of the posterior rami can be used to diagnose and treat pain arising from posterior neck structures.

Since the major structures of the posterior neck are the spinal column and its contents and the supporting musculature, it can be helpful to elicit more detailed history about prior spinal column conditions such as lumbar degenerative disk disease, degenerative joint disease, radiculopathy, or nonspecific low back pain. It can also be helpful to inquire about ergonomic positions of the neck during work or sleep and the effect of positional or postural changes on symptoms. For patients with onset of neck pain after trauma, it is important to obtain a detailed history of the event to help estimate the amount, direction, and location of major forces acting on the neck and any protective or restraint systems such as seat belts or head rests in motor vehicles that may have mitigated the impact of the forces; this detailed data can help determine the likelihood of serious musculoskeletal or neurologic injuries. In patients with potential major trauma to the head or the neck, the neck should be immobilized until the possibility of underlying cervical fracture or spinal instability is ruled out.

Despite a detailed history, it can be difficult to localize neck pain to a specific anatomic source. Neck pain may be referred from multiple organs or areas including the heart, brachial plexus, jaw or esophagus, upper thorax, or the shoulder girdle or upper arm. Even for pain originating from somatic nerves, patients usually present with nonfocal pain making it difficult to pinpoint the inciting anatomic pathology, and degenerative changes on imaging studies have very poor correlation with the presence or severity of patient symptoms. Therefore, diagnostic specificity in the evaluation of neck pain relies on recognition

PATIENT ASSESSMENT

- The history should include the elements of all basic pain histories, plus details about any preceding trauma, a history or risk factors for infection or cancer, and any constitutional or neurologic symptoms.

- The physical examination should screen for neurologic abnormalities of the upper and lower extremities; specialized maneuvers may add additional sensitivity and specificity to the examination.

- The need for and the type of diagnostic testing are determined by the working differential diagnosis after a careful history and physical examination.

- Patients with axial neck pain without neurologic symptoms or signs and who are not suspected of having an emergent or serious underlying condition do not require initial imaging.

- An understanding of cervical spinal anatomy is required to allow interpretation of imaging findings and reports.

of patterns of symptoms, signs, and test results, while excluding emergent or other serious underlying conditions. In particular, patients should be asked about constitutional symptoms and risk factors for infections, history of or symptoms of malignancy, prior trauma, and symptoms suggestive of myelopathy such as clumsiness of the hands, weakness of the arms, bowel or bladder dysfunction, lower extremity weakness or numbness, or gait problems. Pain from tumor or infections is typically constant and progressive and unrelieved by rest or change in position. When morning stiffness is a prominent symptom, a rheumatologic condition such as rheumatoid arthritis, ankylosing spondylitis, or polymyalgia rheumatic should be considered.

Physical Examination

The physical examination of a patient with neck pain should start with general elements such as review of vital signs and observation of patient posture, movement, and gait. Presence of fever should raise suspicion of infection—particularly in IV drug abusers, patients with vascular access devices, or immunocompromised hosts. Abnormal carrying positions of the neck may be due to either a primary underlying musculoskeletal abnormality or a reflex spasm of the posterior neck muscles. In either case, spontaneous movement of the head is typically reduced. It is important to observe for a spastic gait that may originate from cervical spinal cord dysfunction.

Examination should then focus on inspection and palpation of the neck with special attention to the area of maximal symptoms. It is often helpful to have the patients point to the specific area where they are experiencing symptoms and have them point out any abnormalities that they have perceived. Rashes or bruises may suggest zoster or prior trauma, respectively. For patients reporting anterior neck pain, first inspect the anterior cervical triangle bordered by the sternocleidomastoid muscle, mandible, and sternal notch on each side looking for deformities and asymmetry; and then both posterior cervical triangles bordered by the sternocleidomastoid, clavicle, and trapezius. Both areas should then be palpated for localized tenderness. The muscle bodies and their underlying structures should be palpated and the presence of lymphadenopathy or masses determined. For patients with respiratory symptoms or dysphagia, tracheal location, and thyroid size, shape, location, and movement with swallow should be noted. The vessels of the neck should be observed and the carotid pulse palpated. A screening cardiopulmonary examination should also be done since neck pain may be referred from intrathoracic structures.

For patients with posterior neck pain, begin the examination with inspection of the cervical spinous processes by looking at their alignment and noting any deformities. Also look for deformity or asymmetry of the paracervical muscles, scapula, and surrounding muscles. Then palpate the spinous processes and posterior neck soft tissues and musculature from the occipital insertions to the inferior angle of the scapula and laterally out to the shoulders looking for point tenderness and spasm. The associated level of any spinous tenderness, deformity, or step-off should be noted; the prominent C7 spinous process can be used as a point of reference; point tenderness at a particular level warrants further investigation with imaging. For patients with more than one point of muscular tenderness, a search for any trigger points in other body areas is warranted.

The active and passive ranges of motion of the neck should then be observed. Full cervical spine range of motion in young adults is 60 degrees of flexion, 75 degrees of extension, 45 degrees of lateral bend to each side, and 90 degrees of rotation to each side. In patients older than 50 years, extension is reduced to 60 degrees and lateral bend is reduced to 30 degrees (4). Positions that aggravate or alleviate the neck pain or its radiation should be noted. Neck muscle strength testing should then be done. The sternocleidomastoids are the main flexors and rotators of the neck, while the main extensors are the paravertebral muscles

SECTION 2 Regional Pain Syndromes

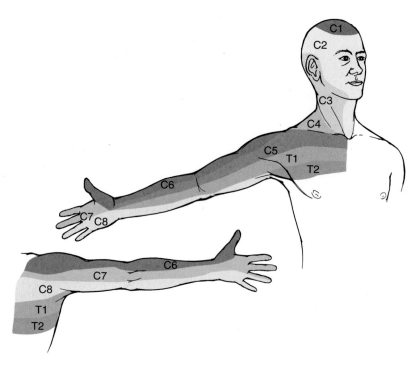

Figure 2.2 Dermatomes of the cervical spine.

and the trapezii. The flexors are tested by putting a hand below the chin; the extensors are tested by placing a hand on the occiput while the other hand holds the shoulder, and the rotators are tested by putting a hand on the side of the chin; the trapezii can be tested by asking the patient to shrug her shoulders against resistance. Reproduction or aggravation of symptoms during strength testing suggests a possible musculoskeletal etiology of the pain.

A detailed neurologic examination of the upper extremities should then be done to help detect an associated radiculopathy or myelopathy. For patients with areas of sensory deficits, dermatome charts can be used to determine the match of the findings to an associated corresponding cervical nerve root level (Fig. 2.2). When testing for myelopathy, include light touch and proprioception testing to assess posterior spinal cord function and temperature and pinprick testing to assess anterolateral spinal cord function. Although the match of cervical nerve roots to individual muscles is very nonspecific, selected motor testing can help localize an involved cervical nerve level, especially if the pattern corroborates a dermatomal pattern of sensory loss (see Table 2.1). Muscle strength should be graded on the standard 0 to 5 scale:

0. No contraction
1. Visible twitch but no joint movement
2. Able to move joint with gravity eliminated
3. Joint movement against gravity but not against resistance
4. Joint movement against some resistance
5. Joint movement against full resistance

Brachioradialis, biceps, and triceps deep tendon reflexes should be checked and graded using the standard scale:

0. Absent
1. Trace
2. Normal
3. Brisk
4. <3 beats clonus
5. Sustained clonus

Table 2.1 Localizing Neurologic Symptoms and Signs Associated with Cervical Nerve Roots

ROOT	PAIN	NUMBNESS	WEAKNESS	AFFECTED REFLEX
C4	Upper neck	Upper posterior and anterior neck	None	None
C5	Neck, scapula, shoulder, anterior arm	Anterolateral aspect of arm	Shoulder abduction	Biceps, brachioradialis
C6	Neck, scapular, shoulder, lateral arm, and forearm into 1st, 2nd digits	Lateral aspect of arm and forearm into thumb	Forearm flexion	Biceps, brachioradialis
C7	Neck, shoulder, lateral arm, medial scapula, extensor surface forearm into 3rd digit	Posterolateral aspect of arm and forearm and dorsum hand into 3rd digit	Triceps, radial wrist extensors, and flexor carpi radialis[a]	Triceps
C8	Neck, medial scapula, medial aspect arm, and forearm into 4th, 5th digits	Distal medial forearm, lateral hand into 4th, 5th digits	Flexor digitorum sublimis to ring finger[b]	Finger flexors

[a]Wrist extensor testing: Flex fingers to eliminate wrist extension by finger extensors and then extend wrist in radial direction. Flexor carpi radialis testing: Extend fingers to eliminate wrist flexion by finger flexors and then flex wrist in radial direction.
[b]Flexor digitorum sublimis to ring finger testing: Stabilize long, index, and little fingers in extension and flex fingers.

SECTION 2 Regional Pain Syndromes

NOT TO BE MISSED

- Spinal instability due to fractures or soft tissue injury due to trauma or inflammatory conditions such as rheumatoid arthritis.
- Spinal cord compression or impending compression due to infection, cancer, and degenerative or congenital conditions.
- Pain that is arising from visceral organs such as the heart, vasculature, lungs, or gastrointestinal tract that is referred to the neck.
- Systemic infectious (e.g., meningitis) or inflammatory (e.g., temporal arteritis) conditions that may present with neck pain as an early symptom.
- Progressive neurologic conditions that may produce symptoms that are similar to those seen with spinal cord compression or spinal nerve compression.

When sensory and motor abnormalities are found but their patterns do not fit well with a specific radicular pattern, common upper extremity peripheral neuropathies should be explored as a potential etiology for the findings. Tests for upper motor neuron signs such as Hoffman's and Babinski's reflexes and an examination of lower extremity motor strength and tone should also be done to screen for cervical myelopathy.

Several specialized maneuvers are often recommended to further evaluate for possible radiculopathy or myelopathy. Spurling's test involves placing the neck in positions that reduce the diameter of the cervical intervertebral foramina which may cause compression of the spinal nerve; the test is considered positive if radicular symptoms are elicited when the patient's neck is extended and rotated toward the symptomatic side. The complementary test that attempts to maximize the foraminal opening is called the "distraction test." The patient is placed supine and the examiner then gently pulls on the head; relief of symptoms suggests underlying cervical radiculopathy. This maneuver should not be done in patients who might have underlying spinal instability. Both tests have low sensitivity, but fair specificity, yielding a positive likelihood ratio of 3 and a negative likelihood ratio of 0.6 (5). A lancinating paresthesia with neck flexion, termed "Lhermitte's sign," may be seen with compression of the spinal cord in patients with spinal stenosis.

Studies

Further diagnostic testing is needed when the history or physical examination uncovers possible emergent or serious underlying conditions; when the pattern or severity of pain or associated symptoms suggest the need for treatments other than analgesics, rest, or physical therapy; or when there may be extenuating nonmedical issues such as work, accident, or disability-related claims. Imaging should be obtained in patients with a history of trauma, constitutional symptoms, underlying systemic illnesses including cancer or infection, or neurologic symptoms, and should be considered in patients older than

50 years with new onset of pain and in patients with chronic pain persisting more than 6 weeks despite conservative therapies.

The type of testing depends on the working differential diagnosis after the history and physical examination, especially for patients presenting with anterior neck pain, since anterior symptoms are not typically caused by spinal-related conditions. In addition to testing related to specific diagnoses suggested by the history and physical examination, if an underlying systemic illness is suspected, a screening CBC with differential, ESR and/or C reactive protein, and alkaline phosphatase should be obtained.

Neck pain patients who report a history of trauma should have further evaluation with imaging. For patients with mild or moderate trauma, high-quality cervical spine plain radiographs have adequate sensitivity to exclude serious underlying fracture, but it is important to remember that sensitivity for fracture detection can be reduced in patients with osteopenia or prior cervical spine surgeries. The full cervical spine series in the neutral position includes lateral and PA views and an odontoid view which is obtained with the mouth open to eliminate teeth overlying the area of C1-C2 and allow adequate visualization of the odontoid process. If fracture is ruled out, left and right oblique views are obtained to complete the series. In some patients, it may be difficult to get adequate views of either C1 or C7; in fact, inadequate visualization of C7 is the most common error made in the x-ray assessment of cervical spine injury. PA and lateral views show the homogeneity, height, and alignment of the vertebral bodies and the intervertebral discs, and the lateral view also shows the spinous processes and facet joints and allows estimation of the prevertebral soft tissue width which may be increased in patients with a related vertebral fracture or prevertebral soft tissue injury; oblique views are better for visualizing the intervertebral foramina. If there are concerns about spinal instability due to soft tissue injury or an underlying inflammatory condition such as rheumatoid arthritis, then lateral flexion and extension views can be obtained if the neutral position views exclude fracture. In general, it is difficult to fully evaluate all elements of the posterior vertebral arch with plain films because of summation effects of overlying shadows. For patients with a history of possibly severe trauma or trauma patients with any neurologic signs suggestive of radiculopathy or myelopathy, the higher sensitivity of cervical computed tomography (CT) or magnetic resonance imaging (MRI) is needed to rule out occult fractures and cervical spinal cord or soft tissue injuries.

For patients with posterior neck pain, the pattern of symptoms and findings can direct the type of subsequent testing. Imaging of chronic pain that has not responded to conservative measures and is localized to the axial and paraspinal area without any radiation or associated symptoms suggestive of radiculopathy or myelopathy should start with a cervical spine series. X-rays will frequently show signs of degenerative disease of the intervertebral discs or facet joints and/or narrowing of the intervertebral foramina. In fact, in asymptomatic patients older than 40 years, cervical degenerative changes (spondylosis) are common, and after the age of 50 years, cervical spondylosis is present in more than 90% of individuals (6). Therefore, these degenerative changes are relevant only if they specifically fit with the rest of the patient's symptoms and signs.

For patients with radicular symptoms and consistent physical examination findings, further testing could be deferred during a period of initial conservative management since symptoms tend to abate over time; however, further initial evaluation is warranted if there is significant weakness. When weakness is present, workup with electromyogram can confirm that the etiology of the weakness is due to cervical radiculopathy and can help confirm the suspected nerve root; however, electromyographic testing will be normal in patients without involvement of the motor part of the spinal nerve. For patients with inconsistent or unclear neurologic examination findings in the upper extremities, electrodiagnostic testing can help uncover an underlying peripheral or entrapment neuropathy.

Patients with possible myelopathy, infection, or malignancy require evaluation with either CT or MRI. Computed tomographic scan provides excellent imaging of osseous structures and requires less time to perform but involves significant radiation exposure. MRI scanning provides excellent soft tissue detail and can provide better detail of spinal cord changes, but it cannot be performed in patients with certain implants or embedded ferromagnetic materials. Noncontrast MRI is adequate for most situations, but contrast MRI has better sensitivity for tumors, infection, and postsurgical epidural fibrosis; however, gadolinium contrast should not be used in patients with significant renal dysfunction because of the possible complication of nephrogenic systemic sclerosis. Computed tomographic myelogram may be necessary if further evaluation is needed to rule out spinal cord compression because computed tomographic or MRI findings are equivocal, when cord compression is suspected at multiple levels, and when surgical decompression is being considered. Unfortunately, as is the case for C spine x-rays, there can be poor correlation of MRI abnormalities with neck pain symptoms. Findings of disc herniation may be seen in up to 50% of asymptomatic older individuals and spinal cord compression in up to 25% (7). Therefore, imaging symptoms must be carefully correlated with the history, physical examination, and other diagnostic testing before making a clinical diagnosis of cervical myelopathy.

Bone scan is rarely done in the evaluation of patients with neck pain, since both CT and MRI have excellent sensitivity for infection and tumor. The physiologic information of bone scan can sometimes be helpful to confirm a specific facet joint as an underlying pain generator; a diagnostic injection of local anesthetic into the suspect joint can then be done to see whether the patient's pain is eliminated. Combined bone and gallium scans are sometimes necessary to evaluate for possible infection in patients with spinal hardware, which distorts computed tomographic and MR images.

Treatment

Initial treatment of neck pain depends on the remaining differential diagnosis after history, physical examination, and indicated diagnostic studies. Treatment is directed at the underlying condition for patients with a specific confirmed diagnosis. For example, patients found to have intervertebral discitis or cervical spinal osteomyelitis are treated with appropriate antibiotics after cultures are obtained. Patients with spinal cord compression due to epidural abscess or cancer should be emergently referred to neurosurgeons, and in the case of malignant tumors appropriate cancer specialists, to help prevent worsening of myelopathy. Patients with cervical spinal fractures or instability due to trauma should also be emergently referred to neurosurgeons for possible spinal stabilization. Patients with spinal cord compression due to cervical spondylosis or spinal stenosis should also be referred to spine surgeons who can present the patient with the benefits and risks of surgical decompression.

Initial treatment for patients without an underlying emergent or serious condition is often aimed at symptom control. Patients with cervical radiculopathy are typically treated conservatively for 6 to 8 weeks. The nonpharmacologic conservative modalities most frequently used are avoidance of aggravating activities and then progressive mobilization and physical therapy exercises once pain is tolerable. Cervical collars may be used in the short term if they provide some symptomatic relief, but long-term use should be avoided, since it can contribute to disuse atrophy of the cervical musculature.

Pharmacologic treatment of cervical radiculopathy typically includes analgesics such as nonsteroidal anti-inflammatories drugs and may also include muscle relaxants in patients with paraspinal muscle spasm detected on examination; neuropathic pain medications should be considered in patients whose radicular symptoms are not controlled with simple analgesics. The selection of

WHEN TO REFER

- Patients with spinal cord compression or instability should be urgently referred to a spinal surgeon.

- Patients with cervical radiculopathy with weakness or persistent symptoms after a course of conservative therapy can be referred for epidural injections or spinal surgery.

- Patients with cervical strain can be referred to physical therapy for instruction in home exercises, posture, ergonomics, and possible activity modifications.

- Patients who are felt to have pain arising from a degenerative facet joint who have persistent pain despite conservative measures can be referred for diagnostic facet joint injection, medial branch block, and/or percutaneous neurotomy.

- Patients found to have systemic conditions presenting with neck pain may need to be referred to appropriate specialists for diagnostic confirmation and management.

which agents to use in each class will depend on patient comorbidities and their other chronic medications. Patients should initially be started on low doses of these medications to help avoid dose-related side effects. Since muscle relaxants and neuropathic pain medicines can be sedating, some patients find that a bedtime dose can help them sleep, but they should be warned to avoid activities such as driving due to possible residual sedation.

Patients with cervical radiculopathy who have persistent symptoms or progressive weakness should be referred to a spine surgeon but may first be offered the option of a trial of epidural injections. A recently published randomized controlled trial suggests that a majority of patients obtain relief after epidural injections of anesthetic either with or without steroid, but without a placebo control group it is difficult to rule out that the observed improvements were not due to the natural course of cervical radiculopathy (8).

Patients with posterior neck pain without radicular or myelopathic symptoms are managed conservatively with nonpharmacologic and pharmacologic measures. In this common clinical scenario, localization of pain to a specific underlying etiology or specific anatomic pain generator is often not possible. Therefore, treatment is aimed at symptom control and maintenance or restoration of function. Physical therapy with patient education, exercises, and possibly ergonomic evaluation and remediation can be particularly helpful in improving neck pain and preventing recurrences. Pharmacologic treatment of patients with nonradicular posterior axial neck pain includes analgesics and may include muscle relaxants in patients with paraspinal muscle spasm on examination. In addition, patients with chronic neck pain, who often have concomitant depressive or fibromyalgia symptoms, may get additional relief with the tricyclic antidepressants amitriptyline or nortriptyline, or the serotonin neuroepinephrine reuptake inhibitor antidepressants venlafaxine, duloxetine, or milnacipran. There is some limited evidence that trigger point injections with lidocaine may also provide partial relief of nonradicular axial chronic posterior neck pain (9).

Many patients with chronic neck pain seek treatment with complementary alternative therapies. Some of the more commonly used therapies include chiropractic or osteopathic manipulation, massage, acupuncture, transcutaneous electric nerve stimulation, or traction. In general, there is little evidence to support or refute the effectiveness of any of these therapies. Some reviews have suggested that these therapies may provide some benefit when used in combination with neck exercises but not when used alone. However, rare but serious complications such as strokes and pathologic fractures have been described in the literature related to manipulations. Therefore, these therapies should be delivered only by qualified practitioners and should not be applied in patients at high risk for these complications (1).

Clinical Course

Patients presenting with neck pain can represent a diagnostic challenge because of an extensive differential diagnosis that includes emergent and serious underlying conditions and the poor correlation of diagnostic test findings to clinical symptoms in patients with chronic, nonurgent conditions. Patients with a history of major neck trauma, or major blunt trauma with altered mental status, or "distracting" injuries (whose pain may supersede pain from a concurrent neck injury) need cervical spine immobilization and emergent imaging to rule out spinal fracture or other spinal cord threatening soft tissue injury. Infection must be ruled out with imaging and blood tests in patients with IV drug abuse, vascular access device, or immunocompromised state, or who have constitutional symptoms or fever on examination; and metastatic cancer must be ruled out in patients with a history of malignancy. Patients with neurologic symptoms or physical examination signs of myelopathy need urgent imaging to rule out spinal cord compression which may require intervention to prevent further loss of neurologic function. Prompt intervention is essential in patients with any of these serious underlying conditions to preserve remaining neurologic function. In many of these cases, the final functional outcome will also depend on the severity of the underlying systemic condition, other patient comorbidities, and the patient's premorbid level of functioning.

Neck pain patients without these urgent or serious underlying conditions typically have good clinical outcomes with control of symptoms and maintenance of neurologic function. Patients with acute cervical strain from trauma or increased muscle use will typically have resolution of symptoms over a few days to weeks with rest and progressive physical therapy. Resumption of normal activities and return to work should be encouraged as soon as possible. Neck pain that develops shortly after sudden flexion–extension movement in the face of normal imaging studies is labeled as "whiplash." The majority of patients with whiplash injuries will gradually improve with conservative measures over the course of a few weeks. However, a subset of patients, often including those with psychosocial risk factors for neck pain or extenuating nonmedical issues such as work, accident, or disability-related claim, may have persistent pain and poorer functional outcomes.

Although degenerative disc disease and degenerative facet joint disease are frequently found on imaging in asymptomatic patients, these structures are felt to be the pain generators in many patients with neck pain. In particular, axial neck pain without neurologic symptoms that has an acute onset is typically attributed to an observed corresponding disc herniation—especially in younger patients, and chronic neck pain is often attributed to observed corresponding facet degenerative joint disease—especially in older patients. The majority of patients diagnosed with acute disc herniation improve over a few weeks. Patients diagnosed with degenerative facet arthritis tend to have chronic symptoms that can be controlled with conservative therapies. For those patients with severe symptoms despite conservative treatments, a diagnostic facet joint injection with local anesthesia can be used to confirm that it is the pain generator. If the patient obtains relief with the targeted diagnostic injection, further measures such as percutaneous radiofrequency neurotomy of the medial branch of the corresponding spinal nerve may provide longer term reduction of symptoms (10).

Similarly, although facet joint osteophytes, intervertebral disc herniations, and thickening of the posterior longitudinal ligament and ligamentum flavum are often seen on computed tomographic or MR images in asymptomatic patients, they are frequently found to cause spinal cord or nerve compression in patients with cervical myelopathy or radiculopathy, respectively. Degenerative changes of the vertebral body and associated soft tissue structures are referred to by the nonspecific term "spondylosis." These degenerative changes are seen more frequently in the lower cervical vertebrae. Consequently, cervical myelopathy and radiculopathy more frequently occur at these levels. Many patients with cervical spondylitic myelopathy have cord compression at more than one level. The majority of patients will improve after surgical decompression, but poorer outcomes are seen in older patients who have longer duration of and more severe symptoms before surgery. Similarly, the majority of patients will improve after surgical decompression of cervical radiculopathy. Cervical radiculopathy patients having surgical decompression have quicker improvement of pain and more improvement in strength than patients managed conservatively, but by 1 year pain symptoms of conservatively managed patients are similar to those patients who had surgical decompression.

In neck pain patients with neurologic symptoms, it is important to consider other etiologies for the observed neurologic symptoms or findings. Diagnoses to consider in the differential for patients with radicular symptoms include peripheral or upper extremity entrapment neuropathies; brachial plexus injuries, degeneration, or inflammation; herpes zoster; and other infectious, inflammatory, or degenerative neuropathies. Additional diagnoses to consider in patients with symptoms of myelopathy include multiple sclerosis, transverse myelitis, viral myelitis, amyotrophic lateral sclerosis, epidural arteriovenous malformations, and spinal cord infarction.

Conclusions

In patients with anterior neck pain, the differential diagnosis can be very broad, since this is a common site for referred visceral pain. Treatment and clinical outcomes will depend on the specific diagnosis uncovered.

Similarly, in patients with neck pain due to other systemic conditions such as rheumatoid arthritis, ankylosing spondylitis, or polymyalgia rheumatica, the specific treatment and eventual clinical outcome is dependent on the underlying condition.

 Refer to Patient Education

ICD9

723.1 **Cervicalgia**
Degeneration, degenerative
> *722.4 cervical, cervicothoracic*
> *722.71 with myelopathy*

Displacement, displaced
> *722.0 cervical, cervicodorsal, cervicothoracic*

729.2 **Radiculitis** *(pressure) (vertebrogenic)*
> *723.4 cervical NEC*

756.11 **Spondylolysis** *(congenital)*
> *738.4 acquired*
> *756.19 cervical*

721.90 **Spondylosis**
> *721.0 with cervical, cervicodorsal*
> *721.1 with myelopathy*

Stenosis *(cicatricial)*
> *723.0 cervical*

References

1. Rindfleisch JA. Neck pain. In: *Integrative Medicine*, 2nd ed. Philladelphia, PA: WB Saunders Company; 2007,697–708.
2. Cameron ID, Rebbeck T, Sindhusake D, et al. Legislative change is associated with improved health status in people with whiplash. *Spine* 2008;33:250.
3. Obelieiene D, Schrader H, Bovim G, et al. Pain after whiplash: a prospective controlled inception cohort study. *J Neurol Neurosurg Psychiatr* 1999;66:279–282.
4. Devin C, Sillay K, Cheng J. Neck pain. In: *Kelley's Textbook of Rheumatology*, 8th ed. Vol. 1. Philadelphia, PA: WB Saunders Company; 2008;571–584.
5. Childs JD, Cleland JA, Elliott JM, et al. Neck pain: clinical practice guidelines linked to the International Classification of Functioning, Disability, and Health from the Orthopedic Section of the American Physical Therapy Association. *J Orthop Sports Phys Ther* 2008;38(9):A1–A34.
6. Elias F. Roentgen findings in the asymptomatic cervical spine. *N Y State J Med* 1958;58:3300.
7. Teresi LM, Lufkin RB, Reicher MA, et al. Asymptomatic degenerative disk disease and spondylosis of the cervical spine: MR imaging. *Radiology* 1987;164:83.
8. Manchikanti L, Cash KA, Pampati V, et al. The effectiveness of fluoroscopic cervical interlaminar epidural injections in managing chronic cervical disc herniation and radiculitis: preliminary results of a randomized, double-blind, controlled trial. *Pain Physician* 2010;13:223–236.
9. Peloso P, Gross A, Haines T, et al. Medicinal and injection therapies for mechanical neck disorders. *Cochrane Database Syst Rev* 2007;2:CD000319.
10. Niemisto L, Kalso E, Malmivaara A, et al. Radiofrequency denervation for neck and back pain. A systematic review of randomized controlled trials. *Cochrane Database Syst Rev* 2003;3:CD004058.

3 Low Back Pain and Lumbar Stenosis

Lisa L. Willett

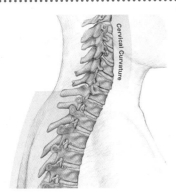

A 62-year-old female presents with complaints of lower back pain and numbness in her feet, intermittently for 8 months. Pain is worse at the end of day and gets better with recumbency; pain is also more noticeable with ambulation and gets better when no longer walking. There is no history of fever, chills, and weight loss. There is no history of trauma or an unusual activity that preceded the onset of these symptoms. There is no history of malignancy or intravenous drug use.

Clinical Presentation

Low back pain is one of the most common reasons that patients seek medical attention. It is estimated that two thirds of adults have experienced low back pain at least once, and approximately 7% have had at least one severe episode within a 1 year period. The typical age of onset of low back pain is between 30 and 50 years, with men and women being equally affected (1,2). Low back pain originates from many spinal structures, and includes ligament strain, degeneration of facet joints, herniated discs, and spinal stenosis (Figs. 3.1A, 3.1B). Symptoms range from mild, self-limiting pain, to severe, incapacitating pain with radicular symptoms, neurologic compromise, and chronic morbidity.

Because of the complexity of the spine anatomy, a precise anatomical diagnosis for patients with low back pain is difficult. It is estimated that only 15% of patients with low back pain are able to be diagnosed with a precise spinal abnormality or specific etiology (1). In an effort to achieve accurate diagnosis and effective therapy, costly imaging and surgical referral is pursued. Despite wide variations in the clinical evaluation and management of low back pain, overall outcomes are similar for patients. Published guidelines exist to guide the clinician on the best approach to evaluate and manage acute and chronic low back pain in the primary care setting.

When taking the medical history, clinicians should attempt to place the patient into a category of risk (2). The three areas of risk are: (a) nonspecific low back pain, (b) pain associated with radiculopathy or spinal stenosis, and (c) pain from a systemic cause. In addition to the pain location, severity, and duration, a prior history of back pain and the clinical course is also important. The first priority is to rule out neurologic compromise. Questions should include the presence of lower extremity motor weakness, fecal incontinence, and urinary retention with overflow incontinence. Of these, urinary retention is the most frequent symptom of cauda equina syndrome.

The next level of questions should evaluate for systematic diseases, especially cancer with spinal metastasis, fractures from osteoporosis or steroid use, and spinal infections. Risk factors for cancer, including multiple myeloma,

CLINICAL POINTS

- Patients with low back pain should be classified into a risk category based on nonspecific low back pain, pain associated with radiculopathy (including herniated disc or spinal stenosis), and pain associated with systemic disease.

- Motor weakness, fecal incontinence, and urinary retention are symptoms of cauda equina syndrome and require immediate surgical evaluation.

- Patients with psychosocial stressors are more likely to develop chronic pain.

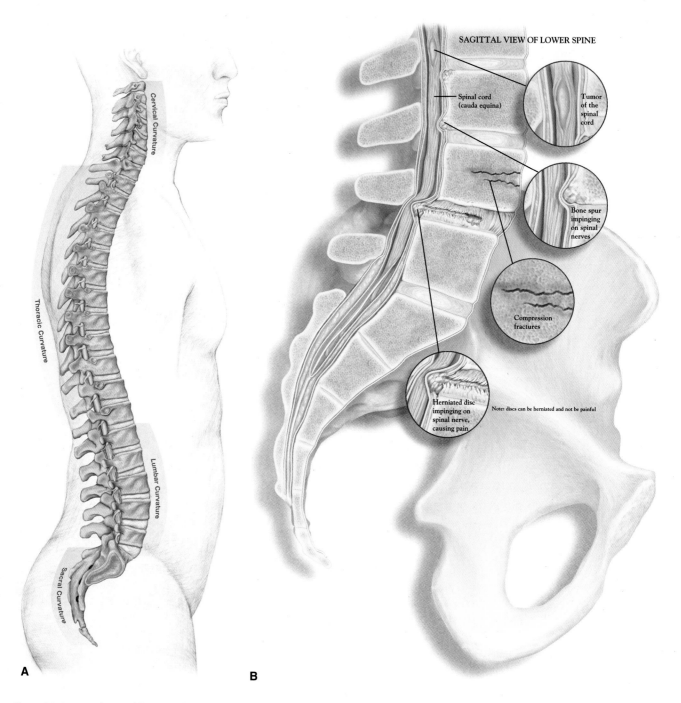

Figure 3.1 A: Sagittal view of the normal spine. Image provided by Anatomical Chart Co. **B:** Causes of low back pain. From Nettina SM. *Lippincott Manual of Nursing Practice,* 9th ed. Philadelphia: Wolters Kluwer Health; 2010.

include the following: age >50 years, a history of cancer, unexplained weight loss, night time pain or pain worsened with recumbent positions, and pain >6 weeks in duration. Risk factors for infection include fever, unexplained weight loss, history of intravenous drug use, indwelling catheters, recent infections, and history of bacteremia.

Of patients who present to primary care with low back pain, spinal stenosis and symptomatic herniated discs account for 3% and 4%, respectively (2). Patients present with neurogenic claudication, or sciatica, the latter being defined as back pain radiating into the buttock and lower leg in a lumbar nerve root distribution. Patients with spinal stenosis are typically over the

• •
PATIENT ASSESSMENT

- Physical examination should evaluate for fever, vertebral tenderness, and neurologic deficits

- Radicular symptoms are seen with herniated discs or spinal stenosis

- Herniated discs cause acute severe back pain, involve L4/L5 and L5/S1, and have a positive straight leg-raising test

- Spinal stenosis occurs in elderly patients with a history of chronic low back pain, worse with walking or standing, improved with bending forward, induced when bending backward, and has bilateral plantar numbness

age of 60 years and have a history of chronic low back pain for months to years. The pain is worse with walking or standing, improved with bending forward, and, at times, induced when bending backward (3,4). In a study of patients presenting to an orthopedic surgeon with pain or numbness in the legs, the most specific symptoms for lumbar spinal stenosis were a history of urinary symptoms, improvement with bending forward, and bilateral plantar numbness (5). Herniated lumbar discs can also present with sciatica, but can be distinguished from spinal stenosis by an acute onset of pain and examination features, such as a positive straight leg-raising, which is suggestive of a herniated disc.

Finally, assessment of psychosocial distress is important. Patients with depression, somatization disorder, substance abuse, job dissatisfaction or disability compensation, and those involved in litigation are more likely to have prolonged back pain and persistent unexplained symptoms (5).

Examination

As with the history, the physical examination for patients with low back pain should focus on the neurologic examination and should ensure that there are no deficits. After assessing for fever and the presence of vertebral tenderness with palpation, a focused neurologic examination should be performed. More than 90% of herniated discs occur at the L4/L5 and L5/S1 levels and the neurologic examination focuses on these nerve roots, and includes the straight leg-raising test (Fig. 3.2), and the motor and sensory function tests (2).

A straight leg-raising test involves having the patient supine on the examination table. The examiner holds the leg straight with one hand and cups the heel with the other. The straight leg is lifted off the examination table from the heel in an effort to reproduce the patient's sciatica. A positive test produces pain that radiates below the knee between 30 and 70 degrees of elevation. A positive test on the ipsilateral side has a sensitivity of approximately 90% for a herniated disc, whereas a positive test when the opposite leg is raised (a crossed test) has a specificity of approaching 90% (2). Further neurologic evaluation includes sensory and motor findings of the L4 through S1 nerve root, and includes assessing knee strength and reflexes (L4), great toe and foot dorsiflexion (L5), foot plantar flexion and ankle reflexes (S1).

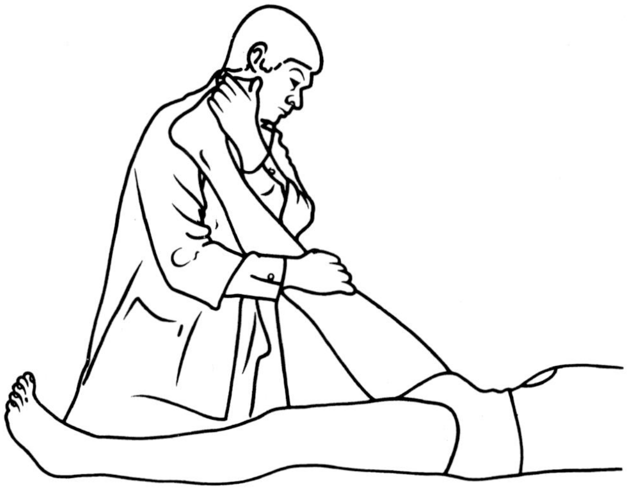

Figure 3.2 The straight leg-raising test. MediClip image copyright © 2003 Lippincott Williams & Wilkins. All rights reserved.

Studies

Findings on radiologic imaging correlate poorly with the severity of symptoms in patients with low back pain. Therefore, routine imaging is not clinically useful for patients with nonspecific low back pain. Imaging is recommended for patients with concerns for cancer, fracture, or infection, and for patients with neurologic findings. Guidelines recommend plain radiography for patients with a possible systemic illness, including patients with fever, unexplained weight loss, a history of cancer, alcohol or drug injection, trauma, focal vertebral tenderness on palpation, and age older than 50 years.

Plain radiography is not sensitive for early cancer or infection. Thus, if the clinical suspicion is high, further testing such as an erythrocyte sedimentation rate (ESR) or C-reactive protein (CRP), a complete blood count (CBC), and a computed tomography (CT) or magnetic resonance imaging (MRI) should be performed. Patients with severe or progressive neurologic deficits should have prompt imaging with a CT or MRI, and emergent evaluation for spinal cord compromise. Delayed diagnosis and treatment for spinal cord compromise from infection, cancer, or cauda equina syndrome has poorer outcomes. MRI is a more sensitive test than CT, and has replaced CT myelography for diagnostic testing.

Elderly patients, specifically those over the age of 65 years, are at increased risk for spinal stenosis, cancer, compression fractures, and aortic abdominal aneurysms (AAA) (1). In these patients, one should have a lower threshold for imaging and should consider alternate studies. For patients with findings suggestive of spinal stenosis, an MRI can confirm the diagnosis; if numbness and weakness are present, an electromyography and nerve conduction study can define the extent of neurologic involvement and rule out a peripheral neuropathy. An abdominal ultrasound can demonstrate an AAA. These patients should have close follow up to ensure that the appropriate diagnosis was made.

Treatment

Treatment for low back pain first involves educating the patient about the expected clinical outcome. Overall, the prognosis is good, and most patients will improve within 4 weeks. For patients with nonspecific low back pain, evidence is limited but suggests that conservative management is effective for symptom relief. Patients should resume normal activities when able to, and should avoid bed rest. Heating pads and blankets may provide relief, but there is insufficient evidence to recommend lumbar supports or ice packs. Heavy lifting and twisting should be avoided.

Medical therapy has been shown to provide short term relief to patients with acute low back pain (1,2). Patients should be prescribed nonsteroidal anti-inflammatory drugs (NSAIDS) and muscle relaxers as first line therapy, unless there is a contraindication such as renal insufficiency or a risk of gastrointestinal bleeding. Acetaminophen is less effective than NSAIDS but a safe and reasonable first-line option for patients who cannot take NSAIDS. There is no data to guide clinicians on the dose and duration of therapy.

For patients with severe pain, unrelieved with NSAIDS and muscle relaxants, opioid analgesics and tramadol can be considered, weighing the risk of chronic usage and abuse potential. Tricyclic antidepressants are effective for chronic low back pain; selective serotonin reuptake inhibitors (SSRIs) and trazodone are not. Gabapentin has limited data showing small short-term benefit in patients with radiculopathy; systemic corticosteroids have not been shown to be effective and are not recommended for patients, with or without sciatica.

Multiple interventions such as spinal manipulation, physical therapy, massage therapy, and acupuncture have been used to treat acute low back pain (1,2). Although evidence is lacking, certain patients may derive relief when used as second line therapy. Traction, facet-joint injections, and transcutaneous electrical nerve stimulation also lack supporting evidence of efficacy. Because the majority of low back pain improves within 4 weeks, referral for such alternate interventions should be delayed until then.

Therapy options for patients with herniated disks are the same as for nonspecific low back pain. Unless there is cauda equina syndrome or progressive neurologic deficits, the majority of patients improve. The pain may be more severe, requiring narcotic analgesia, and epidural corticosteroids may provide additional relief; systemic corticosteroids have not been shown to provide benefit. Patients with severe pain, despite therapy, and those with persistent neurologic deficits should be evaluated with an MRI or CT and referred for surgical evaluation.

Evidence to guide nonsurgical therapy for patients with lumbar spinal stenosis is lacking, and there is wide variation in the methods used. Although data support the benefit of surgical decompression, the benefit of surgery compared to nonsurgical approaches is unknown. Medical therapy is recommended for patients with high surgical risk and mild-to-moderate symptoms (3,4).

NOT TO BE MISSED

- Neurologic compromise and cauda equina
- Metastatic cancer, fracture, or spinal infection
- Focal vertebral tenderness to palpation
- Fever
- Unexplained weight loss
- History of cancer, alcohol, or drug injection
- Trauma
- Age over 50 years
- Pain duration >6 weeks
- Life-threatening conditions outside the spine, such as aortic aneurysm, pancreatitis, and endocarditis

- Neurologic deficits on physical examination, especially cauda equina
- Severe pain unresponsive to medical management
- Spinal stenosis with severe pain or functional limitations

The first line of nonsurgical therapy for spinal stenosis is to modify the patient's activity. Patients can obtain significant pain relief by limiting the activities that induce the pain, such as prolonged walking and standing. Postural adjustment with a cane or walker provides relief by promoting forward flexion of the lumbar spine, relieving the stenosis.

Physical therapy to increase strength and abdominal core muscles provide relief to some patients, and up to 30% of patients may get significant relief (4). Exercise biking and other modalities to increase leg strength, and avoiding sedatives and alcohol are important for fall prevention.

Oral analgesics are given to patients for symptomatic relief, although studies specific to lumbar spinal stenosis are lacking. Gabapentin was shown in one unblinded study to improve pain and walking distance as compared to placebo. Lumbar epidural steroid injections are commonly used, but with no data to support efficacy, it is a second line therapy option.

Surgical intervention with decompressive laminectomy is the traditional first line recommended therapy. Studies support improved outcomes in patients with persistent sciatica, radiologic signs of stenosis, nerve root compression, and no prior back surgery. Surgical techniques have evolved and now include hemilaminectomy and techniques to preserve the interspinous ligaments. Although studies show long term outcomes to be successful in patients with advanced age, even in their 80s, operative risk must be weighed carefully as surgical comorbidities are often present in the elderly (4).

Clinical Course

In patients with acute low back pain, it has been reported that 90% improve within 2 weeks (1). The majority of patients with nonspecific low back pain, and even those with a herniated disc, improve within 4 weeks with conservative treatment. Therefore, patients with pain that persists longer than 4 to 6 weeks, despite conservative therapy, should be reevaluated and have imaging to rule out a systemic process. Some cross-sectional studies of patients followed in primary care show that more than 60% of patients improved within 7 weeks, but recurrence was common, affecting 40% of patients within 6 months (1).

Most patients with spinal stenosis who are managed medically do not have significant clinical progression over the course of a year. Symptoms and neurologic examination should not acutely worsen; likewise, dramatic symptomatic improvement is uncommon. Therefore, patients can be followed clinically over time, and if the patient's pain progresses despite nonsurgical therapy, referral for laminectomy should be considered. Surgery results in better pain relief for several years. However, in cohort studies, 30% of patients had severe pain 4 years after surgery and 10% required reoperation (1).

Chronic low back pain is challenging for both the patient and clinician. In studies, predictors of persistent back pain and worse outcomes at 1 year included the presence of nonorganic signs, maladaptive pain coping behaviors, high baseline functional impairment, psychiatric comorbidities, and low general health status. Depression, job dissatisfaction or disability compensation, and those involved in litigation are also more likely to have prolonged back pain and persistent unexplained symptoms. Baseline pain and the presence of radicular symptoms were not predictive of persistent pain (6).

Conclusions

Low back pain is common and will affect the majority of adult patients in their lifetime. Despite wide variations in the clinical evaluation and management of low back pain, overall outcomes for most patients are good, and even with a herniated disc, clinical improvement is achieved within 6 weeks. Most back pain is nonspecific, although one should evaluate for pain with radiculopathy from a herniated disc or spinal stenosis, and pain from a systemic illness such as cancer or infection. Spinal stenosis is more common in elderly patients with a history of chronic low back pain for months to years, worse with walking or standing, and improved with bending forward. Other causes of back pain, such as referred pain from pancreatitis, AAA, nephrolithiasis, or spondyloarthropathy, should be considered in the differential diagnosis in patients with history or physical examination suggestive of these conditions.

The history and physical examination should focus on ensuring that there is no neurologic compromise or cauda equina syndrome and includes assessing for lower extremity motor weakness, fecal incontinence, and urinary retention. Evidence of systemic illness, such as weight loss and fever, raises concern for malignancy or infection and should be further evaluated. For patients with sciatica, a straight leg-raising test can be sensitive for herniated disc.

Routine imaging is not indicated for the majority of patients with nonspecific low back pain. Imaging is recommended for patients with concerns for cancer, fracture, or infection, and for patients with neurologic findings. Patients with fever, unexplained weight loss, a history of cancer, alcohol or drug injection, trauma, focal vertebral tenderness on palpation, and age over 50 years should have plain radiographs. If the clinical suspicion is high for cancer or infection, laboratory studies and imaging with a CT or MRI should be performed. Patients with severe or progressive neurologic deficits should have an emergent evaluation for spinal cord compromise with an MRI.

First line treatment for patients with nonspecific low back pain is conservative therapy and includes NSAIDS and muscle relaxers, and patient education about the overall good prognosis within 4 to 6 weeks. Patients should resume normal activities and avoid bed rest. Patients with a herniated disc can have severe pain, such that opiate therapy may be required. For patients with progressive severe pain and functional limitations from spinal stenosis, laminectomy should be considered. Psychosocial stressors, including psychiatric conditions or litigation, are predictive of a disabling chronic pain.

ICD9

716.9 **Arthritis, arthritic** *(acute) (chronic) (subacute)*
  721.3 lumbar
724.5 **Backache** *(postural)*
924.9 **Contusion** *(skin surface intact)*
  922.31 With back
Degeneration, degenerative
  722.6 intervertebral disc
  722.70 with myelopathy
  722.52 lumbar, lumbosacral
  722.73 with myelopathy
  722.51 thoracic, thoracolumbar
  722.72 with myelopathy
Displacement, displaced
  722.2 intervertebral disc (with neuritis, radiculitis, sciatica,
    or other pain)
  722.10 lumbar, lumbosacral
  722.73 with myelopathy
  722.11 thoracic, thoracolumbar
729.2 **Radiculitis** *(pressure) (vertebrogenic)*
  724.4 lumbar NEC
  724.2 lumbosacral

ICD9 (Continued)

729.0 **Rheumatism, rheumatic** *(acute NEC)*
   724.9 back
756.12 **Spondylolisthesis** *(congenital) (lumbosacral)*
   738.4 acquired
   738.4 degenerative
   738.4 traumatic
756.11 **Spondylolysis** *(congenital)*
   738.4 acquired
   756.11 lumbosacral region
721.90 **Spondylosis**
   721.3 lumbar, lumbosacral
   721.42 with myelopathy
Sprain, strain *(joint) (ligament) (muscle)*
   846.9 low back
   846.0 lumbosacral
   724.6 chronic or old
Stenosis *(cicatricial)*
   724.00 spinal
   724.02 lumbar, lumbosacral
   724.09 specified region NEC
   724.01 thoracic, thoracolumbar

References

1. Deyo RA, Weinstein JN. Low back pain. *N Engl J Med* 2001;344(5):363–370.
2. Chou R, Qaseem A, Snow V, et al. Diagnosis and treatment of low back pain: a joint clinical practice guideline from the American College of Physicians and the American Pain Society. *Ann Intern Med* 2007;147:478–491.
3. Katz JN, Harris MB. Lumbar spinal stenosis. *N Engl J Med* 2008;358(8):818–825.
4. Markman JD, Gaud KG. Lumbar spinal stenosis in older adults: current understanding and future directions. *Clin Geriatr Med* 2008;24:369–388.
5. Ebell MH. Diagnosing lumbar spinal stenosis. *Am Fam Physician* 2009;80(10):1145–1147.
6. Chou R, Shekelle P. Will this patient develop persistent disabling low back pain? *JAMA* 2010;303(13): 1295–1302.

4 Shoulder Pain

Dennis W. Boulware

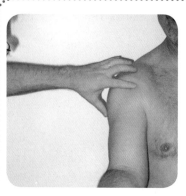

A 26-year-old man presents with a 10-day history of right shoulder and upper arm pain, worse with lifting his arm over his head and interfering with sleep as he cannot find a position of comfort. He has tried rest and acetaminophen without relief. No trauma or precipitating event is recollected, but he had recently completed re-painting his bedroom over the weekend, 2 weeks ago.

Clinical Presentation

Shoulder pain is one of the most common complaints seen in a primary care setting especially with elderly patients. Most causes of shoulder pain are due to soft tissue periarticular problems such as rotator cuff impingement or injury, bursitis, and/or an adhesive capsulitis (frozen shoulder) as opposed to glenohumeral arthritis. The clinical context of the shoulder pain often provides insight into the source of the problem such as a history of a systemic inflammatory or degenerative condition, repetitive use, or recent injury. This chapter addresses the clinical setting of nontraumatic isolated shoulder pain, and for a discussion of shoulder pain due to systemic or generalized diseases such as rheumatoid arthritis, polymyalgia rheumatica, or osteoarthritis, the reader should refer to those specific chapters.

Most causes of shoulder pain can be attributed to soft-tissue structures surrounding the glenohumeral joint, as opposed to those originating from glenohumeral arthritis. An understanding of the anatomy and biomechanics of the shoulder, coupled with a focused physical examination to localize the anatomic source of pain, typically provides the clinician with an accurate diagnosis (Fig. 4.1). Proper and effective management can be implemented only after the source of the pain is identified accurately.

The shoulder is the most flexible and mobile joint in the body. This mobility is achieved by having a bony ball-and-socket joint with a large ball and a relatively small socket. This relatively unstable arrangement is made secure by the surrounding extra-articular structures including the various ligaments, labrum, rotator cuff, bicipital tendon, deltoid muscles, and so on. Typically, shoulder pain is due to dysfunction or disruption of the supporting soft-tissue structures, as opposed to glenohumeral arthritis. The most commonly involved structures causing shoulder pain are the rotator cuff, the subacromial bursa, the bicipital tendon, and the synovial capsule.

The first step in evaluating the patient is to confirm that they are describing a shoulder joint pain or a joint-related problem as they often refer to pain in the trapezius muscle as "shoulder pain." Pain from the shoulder joint or its related periarticular structures is felt in the area over the deltoid muscle or

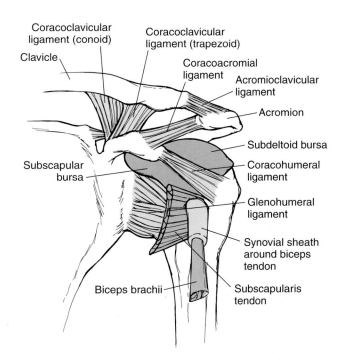

Coracoclavicular ligament (conoid)
Coracoclavicular ligament (trapezoid)
Clavicle
Coracoacromial ligament
Acromioclavicular ligament
Acromion
Subdeltoid bursa
Subscapular bursa
Coracohumeral ligament
Glenohumeral ligament
Synovial sheath around biceps tendon
Biceps brachii
Subscapularis tendon

Figure 4.1 The shoulder joint illustrating the relationship of the glenohumeral joint, the supraspinatus tendon of the rotator cuff, and the long head of the biceps tendon. The area between the humeral head and acromion process is occupied by the subacromial bursa. From Hendrickson T. *Massage for Orthopedic Conditions.* Baltimore: Lippincott Williams & Wilkins; 2002.

the upper brachium. Pain described in the trapezius muscle is likely due to trapezius muscle strain or referred from the cervical spine. If the patient confirms that the pain is localized to the deltoid area and/or the upper brachium, then proceed with an evaluation of the shoulder joint and its periarticular structures.

Historical qualities regarding severity or quality of pain are limited in identifying the cause of pain, whereas precipitating and alleviating factors, recent repetitive nonroutine activities (house painting, wallpaper hanging, etc.), and/ or injuries can provide some insight. Shoulder pain precipitated by use is the most common presenting complaint and certain uses of the affected arm can be helpful. The rotator cuff is typically affected in the external rotators, especially the supraspinatus. Pain felt with forward flexion, abduction, or active external rotation of the shoulder typically suggests involvement of the rotator cuff. Pain on abduction, but not on external rotation or forward flexion of the shoulder suggests the subacromial bursa as the cause of pain. Nocturnal pain during sleep and the inability to find a restful recumbent position in bed are also common complaints of a rotator cuff problem or the subacromial bursa.

Examination

The physical examination of the shoulder is critical in identifying the cause and managing shoulder pain. A systematic routine examination of the shoulder will help the clinician identify the cause of the shoulder pain quickly and effectively. The examination will focus on the range of passive motion in rotation, abduction, and forward flexion as well as provocative maneuvers to attempt to reproduce the pain by active motion, palpation, or resistance. Tenderness present on active motion that is absent on the same motion passively usually suggests a tendinitis as the pain is elicited when tension is placed on the tendon. Typically, the patient will be guarding the painful shoulder voluntarily or involuntarily and the examination will be

CLINICAL POINTS

- Shoulder pain is often due to a soft tissue cause such as tendonitis or bursitis, rather than arthritis.

- The physical examination of the shoulder is essential in identifying the cause.

- The pain frequently radiates into the brachium.

- Exploring recent overuse or trauma may help identify the cause.

- When examination of the shoulder is fruitless in identifying a cause, consider referred pain from a cervical radiculopathy.

SECTION 2 Regional Pain Syndromes

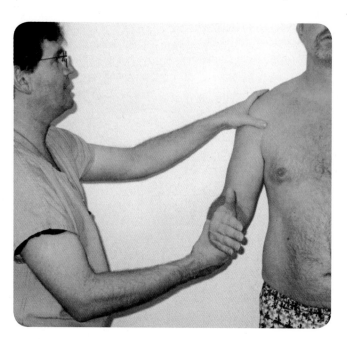

Figure 4.2 Measuring passive rotation. From Berg D, Worzala K. *Atlas of Adult Physical Diagnosis*. Philadelphia: Lippincott Williams & Wilkins; 2006.

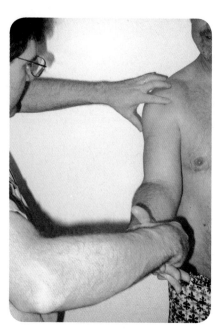

Figure 4.3 Measuring passive glenohumeral abduction and forward flexion. From Berg D, Worzala K. *Atlas of Adult Physical Diagnosis*. Philadelphia: Lippincott Williams & Wilkins; 2006.

insightful only if the patient is relaxed and cooperative. The prudent clinician will examine the non-tender shoulder first to prepare the patient for examination of the painful shoulder.

Start the examination with the patient sitting on the examination table in front of you. Passively flex the elbow to 90 degrees with the patient's elbow to their side and gently use the forearm to rotate the shoulder joint internally, as it typically will not precipitate tenderness and will aid in gaining the patient's confidence, and then test for external rotation (Fig. 4.2). Passive internal rotation to 90 degrees and passive external rotation to 90 degrees are normal, and is typically painless but diminishes slightly with age. Internal rotation is rarely tender or limited, but decreased passive external rotation will suggest structural barriers to full passive motion including bony and soft tissue structures. Osteophytes from degenerative joint disease or a contracted joint capsule from adhesive capsulitis, or a frozen shoulder, are common causes and will require imaging studies to differentiate. Non-tender decreased passive rotation may indicate the later stages of adhesive capsulitis or stable degenerative joint disease. Tenderness on passive external rotation only may indicate an active adhesive capsulitis or active osteoarthritis, whereas tenderness on passive internal and external rotations can suggest active synovitis from infectious or inflammatory causes.

Next, position yourself at the patient's side and stabilize the scapula with your hand closer to the patient's back by placing your fingers on the horizontal scapular spine and your thumb along the scapula's lateral border inhibiting its ability to slide laterally over the ribs. Use your forward hand to grasp the elbow and with the patient relaxed, passively abduct the shoulder to measure glenohumeral abduction (Fig. 4.3). Normal glenohumeral abduction is 90 degrees, but again diminishes with aging. Unless the patient is completely relaxed, the technique may need to be done several times to assess accurately the true range of motion. After measuring glenohumeral abduction, release the scapula and measure full abduction which should approach 180 degrees. Then measure forward flexion by passively flexing the shoulder anteriorly to measure flexion, which should be 180 degrees. The supraspinatus tendon resides in the space between the humeral head and acromion process; a space that decreases in size when the humerus is abducted or flexed forward. Tenderness on passive glenohumeral abduction and forward flexion is very indicative of an inflamed supraspinatus tendon. Tenderness on passive abduction but not flexion suggests subacromial bursitis, which can be confirmed by direct palpation of the subacromial bursa that lies lateral and inferior of the acromion process. These techniques will identify problems with primarily the supraspinatus involvement of the rotator cuff. Active isometric loading to test active rotation will help identify involvement of infraspinatus and teres major muscles as a cause of shoulder pain. To load the shoulder in isometric rotation, have the patient hold their arm at their side with the elbow flexed at 90 degrees. Ask the patient to maintain that position and resist the examiner's attempt to move the forearm. Tenderness when the examiner attempts to move the shoulder in internal rotation indicates a problem with the rotator cuff's external rotators; the supraspinatus, infraspinatus, and/or teres major. Tenderness when the examiner attempts to move the shoulder in external rotation requiring active internal rotation from the patient implicates the internal rotators; the subscapularis. These maneuvers will usually elicit tenderness when the rotator cuff is involved. These maneuvers will not indicate if there is a tear of the rotator cuff, rotator cuff tendinitis, or calcific tendinitis of the supraspinatus tendon, which are all common causes of shoulder pain.

Bicipital tendinitis is a less common cause of shoulder pain than problems with the rotator cuff or subacromial bursitis, and should be suspected if the preceding examination fails to elicit any tenderness. Bicipital tendinitis most commonly occurs as the tendon traverses the humeral head through the bicipital groove on the anterior surface of the humeral head. Bicipital tendinitis at this level can be detected by the presence of tenderness on direct palpation of the tendon within the bicipital groove of the humeral head and/or through Yergason's maneuver, a provocative test. Place your thumb with moderate pressure on the anterior surface of the shoulder and passively rotate the shoulder using the forearm as a lever with the patient holding the elbow at 90 degrees. Your thumb will sense the bicipital groove as it dips into it and the patient will feel tenderness as your thumb rides over the tendon within the bicipital groove. Confirmation can be achieved through Yergason's maneuver, which tests the tendon by active isometric loading. Have the patient place his or her fully flexed elbow at the side with the wrist fully supinated. Grasp the patient's hand and ask the patient to resist your attempt to simultaneously extend the elbow and pronate the wrist. This maneuver actively loads the biceps tendon and should elicit tenderness at the shoulder when an active bicipital tendinitis is present.

Occasionally, shoulder pain is not due to dysfunction or disruption of the shoulder joint or its surrounding supportive soft-tissue structures. If the preceding examination fails to reproduce the patient's complaint and identify the source of the pain within the shoulder area, then a consideration of referred shoulder pain is merited. Pain from a cervical radiculopathy often radiates to the shoulder area. Keeping the shoulder in a neutral non-tender position while testing the cervical spine for passive hyperextension combined with passive lateral bending and/or rotation may precipitate and reproduce the patient's chief complaint of shoulder pain. Less commonly, visceral pathology from the pancreas or gallbladder will refer pain to the shoulder.

Studies

The laboratory is of no help in evaluating the patient with shoulder pain; the physical examination is more enlightening.

In acute shoulder pain, imaging is rarely helpful and should be avoided unless a fracture is a consideration.

SECTION 2 Regional Pain Syndromes

PATIENT ASSESSMENT

- Alleviating and exacerbating factors can be helpful, especially recent overhead use of arm.

- Tenderness on active isometric loading but not passive range of motion suggests tendinitis.

- Tenderness on passive range of motion but not active isometric loading suggests active adhesive capsulitis or active osteoarthritis.

- Reserve imaging studies for recurrent or recalcitrant shoulder pain.

NOT TO BE MISSED

- Pain that is not reproduced on the examination may be referred from the neck.

Treatment

For the nontraumatic causes of shoulder pain discussed earlier, a progressive conservative treatment program is usually successful. This program should start with nonpharmacologic management, including rest and judicious physical therapy. Resting the acutely painful shoulder may require the use of a sling when upright to support the arm. Overhead use of the arm with the shoulder in prolonged abduction is to be avoided as it will certainly aggravate the pain.

Physical therapy in the acutely painful setting should be limited to passive range-of-motion exercises, such as Codman pendulum swinging exercises. Range of motion exercises help avoid the development and complications of adhesive capsulitis, or a frozen shoulder. Passive movements after local heat or cold application, or after analgesic administration, are advisable. These movements should start slowly, with progressively increased range of motion as symptoms subside. A good starting point is the simple pendulum exercise (Fig. 4.4). Instruct the patient to use the unaffected arm for support by placing it on a stable table or chair. The patient can flex the trunk at the hips or waist and suspend the affected arm until approximately 90 degrees of flexion is achieved. The patient can swing the suspended affected arm passively like a pendulum. The exercise should be done in the sagittal plane for flexion–extension, and in the coronal plane for abduction–adduction. With time the degrees of swinging can be increased and the passive swinging can be replaced by an active range of motion exercises, eventually with resistance.

Analgesia can be provided through nonpharmacologic measures such as heat and cold packs, or ultrasonic therapy. If ineffective, then simple analgesics and nonsteroidal anti-inflammatory drugs (NSAIDs) are usually adequate. Narcotic analgesics may be necessary for severe pain but should be used on a limited basis.

If the pain is severe or the preceding basic measures have already failed, then local corticosteroids are usually indicated and can be administered into the subacromial bursa or into the glenohumeral joint.

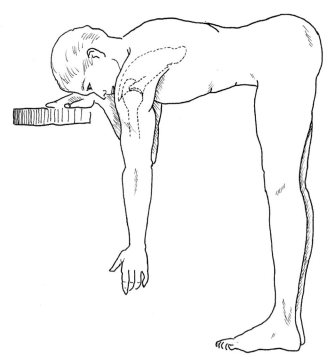

Figure 4.4 The starting position for Codman pendulum exercises for passive motion of the shoulder. From Koopman WJ, Moreland LW, eds. *Arthritis and Allied Conditions A Textbook of Rheumatology*, 15th ed. Philadelphia: Lippincott Williams & Wilkins; 2005.

WHEN TO REFER

- Structural abnormalities like inferior acromioclavicular osteophytes, rotator cuff complete tears, or severe degenerative glenohumeral changes may require referral to an orthopedic surgeon.

In most cases, there will be significant and satisfactory improvement in 1 to 4 weeks. Pain that persists beyond this time or recurs with a resumption of usual activity suggests chronic impingement, instability, or alternative cause. At this time, a referral to a rheumatologist may be advisable.

Clinical Course

In most cases, acute shoulder pain will resolve spontaneously with mild analgesia, passive range of motion exercises, and time. Even with proper treatment, shoulder pain can be recurrent and refractory if an underlying cause of instability or impingement is uncorrected. The patient who returns with recurrent or refractory pain should undergo the same clinical examination initially described to confirm the same diagnosis. At this time, imaging can be helpful and plain radiographs of the shoulder may reveal the underlying cause.

In cases of chronic or recurring pain, imaging studies can identify the cause in cases of chronic rotator cuff pathology or calcific tendinitis. The following are radiographic findings of common causes of recurrent or persistent shoulder pain:

1. Inferior osteophyte of a degenerative acromioclavicular joint. The osteophyte will encroach into the acromiohumeral space and result in a bony impingement of the rotator cuff. This finding may indicate the need for a surgical consultation.
2. Calcific tendinitis. Calcification of the rotator cuff is a consequence of the chronicity of the inflammation and not a cause of the tendinitis. It indicates a more chronic condition and the need for continued therapy. Eventually the calcification may resolve as will the condition.
3. Sclerosis and cystic degeneration of the humeral greater tuberosity. This implies a chronic and severe impingement of the humeral head against the acromion with concurrent impingement of the rotator cuff with consequential joint instability. This finding implies the need for a surgical consultation.
4. Narrowing or obliteration of the acromiohumeral space. This finding can only occur with attrition or a complete tear of the rotator cuff, indicating instability of the joint. If seen on plain radiography, a surgical consultation may be required.

SECTION 2 Regional Pain Syndromes

ICD9

727.3 **Bursitis** *NEC*
  726.10 shoulder
726.90 **Capsulitis** *(joint)*
  726.0 adhesive (shoulder)
Degeneration, degenerative
  718.01 shoulder
Derangement
  718.30 recurrent
  718.31 shoulder region
  718.91 shoulder region
Disorder
  727.9 bursa
    726.10 shoulder region
  733.90 cartilage NEC
    718.01 shoulder region
716.60 **Monoarthritis**
  716.61 shoulder (region)

(Continued)

ICD9 (Continued)

715.91 **Osteoarthrosis/Osteoarthritis shoulder** *(degenerative)*
(hypertrophic)
780.96 **Pain(s)**
  719.40 joint
    719.41 shoulder (region)
726.90 **Periarthritis** *(joint)*
  726.2 shoulder
*726.90–***Tendinitis, tendonitis**
  727.82 calcific
    726.11 shoulder

Additional Reading

1. Husni EM, Donohue JP. Painful shoulder and reflex sympathetic dystrophy syndrome. In Koopman WJ, Moreland LW, eds; *Arthritis and Allied Conditions*, 15th ed. Philadelphia: Lippincott Williams & Wilkins; 2005:2133–2151.
2. Boulware DW. The painful shoulder. In Koopman WJ, Boulware DW, Heudebert GR, eds. *Clinical Primer of Rheumatology*. Philadelphia: Lippincott Williams & Wilkins;2003:43–47.
3. Woodward TW, Best TM. The painful shoulder: part 1. Clinical evaluation. *Am Fam Physician* 2000;61:3079–3088.
4. Woodward TW, Best TM. The painful shoulder: part 2. Acute and chronic disorders. *Am Fam Physician* 2000;61:3291–3300.

CHAPTER 5 Painful Feet

Dennis W. Boulware and Gustavo R. Heudebert

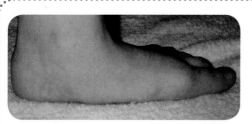

A 42-year-old female marketing executive complains of painful feet that are interfering with her ability to work. Her work involves wearing dress shoes appropriate for her position and often long periods of standing while making presentations. Her business footwear is typically elevated heels and her examination reveals a pes cavus type of foot with numerous hard corns on her toes.

Introduction

Foot pain and loss of function may be caused by a number of problems and can be the manifestation of a large number of defined clinical entities. Foot pain is a symptom, not a diagnosis, and a precise diagnosis should be made to ensure proper treatment, which is specific for that particular problem. If the physician perceives the problem simply as "foot pain," a successful outcome is unlikely and even though foot problems are extremely common, the foot is largely an ignored area.

For practical purposes, the foot is divided anatomically as the forefoot, the midfoot, and the hindfoot. The forefoot comprises the toes, their respective metatarsal bones, and surrounding soft tissues. The hindfoot is defined as the era comprising the calcaneous and the talus with their corresponding surrounding soft tissues. Finally, the midfoot is the area occupied by the cuboid, navicular, and three cuneiform bones (later, intermediate, and medial) and the corresponding surrounding soft tissue. Most of the nontraumatic disorders of the foot will occur in the forefoot and hindfoot area; furthermore, and for the purposes of clarity, we will classify these disorders nosologically as related to mechanical or neurological etiologies.

Clinical Presentation

MECHANICAL PROBLEMS

Forefoot Varus and Valgus Deformities

Forefoot varus or valgus is an abnormality of the foot in which the forefoot is inverted (varus) or everted (valgus) in relation to the hindfoot when the subtalar joint is in the neutral position. The head of the first and fifth metatarsals are no longer in the same horizontal plane of each other with the first metatarsal head dorsal (varus) or ventral (valgus) relative to the fifth metatarsal head. Forefoot varus is a major cause of compensatory subtalar pronation of an abnormal degree during the stance phase of gait.

CLINICAL POINTS

- Foot pain is a symptom and not a diagnosis.
- Careful examination of the foot will provide great insight into the diagnosis.
- Orthoses and proper footwear can provide relief in many cases.

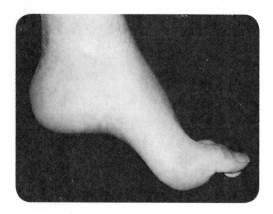

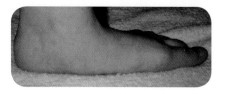

Figure 5.1 Pes planus deformity with loss of the longitudinal arch of the foot. From Berg D, Worzala K. *Atlas of Adult Physical Diagnosis.* Philadelphia, PA: Lippincott Williams & Wilkins; 2006.

Figure 5.2 Severe pes cavus seen in spastic neurological disorders.

Pes Planus

Pes planus, or flat feet, is often asymptomatic but can cause fatigue of the foot muscles and aching with intolerance to prolonged walking or standing (Fig. 5.1). The most common type is the flexible flatfoot although other causes of flatfeet are tarsal coalition, congenital vertical talus, and rupture of the tibialis posterior tendon, which causes the typical unilateral, acquired flatfoot. In pes planus, there is loss of the longitudinal arch on the medial aspect of the foot, the calcaneus is everted (valgus), and on ambulation out-toeing can be seen; these changes are more apparent on weight bearing. This condition is largely inherited and is seen with generalized hypermobility.

Pes Cavus

An unusually high medial longitudinal arch characterizes pes cavus, or claw foot, and in severe cases causes a high longitudinal arch resulting in shortening of the foot (Fig. 5.2). With the abnormally high longitudinal arch, there is relative shortening of the extensor ligaments causing dorsiflexion of the metatarsophalangeal (MTP) joints and plantar flexion of the proximal interphalangeal and distal interphalangeal joints giving the clawing appearance of the toes. The plantar fascia may be contracted and the calcaneus is usually in a varus (inverted) position. In general, the tendency to pes cavus is inherited but can be a clue to an underlying neurologic disorder, such as myelomeningocele, Charcot–Marie–Tooth disease, or Friedreich ataxia. Although pes cavus can cause foot fatigue, pain, and tenderness over the metatarsal heads with callus formation, it can be asymptomatic. Calluses can be present over the dorsum of the toes from increased friction to footwear.

Hallux Valgus

In hallux valgus, deviation of the large toe lateral to the midline and deviation of the first metatarsal medially occur. A bunion (adventitious bursa) of the head of the first MTP joint may be present, often causing pain, tenderness, and swelling. Hallux valgus is more common in women and may result from a genetic tendency, poorly fitted footwear, or secondary to chronic arthritides such as rheumatoid arthritis, chronic gout, or osteoarthritis.

Hallux Rigidus

In hallux rigidus, immobility of the first MTP joint especially on extension is present. Pain is often present at the base of the big toe and is aggravated by walking, especially in footwear with elevated heels. A primary type of hallux rigidus is seen in younger persons, and the acquired form may be secondary to trauma, osteoarthritis, rheumatoid arthritis, or gout. Osteophytes and sclerosis of the first MTP joint can be seen on radiographs. The term *hallux limitus* is sometimes used to denote a milder degree of immobility of the first MTP joint.

Bunionette

A bunionette, or tailor's bunion, is a prominence of the fifth metatarsal head resulting from the overlying bursa and a localized callus. Pressure from shoes can cause pain, and tenderness may be present over the swollen bursa.

Hammer Toe

In hammer toes, the proximal interphalangeal joint is flexed and the tip of the toe points downward. The second toe is most commonly involved and calluses may form at the tip of the toe and over the dorsum of the interphalangeal joints, resulting from friction against the shoe. Hammer toe may be congenital, acquired secondary to hallux valgus or improper footwear. When hammer toes are associated with hyperextension of the MTP joints, the deformity is known as "cocked-up toes." This may be seen in rheumatoid arthritis.

Metatarsalgia

Pain arising from the metatarsal heads, known as metatarsalgia, is a symptom resulting from a variety of conditions. Pain on standing and tenderness on palpation of the metatarsal heads are present. Calluses over the metatarsal heads are usually seen. The causes of metatarsalgia are many, including foot strain, use of high-heel shoes, an everted foot, trauma, sesamoiditis, hallux valgus, chronic arthritis, foot surgery, or a foot with a pes cavus deformity.

Metatarsal Stress Fracture

Pain, swelling, tenderness, and occasional erythema develop over the metatarsal area, usually without any clear history of trauma. The neck of the second metatarsal bone is most frequently involved, but all metatarsals can be sites of fracture (Fig. 5.3). While overuse such as jogging are common causes, stress fractures can be seen in rheumatoid arthritis or generalized osteoporosis or the elderly without a precipitating identifiable event or activity. The key to diagnosis of stress fractures of the foot is to have a high index of suspicion. The difficulty in making the diagnosis is that initial radiographs usually show no abnormalities requiring a repeat radiograph several weeks later to demonstrate healing with callus formation. Bone scans can be helpful to establish an early diagnosis as they show an increase in uptake over the fracture site.

Sesamoid Injuries

Lesions of the sesamoid bones of the big toe may exhibit local pain and tenderness under either the medial or lateral sesamoid. The pain may have a gradual onset or begin abruptly following acute trauma and is exacerbated by dorsiflexion of the big toe or upon weight bearing. Recognized causes of sesamoid pain, which has loosely been called sesamoiditis, are repetitive strain from activities such as dancing or long-distance running, stress fracture, traumatic fracture, bipartite sesamoid, and osteochondritis.

Freiberg Disease

Freiberg disease is an osteochondrosis of the second metatarsal head, primarily affecting girls around 12 years of age. Pain, tenderness, and swelling of the metatarsal are present. Radiographs reveal fragmentation, sclerosis, and deformity of the metatarsal head.

Achilles Tendinitis

Achilles tendinitis usually results from trauma, athletic overactivity, or improperly fitting shoes with a stiff heel counter, but it can also arise from inflammatory conditions such as ankylosing spondylitis, Reiter syndrome, gout, rheumatoid

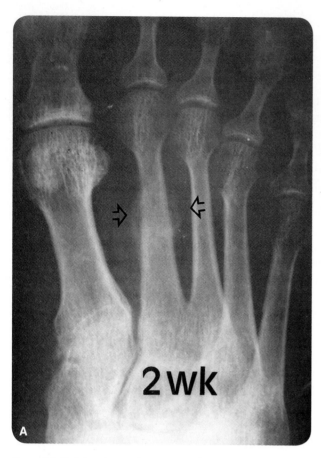
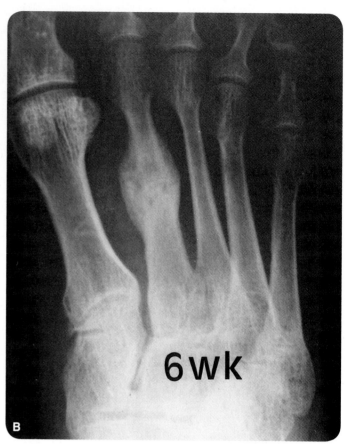

Figure 5.3 Metatarsal stress fracture 2 weeks **(A)** after injury and 6 weeks **(B)** later demonstrating early periosteal reaction at 2 weeks and callus formation at 6 weeks. With permission from Daffner RH. *Clinical Radiology: The Essentials,* 3rd ed. Philadelphia, PA: Lippincott Williams & Wilkins; 2007.

arthritis, and calcium pyrophosphate deposition disease. Pain, swelling, and tenderness occur over the Achilles tendon at its attachment and in the area proximal to the attachment. Crepitus on motion and pain on dorsiflexion may be present.

Achilles Tendon Rupture
Spontaneous rupture of the Achilles tendon is well known and occurs with a sudden onset of pain during forced dorsiflexion. An audible snap may be heard, followed by difficulty in walking and standing on one's toes on the affected foot. Swelling and edema over the area usually develop. Diagnosis can be made with the Thompson test, in which the patient kneels on the chair with the feet extending over the edge and the examiner squeezes the calf and pushes toward the knee. Normally, this produces plantar flexion, but in a ruptured tendon, no plantar flexion occurs. Achilles tendon rupture is generally due to athletic events or trauma from jumps or falls. Magnetic resonance imaging (MRI) can aid in the diagnosis and can distinguish a complete rupture from a partial one. The tendon is more prone to tear in those having preexisting Achilles tendon disease or taking corticosteroids.

Retrocalcaneal Bursitis
The retrocalcaneal bursa is located between the inside surface of the Achilles tendon and the calcaneus; inflammation of this structure is known as an enthesitis. The bursa's anterior wall is fibrocartilage where it attaches to the calcaneus, whereas its posterior wall blends with the surface of the Achilles tendon. Manifestations are pain at the back of the heel, tenderness of the area

anterior to the Achilles tendon, and pain on dorsiflexion. Local swelling is present, with bulging on the medial and lateral aspects of the tendon. Retrocalcaneal bursitis may coexist with Achilles tendinitis, and distinguishing the two is sometimes difficult. This condition may be secondary to rheumatoid arthritis, spondylitis, Reiter syndrome, gout, and trauma.

Subcutaneous Achilles Bursitis
A subcutaneous bursa posterior to the Achilles tendon may become swollen in the absence of systemic disease. This bursitis, known as "pump-bumps," is seen predominantly in women and results from pressure of shoes, although it can also result from bony exostoses.

Plantar Fasciitis
Plantar fasciitis occurs primarily between 40 and 60 years of age but can be seen in all ages. A gradual onset of pain in the plantar area of the heel usually occurs but may occur following trauma or from overuse after activities such as taking part in athletics, walking for a prolonged time, wearing improperly fitting shoes, or striking the heel with some force. The pain is characteristically most severe in the morning upon arising especially with the first few steps from bed. After an initial improvement, the pain may get worse later in the day especially after prolonged standing or walking, or after prolonged periods of inactivity again. Palpation typically reveals tenderness anteromedially on the medial calcaneal tubercle at the origin of the plantar fascia. Most patients with heel pain have calcaneal spurs, but the spur itself is not likely the cause of pain.

Posterior Tibial Tendinitis and Rupture
Pain, swelling, and localized tenderness just posterior to the medial malleolus occur in posterior tibial tendinitis. Extension and flexion may be normal, but pain is present on active inversion against resistance or passive eversion. The discomfort is usually worse after athletic events.

Rupture of the posterior tibialis tendon, which is not commonly recognized, is a cause of a progressive flatfoot. It may be caused by trauma, chronic tendon degeneration, or rheumatoid arthritis. An insidious onset of pain, swelling, and tenderness occurs along the course of the tendon just distal to the medial malleolus. The unilateral deformity of hindfoot valgus and forefoot abduction is an important finding. The forefoot abduction can be seen best from behind; more toes are seen from this position than would be seen normally. The result of the single heel rise test is positive when the patient is unable to rise onto the ball of the affected foot while the contralateral foot is off the floor. Computed tomography (CT) and MRI are helpful in the diagnosis of tendon rupture.

Peroneal Tendon Dislocation and Peroneal Tendinitis
Dislocation of the peroneal tendon may occur from a direct blow, repetitive trauma, or sudden dorsiflexion with eversion. Sometimes a painless snapping noise is heard at the time of dislocation. Other patients report more severe pain and tenderness of the tendon area where it lies over the lateral malleolus. The condition may be confused with an acute ankle sprain. Peroneal tendinitis is manifested as localized tenderness and swelling over the lateral malleolus.

NEUROLOGICAL PROBLEMS
The foot is a frequent site of neurologic symptoms, some of which are common and others of which are rare. The usual symptom is numbness of some portion of the foot, but this complaint is often ignored as being nonspecific. The symptoms of numbness, tingling, paresthesias, burning pain, or pins and needle sensation should first point to a possible neurologic lesion. The most common cause of numbness of the feet is peripheral neuropathy, although a number of

SECTION 2 Regional Pain Syndromes

other local clinical conditions causing numbness of the foot should also be considered.

Morton Neuroma

Middle-aged women are most frequently affected by Morton neuroma, an entrapment neuropathy of the interdigital nerve occurring most often between the third and fourth toes. Paresthesias and a burning, aching type of pain are usually experienced in the fourth toe. The symptoms are made worse by walking on hard surfaces or wearing tight shoes or high-heel shoes. Tenderness may be elicited by palpation between the third and fourth metatarsal heads. Occasionally, a neuroma is seen between the second and third toes. Compression of the interdigital nerve by the transverse metatarsal ligament and possibly by an intermetatarsophalangeal bursa or synovial cyst may be responsible for the entrapment.

Tarsal Tunnel Syndrome

In tarsal tunnel syndrome, the posterior tibial nerve is compressed at or near the flexor retinaculum, which is located posterior and inferior to the medial malleolus. Numbness, burning pain, and paresthesias of the toes and sole extend proximally to the area over the medial malleolus with nocturnal exacerbation reported. The patient usually gets some relief by leg, foot, and ankle movements. A positive Tinel sign is elicited on percussion posterior to the medial malleolus, and loss of pinprick and two-point discrimination may be present. Women are more often affected, and trauma to the foot, especially fracture, valgus foot deformity, hypermobility, occupational factors, and synovitis, may contribute to development of the tarsal tunnel syndrome. An electrodiagnostic test may show prolonged motor and sensory latencies and slowing of the nerve conduction velocities. In addition, a positive tourniquet test and pressure over the flexor retinaculum can induce symptoms.

Anterior Tarsal Tunnel Syndrome

The anterior tarsal tunnel syndrome (or deep peroneal nerve entrapment) is an entrapment neuropathy of the deep peroneal nerve at the level of the inferior extensor retinaculum on the dorsum of the foot. The symptoms consist of numbness and paresthesias over the dorsum of the foot, especially at the web space. A tight feeling may be described over the anterior aspect of the ankle. The symptoms may arise following the wearing of tight shoes or high heels. Other causes include contusion of the dorsum of the foot, metatarsal fracture, talonavicular osteophytosis, and ganglion. Symptoms also tend to occur in bed at night and are relieved by standing or walking. Hypesthesia and hypalgesia may be present in the first dorsal web space, and a Tinel sign may be elicited on percussion just anterosuperior to the medial malleolus. The extensor digitorum brevis may be atrophied and weak.

A diagnosis of anterior tarsal tunnel syndrome may be confirmed by electrodiagnostic studies.

Superficial Peroneal Nerve Entrapment

The superficial peroneal nerve bifurcates into the intermediate dorsal cutaneous and the medial dorsal cutaneous terminal nerves. The lateral aspect of the foot is usually innervated by a branch of the sural nerve, the lateral dorsal cutaneous nerve. When this branch is absent, the intermediate branch of the superficial peroneal nerve supplies the innervation to the lateral foot.

The symptoms are pain, numbness, or tingling over the lateral aspect of the dorsum of the foot, worsened by exercise and often becoming more severe at night. The intermediate dorsal cutaneous branch, being very superficial, can be observed and palpated upon plantar flexing and inverting the foot. If this branch of the nerve is entrapped, then compression at this site will reproduce

PATIENT ASSESSMENT

- The location of pain and the presence of calluses will offer clues as to the cause of pain.

- Anatomic variances such as pes planus or cavus deformities are important clues to the diagnosis.

- Palpation can often reproduce the chief complaint to identify the cause of pain.

- Young athlete with foot pain should be evaluated for the possibility of stress fracture.

symptoms and a Tinel sign will be present. A decrease in sensation to light touch and pinprick may be present in the cutaneous distribution of the nerve.

The most common cause of this neuropathy is acute and chronic ankle sprains. Other causes include osteoarthritis of the tarsal bones and muscle herniation in the anterior compartment. Since the intermediate branch is so superficial, it is very susceptible to trauma and may be the source of chronic trauma ankle and foot pain. Electrodiagnostic studies with abnormal sensory conduction velocity and prolonged distal latency help confirm the diagnosis.

Sural Nerve Entrapment

Entrapment of the sural nerve, although uncommon, may be overlooked because of its limited cutaneous distribution. This nerve, which is formed from branches of the posterior tibial and common peroneal nerves, descends lateral to the Achilles tendon, and after passing the lateral malleolus, the nerve turns anteriorly and continues as the lateral dorsal cutaneous nerve along the lateral side of the foot and the fifth toe.

The manifestations are numbness and a burning pain along the lateral side of the dorsum of the foot, which may be worse at night. A decrease in sensation and a Tinel sign may be present. Trauma, scar tissue, and ganglia have been reported as causes of entrapment.

Examination

A proper physical examination of the foot leads to the anatomic localization of the source of the pain symptoms, helps to identify the static and mechanical abnormalities of the foot, and aids in detecting an underlying disease. Look at the shoes for excessive wear on the heels and soles. Extreme lateral heel wear can signify hindfoot (calcaneal) varus. An examination of gait is valuable in diagnosing and treating many foot problems. The patient walks barefooted with the feet and ankles exposed, and the hindfoot, midfoot, and forefoot are viewed separately.

Observe the foot for swelling, deformity, and erythema or other skin changes. Palpation to detect tenderness is important for diagnosis. Palpate the subtalar joint in the neutral position for tenderness and alignment. Look for forefoot varus or forefoot valgus. Examine the midtarsal area for tenderness and mobility. Examine for range of motion and tenderness or swelling of the MTP joints. Check for hammer toes, cocked-up toes, and tenderness or swelling of toes. Observe the toenails for abnormalities. Check the calcaneus on the plantar surface for tenderness. Examine the Achilles tendon, retrocalcaneal bursa, posterior tibial tendon, and peroneal tendon for swelling, tenderness, subluxation, or rupture.

Identify calluses to reveal areas of excessive stresses on the foot. Describe the location of calluses. Identify corns, which are hyperkeratotic lesions secondary to pressure. Hard corns occur over bony prominences and typically are found on the lateral aspect of the fifth toe. Soft corns occur between the toes.

NOT TO BE MISSED

- Metatarsal stress fractures

- Rupture of the Achilles tendon or posterior tibial tendon

Studies

The standard plain radiograph views include standing anteroposterior, standing lateral, and oblique (pronated), depicting the medial aspect of the foot. It is important to obtain the anteroposterior and lateral radiographs in the standing position to demonstrate the anatomic relationships of the foot in their functional position. In the lateral view, the x-ray beam passes from lateral to medial. Other special views are the lateral oblique (supinated) to visualize an accessory navicular bone; sesamoid view, which is an axial, oblique position (tilted lateral of sesamoids); and axial view of the heel (Harris) for calcaneal fractures.

CT scanning is helpful in imaging the hindfoot, especially for subtalar joint pathology and fractures of the calcaneus. CT is beneficial in the diagnosis of fibrous and cartilaginous coalition, calcaneonavicular bony coalition, and talocalcaneal coalition. MRI may be used to help diagnose tarsal coalition, osteomyelitis, osteonecrosis, tendinitis, tendon rupture, ligamentous injury, and osteochondral injuries of the talar dome. MRI is helpful in identifying soft tissue masses, such as ganglia, fibromatosis, Morton neuroma, and pigmented villonodular synovitis of the tendon sheath. Technetium bone scans can be used to determine stress fractures, especially of the metatarsals or calcaneus. Diagnostic ultrasonography can help identify tendinitis and partial or complete tears of tendons of the foot, especially the Achilles tendon and the posterior tibial tendon.

Treatment

ORTHOSES

Orthotics is the field of correcting foot deformities by means of external support, and devices used for this task are known as orthoses. These orthoses are used to relieve and/or cushion an area of pressure, support an area of collapse, or convert a biomechanically abnormal foot into a biomechanically functional foot during the stance phase of gait. In short, these mechanical devices help restore lost function or help maintain optimal function by altering biomechanics. Orthoses may provide pain relief and compensate for muscle and ligament weakness by decreasing forces passing through painful weight-bearing areas, stabilizing or immobilizing subluxing joints, and repositioning toes.

The range of these orthotic devices varies from simple inexpensive pads available in drugstores to complex, expensive, custom-made orthoses. The importance and value of foot orthoses in the treatment of foot disorders is often under recognized. The physician should establish a relationship with a pedorthotist (an orthotist who is trained in foot devices), an orthotist, or a trained therapist who can fabricate orthoses that are specific for the problem.

Foot orthoses can be divided into three types: devices that relieve pressure on various parts of the foot; those that cushion the foot and decrease impact; and those that are custom made to correct abnormal biomechanics and restore better function of the foot. Orthoses that relieve pressure on specific areas of the foot are generally foam or felt with an adhesive backing. These can be shaped specifically for pressure areas such as under the first, second, or fifth metatarsal heads. The pad is placed just proximal to the area of pressure.

The second type of orthosis, which reduces impact and cushions the foot, is constructed of material composed of microcellular rubber. These are transferable to different shoes and are used in mild cases. Additional materials used in orthoses that reduce impact and cushion the foot are closed-cell thermoplastic, polyethylene foam devices, and viscoelastic material. These materials can be molded to the contour of the foot.

The third type of orthosis is the biomechanical custom-fabricated type, which attempts to restore the subtalar joint to a neutral position. These may be rigid, semiflexible, or soft, depending upon the need. The thermoplastic materials are the semiflexible types. The rigid type is usually composed of an acrylic, rigid polyurethane foam, or polypropylene. As part of this type of orthosis, a "post," which is a wedge, can be incorporated to support the foot and correct the abnormality. If forefoot varus is present, then a medial post is used; and if forefoot valgus is present, then a lateral post is devised. Likewise, a medial post is used to correct pronation (eversion) of the hindfoot, whereas a lateral post is used to correct hindfoot supination (inversion). Typically, a custom-made orthosis may incorporate several features to address the foot problems, and if needed, all three types of foot orthoses can be combined into one orthosis. A depression can be made in the orthosis to relieve pressure in a specific area. Larger-than-normal or extra-depth shoes are needed for the orthosis to fit comfortably.

Ligament laxity is common in many inflammatory rheumatic diseases, often resulting in subluxation of joints. Subluxation of the MTP joint results in broadening of the forefoot, clawing of toes, and painful weight bearing on MTP heads. Callous, a protective reaction of the skin to stress, may be seen on the bottom of the foot. An internal or external metatarsal bar or pad can be placed in, or on, the shoes just behind the metatarsal heads to redistribute the weight away from this area to the metatarsal shafts. Alternatively, a metatarsal corset (a metatarsal pad attached directly to a toe with a strap, inside the sock) may be used in any shoe. Joint subluxation also results in loss of foot arches, uneven weight distribution, and pain. Arch supports, such as a medial longitudinal arch support, placed in the shoe can reform these arches. Spacers can be placed between toes to prevent overlapping and secondary calluses.

SHOE MODIFICATION

It is important to have a general understanding of shoe construction and available shoe modifications to help treat foot problem. As a start, one can simply examine shoe bottoms for wear and tear to determine the abnormal forces involved. A variety of modifications can be made. Extra-depth shoes with a large toebox should be used to accommodate fixed deformities such as clawed toes and to provide room for foot and ankle–foot orthoses. Otherwise, corns may develop where the proximal interphalangeal joints of the toes or other parts of the foot rub on the superior part of the shoe. For patients with toe deformities, shoe closures can be modified. Traditional shoelaces can be changed to Velcro closures. Elastic laces can replace regular laces, effectively turning the shoe into a loafer type. Shoes with proper closures are generally preferred over loafers, however, as loafers maintain their place on the foot by tension.

A Thomas heel, which is a medial extension of the heel, may be added to support the longitudinal arch. Replacing the regular shoe heel with a "solid ankle cushion heel" may be helpful for heel pain or a fused ankle, as this heel can simulate ankle plantar flexion while walking. A rocker bottom sole may be helpful for a fused ankle, hallux rigidus, or other toe deformities by substituting for the push-off and heel-strike phase of walking.

Lighter shoes are easier to wear but have less stability and durability. Heavier shoes may have greater stability and durability but are more difficult to carry. Ultimately, the shoe must be comfortable, have a good fit, and be aesthetically appealing. Otherwise, it will not be used. One can always advise patients to wear their special shoes at home and on the way to work, and to change when they get there.

In a leg length discrepancy, a lift can be attached to the outside of the whole shoe of the short leg and not just to the sole or heel. The shoe raise should be one half to three fourths of the leg length discrepancy. The difference should probably be >1 cm to consider correcting. However, if the leg length discrepancy is not a recent event, and especially if it is asymptomatic, it is probably best left untreated, since changing walking biomechanics after years of compensation may result in new symptoms.

BRACES

A patellar tendon–bearing orthosis is helpful for the problem of pain and limitation in ambulation due to destructive changes of the ankle or subtalar joint subsequent to rheumatoid arthritis or other inflammatory arthritis. This patellar tendon–bearing brace, which provides weight bearing on the patellar tendon

SECTION 2 Regional Pain Syndromes

and tibial condyles through a molded upper-calf band, has a fixed ankle and a rocker bottom sole. Thus, weight of the upper body can be directly transmitted from the knee region and calf to the floor, bypassing the ankle. This patellar tendon–bearing brace is also used to decrease stress on the ankle or subtalar joints in other conditions such as severe osteoarthritis, Charcot joint, and non-united fractures of the lower limb.

MODALITIES

The most commonly used modalities are heat and cold. Methods of superficial heating for the feet include hot packs, heating pads, hydrocollator packs, hot water bottles, heated whirlpools, and infrared lamps. Hydrotherapy in a whirlpool can provide superficial heat to the whole foot. At home, hot baths and foot soaks, especially in the morning, can be used for relief. Ultrasound may be used to heat tendons and deeper structures.

Cooling of tissues can be obtained with coolant sprays, ice packs, basins of ice water, and frozen food packages. Cooling also causes vasoconstriction, with a reduction of blood flow and a decrease in metabolic activity in the region treated. In general, patients seem to prefer heat; however, both heat and cold may be used alternatively as a contrast bath.

THERAPEUTIC EXERCISES

Therapeutic exercise may be broadly classified into three groups: (a) range of motion or stretching, (b) strengthening (resistive), and (c) aerobic (endurance). In many cases, a simple home exercise program is adequate and may be taught to the patient by the physician. Other cases require the prescription of a more formal physical therapy program. An exercise prescription should include the exercise frequency, intensity, type, and duration.

Range-of-motion exercises are important during the active phase of an inflammatory arthritis to maintain mobility of the ankle, subtalar, tarsal, and MTP joints. Ankle exercises include foot circles, active dorsiflexion, and plantar flexion. Writing the alphabet with the toes and cloth tugs with the toes and foot provide range of motion to the joints of the foot. After the acute phase has resolved, strengthening exercises against a resistance can be used. The ankle may be stretched with rubber tubing. Patients can be asked to push their feet against a board attached to the bed. Bicycle riding, swimming, and a rowing machine are non–weight-bearing exercises that can help maintain cardiovascular conditioning.

STEROID INJECTIONS

Local steroid injections can be helpful in certain entrapment neuropathies (Morton neuroma, superficial peroneal nerve, sural nerve, and anterior tarsal tunnel syndromes) and local inflammatory conditions such as a retrocalcaneal bursitis, posterior tibial tendonitis, or plantar fasciitis. Steroid injections of an Achilles tendonitis are to be avoided, as they are linked with rupture of the tendon.

Clinical Course

Through judicious use of nonsteroidal anti-inflammatory drugs, rest, orthoses when indicated, and local steroid injections when indicated, these conditions can be managed effectively. In cases involving tendon rupture or bony deformity that contributes to the painful condition, then a surgical referral is indicated.

WHEN TO REFER

- Tendon ruptures should be referred to an orthopedic surgeon.
- Custom orthoses are required.
- When an inflammatory arthritis is identified requiring disease modifying antirheumatic drugs.

ICD9

727.3 **Bursitis** *NEC*
  726.79 ankle
  726.79 foot
924.9 **Contusion** *(skin surface intact)*
  924.21 ankle
  924.20 foot (with ankle) (excluding toe(s))
Derangement
  718.97 ankle (internal)
  718.90 joint (internal)
    718.97 ankle
    718.97 foot
  718.30 recurrent
    718.37 ankle
    718.37 foot

Disorder
  733.90 cartilage NEC
    718.07 ankle
    718.07 foot
716.60 **Monoarthritis**
  716.67 ankle
  716.67 foot (and ankle)
715.9 **Osteoarthrosis/Osteoarthritis** *(degenerative) (hypertrophic)*
  715.97 ankle and foot
780.96 **Pain(s)**
  719.40 joint
    719.47 ankle
    719.47 foot
848.9 **Sprain, strain** *(joint) (ligament) (muscle) (tendon)*
  845.00 ankle
    845.00 and foot
  845.10 foot
782.3 **Swelling**
  719.07 ankle
  729.81 foot

SECTION 2 Regional Pain Syndromes

Additional Reading

1. Biundo JJ, Rush PJ. Painful feet. In: Koopman WJ, Boulware DW, Heudebert GR, eds. *Clinical Primer of Rheumatology*. Philadelphia, PA: Lippincott Williams and Wilkins; 2003:48–61.
2. Espinosa N, Brodsky JW, Maceira E. Metatarsalgia. *J Am Acad Orthop Surg* 2010;18:474–485.
3. Barton CJ, Munteanu SE, Menz HB, et al. The efficacy of foot orthoses in the treatment of individuals with patellofemoral pain syndrome: a systematic review. *Sports Med* 2010;40:377–395.
4. Simpson MR, Howard TM. Tendinopathies of the foot and ankle. *Am Fam Physician* 2009;80:1107–1114.
5. Thomas JL, Christensen JC, Kravitz SR, et al. American College of Foot and Ankle Surgeons heel pain committee. The diagnosis and treatment of heel pain: a clinical practice guideline-revision 2010. *J Foot Ankle Surg* 2010;49:S1–S19.

6 Mechanical Disorders of the Knee

Dennis W. Boulware

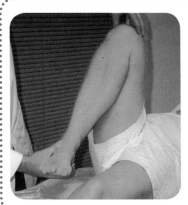

A 25-year-old man presents with a 3-day history of right knee after playing soccer with friends in the past weekend. Despite rest and acetaminophen, he is still in pain, unable to straighten his knee completely and his knee occasionally buckling.

Introduction

Mechanical disorders of the knee include clinical conditions caused by malfunction, trauma, or degeneration of a specific intra-articular and/or extra-articular component of the knee interfering with normal knee function. An internal derangement of the knee commonly refers to a disorder of the intra-articular components, more commonly the articular cartilage, meniscus fibrocartilage, collateral ligaments, or cruciate ligaments (Fig. 6.1). Disorders of extra-articular components of the knee joint include patellofemoral malalignment and insufficiency of the quadriceps or hamstring muscle groups, and are considered as mechanical disorders too.

Significant mechanical disorders of the knee causing instability, if continued unabated, eventually lead to osteoarthritis. Experimental animal models of osteoarthritis typically involve initiating an internal derangement of the joint, followed by continued use of the limb. The most common models of experimental osteoarthritis include partial medial meniscectomy or transection of the anterior cruciate ligament. Injuries of the medial meniscus and anterior cruciate ligament are common and as our population ages and becomes more engaged in recreational and sports-related activities, mechanical disorders of the knee will become more prevalent and, if not recognized early, will result in an increased prevalence of osteoarthritis of the knee.

Clinical Presentation

Most knee pain results from disruption of one of the many components that comprise a functional knee joint. These components include the articular hyaline cartilage, the supporting meniscal fibrocartilage, and the various ligaments. An understanding of the anatomy and biomechanics of the knee coupled with a focused physical examination of various components of the knee usually identify the cause of pain. This chapter focuses on derangements of the menisci, ligaments, and patellofemoral alignment as a cause of knee pain since they are the most common mechanical disorders of the knee.

In general, patients complain of knee pain primarily with use and further history is of limited value in identifying the mechanical disorder other than the

CLINICAL POINTS

- Mechanical disorders can lead to knee instability and premature osteoarthritis.

- The physical examination of the knee is essential in identifying the cause.

- Buckling of a painful knee is common and not always associated with a torn meniscus.

- Chronic meniscal tears are commonly associated with osteoarthritis.

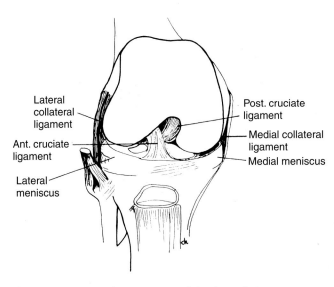

Figure 6.1 Anatomical components of the knee that can cause a mechanical disorder of the knee. From Koopman WJ, Moreland LW, eds. *Arthritis and Allied Conditions: A Textbook of Rheumatology*, 15th ed. Philadelphia: Lippincott Williams & Wilkins; 2005.

acuity of the pain and an identifiable precipitating event. Buckling of the knee with weight-bearing is associated with all types of internal derangements and more commonly occurs as a reflexive muscular relaxation to the sudden onset of pain, causing the knee to "give way." True locking of the knee, though, should focus the clinician on a torn and displaced meniscus getting entrapped within the joint.

Acute injuries with identifiable precipitating events such as trauma or injury commonly involve meniscus or ligament damage with immediate pain, and continued pain with weight-bearing or use of the limb and often limited range of motion secondary to the pain. If the acute injury resulted in a displacement of the torn meniscus, patients often complain of a painful "catching" or "popping" sensation in the knee. Large sudden effusions suggest a hemarthrosis that is more commonly seen with torn ligaments as opposed to a torn meniscus. Ligaments are vascularized structures, and damage to the ligament usually results in a hemarthrosis. Effusions that occur later can be seen in either ligament or meniscus damage. An examination of the joint will help identify the source of damage.

The absence of an identifiable precipitating event suggests a degenerative process that eventually reached a tipping point causing clinical symptoms. Particularly with a chronic tear of the meniscus, there is usually less pain than an acute tear, and there is frequently a lack of any recognizable precipitating event. Chronic meniscal tears are typically associated with osteoarthritis, and a precipitating cause may be as simple as a squatting and twisting maneuver or a simple misstep. Chronic pain with use of the knee and episodic effusions of the knee often precede the patient's eventual visit to see the physician. With chronic derangements, limitation in range of motion is less of a prominent feature than with acute and displaced tears.

Complaints of pain with use are common in all mechanical disorders of the knee, but pain felt in the anterior of the knee or with descending stairs or inclined surfaces as opposed to ascending stairs or descending surfaces are common complaints of patellofemoral compartment problems. Patients with patellofemoral pain often complain of pain after prolonged periods of immobility with the knee in flexed positions such as sitting at a desk or riding in an automobile; when resuming activity again, the condition will often cause pain for a brief period of time, such as the first few steps after resuming a standing position.

Pain felt in the popliteal area is typically due to effusions distending the joint capsule or due to an effusion causing a popliteal cyst to fill, causing pain from distention of the cyst. Popliteal pain does not often identify the source of the mechanical disorder causing the increased synovial fluid to accumulate as much as reflect distention of the popliteal cyst or joint capsule. Popliteal cysts are common in many individuals and communicate with the joint space, but typically are not fluid-filled except when the pressure in the synovial space increases and synovial fluid is pumped from the joint into the popliteal cyst. The communication between the cyst and joint space does not always allow the fluid to return to the joint space, but will eventually be reabsorbed when the joint space pressure returns to normal and no further fluid is pumped in the popliteal cyst.

Physical Findings

The physical examination is the most helpful in the clinical evaluation of the patient as various maneuvers allow the clinician to test each component of

PATIENT ASSESSMENT

1. Worse pain with descending stairs or declining surfaces suggests patellofemoral disease.

2. Testing for instability is critical in ligamentous lesions.

3. Displaced meniscal fragments can become entrapped and lock the knee.

4. Reserve imaging studies for recurrent or recalcitrant knee pain.

SECTION 2 Regional Pain Syndromes

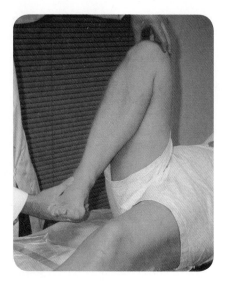

Figure 6.2 McMurray test. From Berg D, Worzala K. *Atlas of Adult Physical Diagnosis.* Philadelphia: Lippincott Williams & Wilkins, 2006.

the knee, allowing identification of a dysfunctional component or source of the pain. In addition to these provocative maneuvers, the examination should assess for passive ranges of motion and the presence of effusions.

Positioning the patient in a supine posture will aide in getting the patient to relax which will be essential in measuring the full passive range of motion. In measuring passive range of motion, the femur is used as the reference arm of the knee and the normal range of extension is measured as 0 degree with the knee extending the same trajectory as the femur. The inability of the knee to position into full extension should be recorded in degrees relative to the femur. An acute loss of full extension may reflect a displaced meniscus, a large joint effusion distending the knee joint capsule, or a distended popliteal cyst. A chronic loss of full extension typically reflects a longstanding osteophyte suggesting a degenerative process. With the patient relaxed as much as possible, passive full flexion in the patient should be measured. Normally, the knee will have 0 degree of extension and 140 degrees of flexion. As in measuring extension, the acute loss of full flexion may reflect a displaced meniscus; a large joint effusion distending the knee joint capsule or a distended popliteal cyst and a chronic loss will suggest an osteophyte indicating a degenerative process. Joint effusions often impair full passive range of motion and usually correlate with the severity of inflammation within the knee joint.

A torn and displaced meniscus can cause limitation in passive range of motion when the displaced meniscal tear causes entrapment of the displaced fragment to impede the full flexion or extension of the knee. The McMurray test (Fig. 6.2) is a specific test to induce entrapment of a meniscal tear. With the patient supine and relaxed, the examiner grasps the affected leg and passively flexes the knee and hip maximally to position the knee as close to the chest as possible. At the point of maximal passive flexion, the knee is rotated fully using the foot as a lever to attempt impingement of the torn lateral or medial meniscus. With the knee held in passive internal rotation in flexion, the knee is extended to detect a palpable or audible snap in the joint. The maneuver is repeated with the flexed knee held in full, passive, external rotation. Pain is not always present, particularly in an older degenerative tear. The Apley grind test (Fig. 6.3) is also used to detect possible meniscal derangement. This test is performed with the patient in a prone position and the knee flexed at 90 degrees. In this position the examiner uses the plantar surface of the foot to manually load the knee joint while rotating the knee in internal and external rotations. Tenderness elicited during the Apley grind test is not specific for a meniscal injury, as an articular cartilage lesion will also produce tenderness. The combined presence of a "snap" and an abnormal Apley grind test is consistent with a torn meniscus. Because of the anatomic location of the menisci near the medial and lateral joint lines, joint line tenderness to direct palpation is the hallmark of a meniscal injury. The menisci are in close congruity with the peripheral joint capsule, which has a rich nerve supply, accounting for the localized tenderness. Joint line tenderness to palpation is also seen in osteoarthritis of the knee and its presence should suggest a meniscal lesion only when combined with the McMurray and/or Apley signs. A combination of joint line tenderness with a positive McMurray and/or Apley sign correlates well with a clinically torn meniscus.

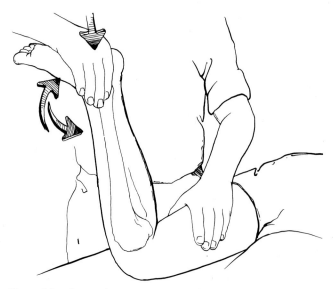

Figure 6.3 Apley grind test.

Most serious and dysfunctional ligament disorders are detected by simple physical examination. There are two sets of opposing ligaments to be examined: the medial and lateral collateral ligaments and the anterior and posterior cruciate ligaments. Normal knee stability and range of motion depend on intact ligaments to restrict the knee to primary flexion and extension. The collateral ligaments reside on the medial and lateral aspect of the knee and restrict the knee from varus or valgus motion. The anterior and posterior cruciate ligaments function to retard anterior and posterior displacement of the tibia relative to the femoral condyles during flexion and extension.

Medial and lateral collateral ligament injury is best tested when the patient is seated or is supine and relaxed. After passively placing the relaxed knee in 30 degrees of flexion, the patient's ankle should be grasped with one hand and the knee stabilized with the other to apply passive stress to attempt to displace the distal leg in a valgus and then a varus direction. Normally there should be no motion to displacement in either valgus or varus deviations of the knee. The ability to displace the knee in a valgus direction would indicate a medial collateral ligament tear or instability. In a partial tear, especially an acute one, there will be tenderness in the medial compartment as stress is placed in the displacement. A complete tear will deviate significantly and may not have significant associated tenderness. Since the medial collateral ligament is firmly attached to the medial meniscus, and disruption of one structure often leads to injuries to the other structure in the medial compartment, a torn medial collateral ligament frequently has an associated torn medial meniscus involved. Conversely, varus force applied to the distal leg still held in this position can be used to detect similar signs in the lateral compartment, implicating a lateral collateral ligament injury and can be followed by palpation along the lateral joint line for tenderness. Most collateral ligament abnormalities can be quantified by the degree of displacement. A grade I laxity would represent up to 5 mm of additional motion; grade II, 6 to 10 mm; grade III, 11 to 15 mm; and grade IV, >15 mm of additional displacement. Caution should be exercised in interpreting this maneuver because "relative" laxity of the collateral ligaments is often seen in knees with loss of full articular cartilage thickness due to chronic osteoarthritis.

A torn anterior cruciate ligament is best tested by the anterior drawer sign or Lachman test. This maneuver is performed with the patient seated comfortably or supine. The knee is passively flexed to 25 degrees and the foot fixed in place with one hand and anterior force placed on the tibia relative to the femoral condyles drawing the tibial plateau toward the clinician. Normally there is no more than 5 mm of displacement and anterior displacement of the tibial plateau relative to the femoral condyle >5 mm indicates a torn or lax anterior cruciate ligament. Tenderness elicited by this maneuver in the absence of displacement suggests an incomplete tear of the anterior cruciate ligament. The posterior cruciate ligament is best tested by the posterior drawer sign, which is performed with the knee in 90 degrees of flexion. Fixing the patient's foot with one hand and displacing the tibial plateau posteriorly, relative to the femoral condyles should result in no more than 5 mm of displacement. Posterior cruciate ligament problems are much less commonly seen than anterior cruciate ligament issues. Again, caution should be exercised in interpreting these tests in patients with chronic osteoarthritis and relative laxity of the ligaments due to articular cartilaginous loss.

If the examination has not determined a cause for the pain thus far, the clinician should consider patellofemoral involvement. In patellofemoral malalignment, the end result is a damaged patellar articular surface causing pain with use. Joint effusions are not commonly seen in patellofemoral disease, but all effusions correlate with the degree of inflammation and histopathology of the articular cartilage and severe lesions of the patellar articular cartilage can cause an effusion. In patellofemoral disease, the passive range of motion is preserved, but motion of the knee in flexion and extension frequently causes crepitus confined to the patellofemoral compartment. The patellofemoral compartment as a source of knee pain can be confirmed by reproducing the complaints by patellofemoral compression or grinding. With the patient supine and the knee relaxed, compression of the patella against the femoral intercondylar groove while passively moving the patella superiorly and inferiorly within the intercondylar groove will reproduce tenderness. Tenderness on patellar inhibition is more sensitive but less specific for patellofemoral disease as the absence of tenderness excludes the patellofemoral compartment as a source of pain, but can cause tenderness in the absence of significant patellofemoral disease. With the patient still supine and the knee relaxed, passively displace the patella inferiorly and hold it there while asking the patient to contract the quadriceps muscles. The quadriceps contraction will pull the patella superiorly beneath the examiner's fingers holding the patella inferiorly and cause tenderness.

An abnormal degree of patellar laxity can be a cause of patellofemoral malalignment and subsequently a mechanical disorder of the knee. To test for laxity, the patient is still supine and the knee relaxed. The examiner passively displaces the patella laterally with the knee in passive full extension and the ability to displace the patella more than half of its total width suggests laxity of the medial retinacular restraints. Medial retinacular laxity is a common cause or patellofemoral malalignment and can result in patellofemoral disease.

STUDIES

The laboratory is of no help in evaluating the patient with knee pain from a mechanical disorder of the knee; the physical examination is more enlightening.

Plain radiography is a poor diagnostic modality for soft-tissue injury. The only utility of plain radiography would be to assess the severity of coexisting osteoarthritis, a common comorbid feature of a degenerative or chronic tear. Cross-sectional imaging such as CT and/or MRI has higher levels of sensitivity for lesions of the menisci or ligaments, but should be reserved for lesions suspected of requiring surgical intervention such as high grade instability of the ligaments and displaced menisci causing true locking or in cases that fail conservative management and observation. MRI is an excellent modality to evaluate soft-tissue injuries, but is limited by the difficulty in differentiating a degenerative intact meniscus from a chronic or degenerative meniscal tear. The greatest utility of MRI is in a negative study, because of its high negative predictive value. Computerized tomography is of limited value in evaluating meniscal injury when compared with the ability of MRI to differentiate soft-tissue lesions. Invasive imaging, including arthroscopy and arthrography, carries a higher accuracy and is better left for the subspecialist's domain.

NOT TO BE MISSED

1. The patellofemoral compartment is a common source of knee pain.

TREATMENT

In primary care the initial treatment consideration is to determine the need for surgical treatment, particularly in cases of ligamentous and meniscal lesions. In general the greater the severity grade the more likely surgical intervention will be required. This guideline is particularly true for individuals who wish to resume an active lifestyle, as internal derangement followed by active use is the experimental model for inducing osteoarthritis. Lesions of the cruciate and collateral ligaments with more than a grade II lesion (over 10 mm of motion) are at greater risk of future premature osteoarthritis and should be referred to orthopedic surgery for consideration of repair. For meniscal injuries that have locking of the knee from a displaced fragment, referral to orthopedic surgery is recommended. Meniscal tears that are not displaced or do not result in entrapment can be treated conservatively.

For all other injuries and lesions treated by the primary care clinician, conservative general management should start with rest, ice, compression, and elevation. Although well designed controlled trials are lacking to assess efficacy of the components of this common recommendation individually or in combination, the recommendation makes good sense and is used widely. Resting the area of pain combined with cyclic icing the area of pain for 15 to 20 minutes followed by 15 to 20 minutes without ice will provide good analgesia. Compression using an elastic wrap bandage around the knee provides symptomatic relief and has the advantage of inhibiting full range of motion and reminding the patient to rest the affected limb. Elevation is felt to assist in reducing swelling, but has the additional value of reinforcing the patient to rest the knee.

Pharmacologic analgesia with nonsteroidal anti-inflammatory drugs should suffice when added to rest, ice, compression, and elevation. Physical therapy can be instituted later after the pain is managed as its success will be dependent on the patient's ability to participate in the prescribed therapy. Use of a neoprene brace or hinged splint which limits valgus and varus stress on the knee can provide relief and support, especially for patients with mild instability of the knee during rehabilitation. In cases of patellofemoral disease, the use of external support such as elastic knee supports and orthotics, particularly neoprene sleeves with a patellar window, are often helpful.

Supervised rehabilitation is an important modality of treatment for all knee injuries, but particularly with cruciate ligamentous injuries where the goal of strengthening the hamstring muscle relative to the quadriceps depends on the type of ligamentous injury. After anterior cruciate ligament injuries, physical therapy should be directed toward achieving hamstring and quadriceps muscles of relatively equal strength. This is unlike the normal situation where the quadriceps muscle is roughly 50% stronger than the hamstring. In posterior cruciate ligament injuries, the quadriceps muscles are strengthened maximally to ensure knee stability. Each patient must have a physical strengthening regimen specifically tailored to the injury. In cases of patellofemoral disease from patellar malalignment, supervised physical therapy is indicated to stretch the lateral retinaculum, hamstring, and iliotibial band in concert with strengthening exercises of the quadriceps muscles, particularly the vastus medialis. Quadriceps-strengthening exercises utilizing the last 30 degrees of extension to strengthen the vastus medialis muscle are pivotal in patellar laxity to enhance the vector force of the quadriceps muscles in keeping the patella within the intercondylar groove and limiting lateral motion and deviation. Heavily loaded isotonic exercises with full range of motion (i.e., full squats with weights) should be avoided in patellofemoral disease.

Arthrocentesis and aspiration of synovial fluid for large effusions can help decompress a large tense effusion and provide immediate relief. Instilling intra-articular corticosteroids can relieve pain in cases associated with osteoarthritis with patellofemoral disease or small meniscal tears.

Clinical Course

In cases of mild derangement without instability of the knee or a displaced meniscal fragment, the outcome is good with a return to full activity in weeks. In patients with a strong family history of osteoarthritis and/or obesity, a derangement of the knee with instability may lead to an increased likelihood of osteoarthritis. The risk of premature osteoarthritis varies directly with the severity of the knee instability and severe lesions should be referred to orthopedic surgery for consideration of stabilization repair. Patients with an increased risk from family history of osteoarthritis, obesity, and/or instability should be advised strongly to continue physical conditioning of the knee as prescribed by physical therapy and to lose weight when appropriate to ideal body weight as much as possible.

In recurrent knee pain or pain failing to improve after several weeks of conservative therapy, referral to orthopedic surgery may be warranted.

WHEN TO REFER

1. Ligamentous tears with high grade instability require referral to an orthopedic surgeon.

2. Displaced meniscal fragments that cause entrapment require referral to an orthopedic surgeon.

ICD9

Baker's
  727.51 cyst (knee)
727.3 **Bursitis** *NEC*
  726.60 knee
  726.61 pes anserinus
  726.65 prepatellar
924.9 **Contusion** *(skin surface intact)*
  924.11 knee
  924.5 leg
    924.10 lower (with knee)
Cyst *(mucus) (retention) (serous) (simple)*
  727.51 Baker's (knee)
Degeneration, degenerative
  718.0 articular cartilage NEC
    717.5 knee
    717.7 patella
Derangement
  718.0 cartilage (articular) NEC •
    717.9 knee
      718.36 recurrent
  718.90 joint (internal)
    717.9 knee
  718.30 recurrent
    718.36 knee
  717.9 knee (cartilage) (internal)
Disorder
  733.90 cartilage NEC
    717.9 knee
715.96 **Osteoarthrosis/Osteoarthritis** *(degenerative) (hypertrophic) knee*
780.96 **Pain(s)**
  719.46 knee
848.9 **Sprain, strain** *(joint) (ligament) (muscle) (tendon)*
  844.9 knee
    844.9 and leg
    717.5 old
726.90 **Tendinitis, tendonitis**
  726.61 pes anserinus

Additional Reading

1. Husni EM, Donohue JP. Painful shoulder and reflex sympathetic dystrophy syndrome. In Koopman WJ, Moreland LW, eds. *Arthritis and Allied Conditions*, 15th ed. Philadelphia: Lippincott Williams and Wilkins; 2005; 2133–2151.
2. Boulware DW. The painful shoulder. In Koopman WJ, Boulware DW, Heudebert GR, eds. *Clinical Primer of Rheumatology*. Philadelphia: Lippincott Williams & Wilkins; 2003; 43–47.
3. Woodward TW, Best TM. The painful shoulder: part 1. Clinical evaluation. *Am Fam Physician* 2000;61: 3079–3088.
4. Woodward TW, Best TM. The painful shoulder: part 2. Acute and chronic disorders. *Am Fam Physician* 2000;61:3291–3300.

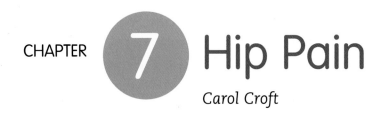

CHAPTER 7 Hip Pain

Carol Croft

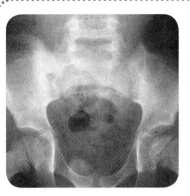

A 45-year-old man is seen for left hip pain that had progressed in severity for the last month. The pain especially bothers him at night making it difficult to lie on his side, which is his preferred sleeping position. On examination, he has a normal gait with full nontender, passive motion including rotation. Moderate tenderness is detected on palpation of the left greater trochanter.

Hip pain is a common complaint in primary care and it has many possible causes. The regional anatomy of the hip and pelvis is complex, encompassing the hip and the sacroiliac (SI) joints, different groups of muscles, tendons and bursae, and the various vascular and neural structures that cross the hip joint. Referred pain can arise from the iliopsoas region, lumbosacral spine, or retroperitoneal space. Thus, the differential diagnosis is broad and includes intra-articular pathology, extra-articular pathology, and mimickers. The history and examination are critical to narrow the broad differential diagnosis.

Clinical Presentation

CLINICAL POINTS

- Correct diagnosis depends on understanding the hip anatomy.

- Careful history and examination.

- Cognizance of past hip pathology including developmental hip dysplasia and childhood diagnoses.

- Magnetic resonance imaging is becoming the standard for evaluation of soft tissue and cartilage structures around the hip joint.

- Early diagnosis of structural hip disease may prevent development of severe osteoarthritis and the need for total hip replacement.

Patients frequently describe pain in the groin, upper thigh, or buttock as "hip" pain. Pain in the groin or medial thigh region is more often due to hip pathology and arises from irritation of the joint capsule, synovial lining, or both. Lumbosacral spine pathology can cause referred pain to the buttocks, lateral thigh, or groin. Lateral thigh pain is often attributed to trochanteric bursitis or adductor tendinitis.

Evaluation of the patient should begin with consideration of age, level and type of activity, past injuries, past surgeries, and comorbidities. Pointed questioning about childhood hip problems, such as hip dysplasia, slipped capital femoral epiphysis (SCFE), and Legg-Calve-Perthes disease is important to determine the likelihood of early degenerative arthrosis. Directed questioning should address any limitations of patient function including impairment in activities of daily living, such as donning socks, getting in and out of the car, jogging, walking, and climbing stairs. Symptoms that refer to the spine, lower abdomen, and neuropathic pain should be questioned. Comorbidities can be an important clue to the likelihood of avascular necrosis (AVN) including clotting disorders, hyperlipidemia, use of alcohol and tobacco, and previous treatment with corticosteroids. The social history including type of work and recreational exercise and exposure to altitude can also provide guidance as to the pretest probability of serious hip pathology.

Hip pain in children is often acute and a result of one of the three common disorders of the hip joint: acute transient synovitis, Legg-Calve-Perthes' disease, and SCFE (1). The typical presentation of hip pain in children is

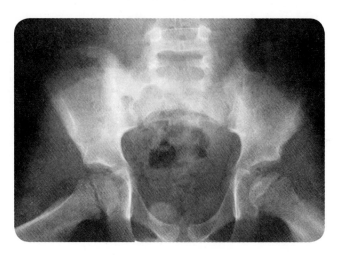

Figure 7.1 Legg-Calve-Perthes disease of left hip. Epiphysis is narrowed and radiodense. A subchondral fracture is also visible. (With permission from Fleisher GR, Ludwig S, Baskin MN. *Atlas of Pediatric Emergency Medicine.* Philadelphia, PA: Lippincott Williams & Wilkins; 2004.)

referred pain to the anterior thigh and knee joint with limping and refusing to walk. Transient synovitis is a self-limited, inflammatory condition with effusion of the hip joint. In about half the cases, a history of preceding upper respiratory infection or mild trauma can be elicited. Perthes' disease is a result of ischemic necrosis of the femoral head that leads to collapse of the epiphysis followed by remodeling. Boys are more often affected and the age range for onset is between ages 2 and 13 years. Medical treatments include anti-inflammatory drugs, physical therapy (PT), and bracing to achieve optimal positioning of the femoral head in the acetabular cup. Surgery for proximal femoral osteotomy is sometimes performed. About half of untreated patients will go on to develop early onset osteoarthritis (OA) of the hip. SCFE is a disease of adolescence and is also more common in boys. It is felt to result from softening of the epiphyseal cartilage at adolescence and is more common in children with endocrinopathies, such as hypogonadism, hypopituitarism, and hypothyroidism. Surgical treatment is warranted early as only acute slipped epiphysis can be reduced, and it is usually performed bilaterally because of high risk of recurrence on the unaffected side. Congenital dysplasia of the hip joint is common and often detected with routine newborn screening. When diagnosis is delayed, limping and weakness of the surrounding muscles are the typical clinical signs. X-rays are usually diagnostic, and referral to an orthopedic surgeon for age appropriate treatments is appropriate (Fig. 7.1).

Hip pain in adolescents and young athletes may represent avulsion fractures at the site of the bony insertion of the tendons of the rectus femoris, iliopsoas, sartorius, or other regional musculature. Treatment is usually rest and nonsteroidal anti-inflammatory medications (Fig. 7.2).

Hip Pain in Adults

Acute hip pain located in the groin region in the setting of acute trauma in adults is most often due to fracture of the femoral head or acetabulum. Other common causes include stress fractures, AVN, muscular strain of the adductor or iliopsoas muscles and tendons, and iliopectineal bursitis. Labral tears, femoroacetabular impingement, and OA can all be signs of residual sequelae of developmental disorders of the hip joint. Inflammatory arthropathies, such as rheumatoid arthritis, calcium pyrophosphate dihydrate deposition disease, and septic arthritis should be entertained in the correct clinical circumstances.

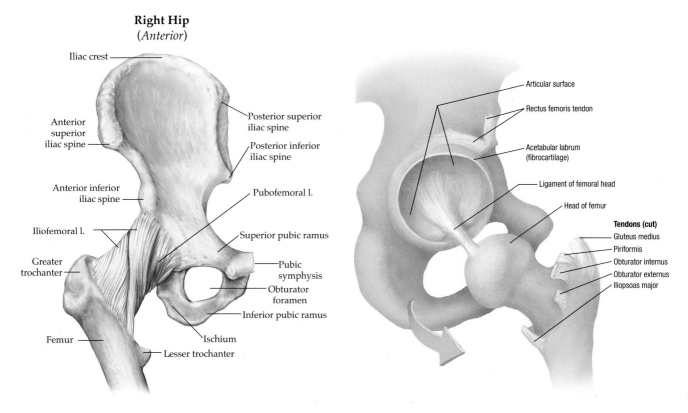

Right Hip
(*Anterior*)

Iliac crest

Anterior superior iliac spine

Anterior inferior iliac spine

Iliofemoral l.

Greater trochanter

Femur

Posterior superior iliac spine

Posterior inferior iliac spine

Pubofemoral l.

Superior pubic ramus

Pubic symphysis

Obturator foramen

Inferior pubic ramus

Ischium

Lesser trochanter

Articular surface

Rectus femoris tendon

Acetabular labrum (fibrocartilage)

Ligament of femoral head

Head of femur

Tendons (cut)
Gluteus medius
Piriformis
Obturator internus
Obturator externus
Iliopsoas major

Figure 7.2 Anterior right hip ligaments. (Asset provided by Anatomical Chart Co.)

The orthopedic literature has long attributed much of the OA in the hip joint to anatomical deformities. Osteoarthritis of the hip is often secondary to congenital or developmental abnormalities such as developmental dysplasia of the hip, Perthe's disease and SCFE. Primary osteoarthritis was presumed to be idiopathic (due to developmental abnormalities of the articular cartilage), but more recent information suggest the mechanism in these cases is femoroacetabular impingement rather than excessive contact stress (2). Acetabular dysplasia is a shallowness of the acetabulum that leads to unequal distribution of stress on the acetabular cartilage, labral tears, and OA. It is often a component of developmental dysplasia of the hip, which predominantly affects women. Other anatomical abnormalities of the acetabulum such as protrusion result in overcoverage and resultant impingement between the acetabular rim and the femoral head–neck junction. Acetabular protrusion may be seen in Marfan syndrome and rheumatoid arthritis, but most cases are idiopathic.

Anatomic variations in the femur can also lead to significant abnormalities in hip joint mechanics. The most commonly recognized femoral abnormality is called "a pistol grip deformity" and is felt to be a major cause of OA of the hip in men. The deformity resembles mild SCFE and may be a developmental variant that is related. Tears of the acetabular labrum have been described in patients with developmental hip dysplasia, Perthes' disease, previous SCFE, previous trauma, and in association with femoroacetabular impingement. Patients will generally report gradual onset of symptoms but occasionally relate the onset of pain to trauma of some kind. The pain is generally both dull and sharp groin pain and occasionally is also present in the buttock and worsened with activity or prolonged sitting (3).

Intra-articular loose bodies result from various causes including OA, AVN, pigmented villonodular synovitis, osteochondritis dissecans, and prior trauma to the hip, such as dislocation with reduction. Mechanical symptoms like clicking, locking, catching, or giving way are common along with groin pain and stiffness.

SECTION 2 Regional Pain Syndromes

Some patients describe a popping or snapping sensation in association with pain around the hip joint. So-called "snapping hip" syndrome presents in three ways. Intra-articular snapping can result from loose bodies and labral pathology. Internal snapping is caused by the iliopsoas tendon moving over a bony prominence. Pain or discomfort associated with internal snapping indicates iliopsoas tendonitis. External snapping hip is less common and results from the iliotibial (IT) band or gluteus maximus tendon snapping over the greater trochanter. The friction of the tendon moving over surrounding bursae can result in trochanteric bursitis.

Pain overlying the trochanteric bursa is another common form of "hip pain." The recent literature provides greater understanding of lateral hip pain or greater trochanteric pain syndrome and the contributing diagnoses. Greater trochanteric pain syndrome was originally defined as "tenderness to palpation over the greater trochanter with the patient in the side-lying position." The typical presentation is pain and reproducible tenderness in the region of the greater trochanter, buttock, or lateral thigh. It affects between 10% and 25% of the general population. Some investigators suggest that it is more common in patients with musculoskeletal low back pain and in women compared with men.

The anatomy of the region bears review, as understanding is critical for accurate diagnosis. The greater trochanter arises from the junction of the femoral neck and shaft. Five muscles attach to it, the gluteus medium and gluteus minimus laterally and the piriformis, obturator externus, and obturator internus more medially. Superficial to the gluteus medius and minimus tendons lies a fibromuscular sheath composed of the gluteus maximus, tensor fascia lata, and IT band (Fig. 7.3) (4).

Trochanteric bursitis is a commonly diagnosed inflammatory condition with pain around the greater trochanter that radiates down the lateral thigh or into the buttock. It is believed to arise from friction created between the IT band and the greater trochanter with repeated hip flexion and extension. It can be associated with overuse, trauma, or abnormal gait patterns. Schapira et al. reported that 91.6% of patients diagnosed with trochanteric bursitis had associated pathology affecting adjacent areas, such as the ipsilateral hip or lumbar spine. Previously thought to affect primarily middle-aged women, the diagnosis is now increasing common in younger active patients of both sexes, particu-

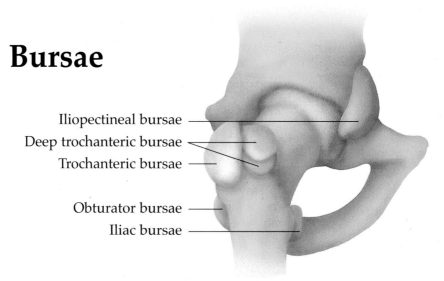

Bursae

Iliopectineal bursae

Deep trochanteric bursae

Trochanteric bursae

Obturator bursae

Iliac bursae

Figure 7.3 Hip bursae. (Asset provided by Anatomical Chart Co.)

larly runners. Characteristic description of the pain includes activity-related pain and symptoms lying on the affected side, as well as discomfort with prolonged standing or sitting with the affected leg crossed. The examination reveals tenderness to palpation and worsened pain on hip abduction against resistance that radiates down the lateral thigh. The FABER and Ober test are often positive as well (5).

Examination

The clinical examination can begin as the patient walks to the examination room. The examiner should note the walking speed and evidence of any limp. After taking the history, observe the patient rising from the chair and ask him or her to identify the location of the pain using one finger. Often, patients with intra-articular hip pain will demonstrate the "C sign." The patient holds his or her hand in the shape of a C and places it above the greater trochanter with the thumb posteriorly and the fingers wrapping toward the groin. Intramedullary lesions of the femoral head can result in pain referred to the ischial tuberosity. Posterior–superior pain requires attention to differentiating hip and spine pathology.

The Multicenter Arthroscopy of the Hip Outcomes Research Network group identified common practice among specialists in the examination of the hip (reference 25, Martin article) (6). Beginning with the standing position the examiner should assess the height of the shoulders and iliac crests on each side, observe spinal alignment including flexion to detect scoliosis, and perform single leg stance testing. Weakness on the affected side will result in a drop in the contralateral buttock when standing on the painful leg. Gait abnormalities often help to detect pathology owing to the transfer of dynamic and static loads to the ligaments and osseous structures (Figs. 7.4 and 7.5).

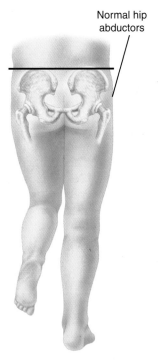

Normal hip abductors

Figure 7.4 Trendelenburg sign. (With permission from Bickley LS, Szilagyi P. *Bates' Guide to Physical Examination and History Taking*, 8th ed. Philadelphia, PA: Lippincott Williams & Wilkins.)

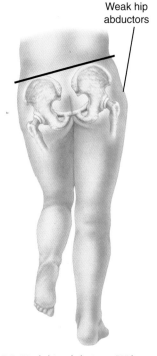

Weak hip abductors

Figure 7.5 Weak hip abductors. (With permission from Bickley LS, Szilagyi P. *Bates' Guide to Physical Examination and History Taking*, 8th ed. Philadelphia, PA: Lippincott Williams & Wilkins, 2003.)

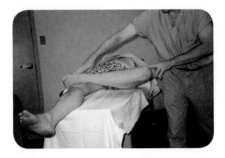

Figure 7.6 Technique for FABER maneuver. (With permission from Berg D, Worzala K. *Atlas of Adult Physical Diagnosis.* Philadelphia, PA: Lippincott Williams & Wilkins; 2006.)

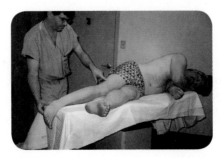

Figure 7.7 Technique for Ober's maneuver useful to assess for tightness in the iliotibial band. (With permission from Berg D, Worzala K. *Atlas of Adult Physical Diagnosis.* Philadelphia, PA: Lippincott Williams & Wilkins; 2006.)

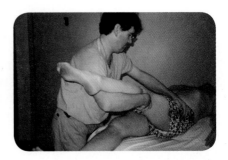

Figure 7.8 Technique for greater trochanteric bursa assessment: passive hip forward flexion and internal rotation. (With permission from Berg D, Worzala K. *Atlas of Adult Physical Diagnosis.* Philadelphia, PA: Lippincott Williams & Wilkins; 2006.)

Testing of range of motion including flexion, extension, adduction, abduction, and internal rotation in extension and external rotation in extension is performed in the supine position. Hip flexion is best tested with the knee flexed to remove tension in the hamstring and is normally 100 to 135 degrees. Motion is often limited in cases of deformity and advanced OA. Hip flexion contracture can be qualified with the Thomas test in which both thighs are brought to the chest in the supine position. Then the affected leg is allowed to extend to neutral, and inability to reach neutral demonstrates flexion contracture. The Ober test can be performed to measure tightness in the IT band, and Ely's test is performed to detect tight rectus femoris muscles. Internal rotation and abduction are limited earlier than other range of motion in OA. More complete testing of extension is best done in the prone or lateral position by passively extending the straightened leg (Figs. 7.6 to 7.8).

Impingement testing includes several common testing maneuvers. Begin with actively then passively flexing the hip as far as possible with the knee in flexion, observing the contralateral hip for movement. With the leg fully extended hold the contralateral anterior superior iliac spine to stabilize the pelvis and then passively abduct and adduct the leg. Further impingement testing is performed with the hip and knee flexed to 90 degrees followed by internal and external rotation of the hip joint. The FABER or Patrick's test includes applying downward pressure on the flexed knee and the contralateral anterior superior iliac spine during the test. Pain radiating to the buttock is consistent with SI pathology, whereas pain in the groin indicates hip pathology. The Straight Leg Raise Against Resistance Test (Stinchfield test) is an assessment of hip flexor/psoas strength and can elicit signs of intra-articular pathology by increasing compressive force across the hip joint or psoas placing pressure on the labrum. With the knee in extension, the patient carries out active straight leg raise up to 45 degree at which point the examiner's hand is placed distal to the knee, while applying a downward force. A positive test is noted when this maneuver causes pain or demonstrates focal weakness.

Palpation of the bony landmarks including the iliac crest, anterior superior iliac spine, posterior superior iliac spine, SI joints, ischial tuberosity, coccyx, and greater trochanter should be performed. The femoral neck is located three fingerbreadths below the anterior superior iliac spine.

Studies

Plain radiographs are the first choice for initial imaging of the hip joint. The standard screening series usually includes supine anteroposterior hip view for a qualitative assessment of acetabular coverage, femoral head shape, and extent of OA. Functional radiographs such as a frog lateral view and cross table

NOT TO BE MISSED

1. Fever
2. Acute pain
3. Deformity and/or inability to bear weight
4. Risk factors for septic arthritis including immunosuppression, bacteremia
5. Risk factors for AVN such as previous steroid use, exposure to altitude, thrombophilia

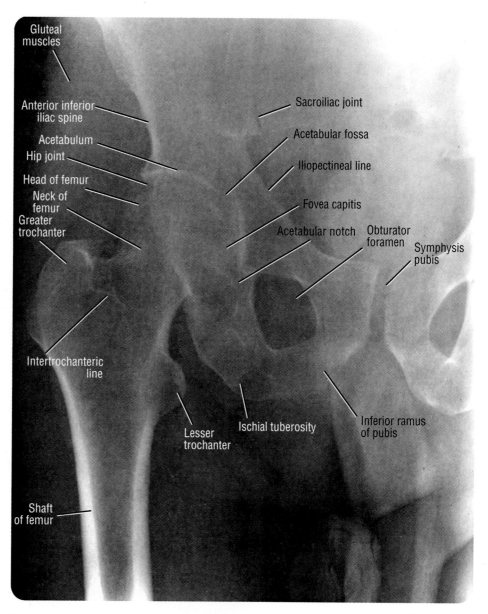

Gluteal muscles

Anterior inferior iliac spine

Acetabulum

Hip joint

Head of femur

Neck of femur

Greater trochanter

Intertrochanteric line

Lesser trochanter

Shaft of femur

Sacroiliac joint

Acetabular fossa

Iliopectineal line

Fovea capitis

Acetabular notch

Obturator foramen

Symphysis pubis

Ischial tuberosity

Inferior ramus of pubis

Figure 7.9 Anteroposterior radiograph of the hip joint. (With permission from Snell RS. *Clinical Anatomy*, 7th ed. Philadelphia, PA: Lippincott Williams & Wilkins; 2003.)

lateral views help visualize the proximal femur and femoral head sphericity and assess the prominence in the anterior head–neck junction characteristic of femoroacetabular impingement (7). These views are also used in assessing advance OA. Quantitative assessment of OA using joint space width should be done with a standing radiograph. Note that in trochanteric bursitis the imaging studies are frequently unrevealing although calcification may occasionally be visible within the bursal space (Figs. 7.9 and 7.10).

Computed tomography is primarily used for assessment of acetabular fractures, femoral head fractures, femoral neck fractures, and assessment of bone in the setting where revision of total hip arthroplasty is considered. Magnetic resonance imaging (MRI) is the superior modality for evaluating the soft tissues around the hips joint and thus has largely replaced computed tomography for this purpose.

Radionuclide scintigraphy with technetium, gallium, and indium-labeled white blood cells can be useful in detecting metastatic lesions, Paget's disease, acute and chronic osteomyelitis, and prosthetic joint infections.

SECTION 2 Regional Pain Syndromes

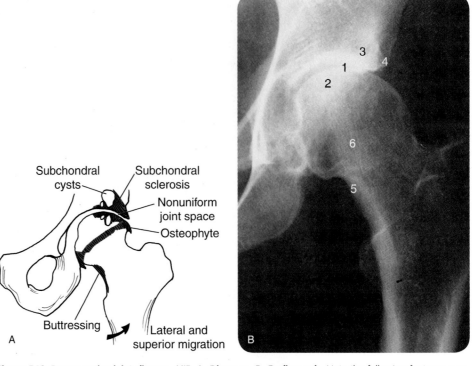

Figure 7.10 Degenerative joint disease: HIP. A. Diagram. B. Radiograph. Note the following features: non-uniform loss of joint space (*1*), subchondral sclerosis (*2*), subchondral bone cysts (*3*), osteophytes (*4*), cortical buttressing (*5*), and thickened weight-bearing trabeculae (*6*). (With permission from Yochum TR, Rowe LJ. *Yochum and Rowe's Essentials of Skeletal Radiology*, 3rd ed. Philadelphia, PA: Lippincott Williams & Wilkins; 2004.)

Dynamic sonography of the bursae around the hip may be helpful, though MRI is more sensitive for detecting inflamed bursae and muscular tears.

MRI is particularly effective at detecting AVN and is the gold standard since significant joint destruction can occur prior to evidence of radiographic abnormalities on plain radiographs. Likewise, MRI can detect soft tissue abnormalities, such as pigmented villonodular synovitis (Figs. 7.11 to 7.13) (8).

Medical and surgical treatment options for OA in the last decade can be offered to patients before advanced joint involvement requiring total joint

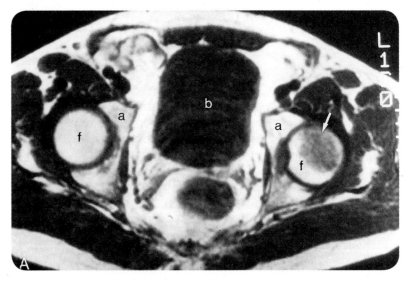

Figure 7.11 A: Transverse t1-weighted image of a patient (supine) with hip pain on long-term steroid therapy for lupus erythematosus shows nonspecific marrow edema (arrow) in the left femoral head (f). The location and clinical context of this finding are suggestive of avascular necrosis, but the imaging appearance is otherwise nonspecific. *a*, acetabulum; *b*, bladder. (From Koopman WJ, Moreland LW. *Arthritis and Allied Conditions: A Textbook of Rheumatology*, 15th ed. Philadelphia, PA: Lippincott Williams & Wilkins; 2005.)

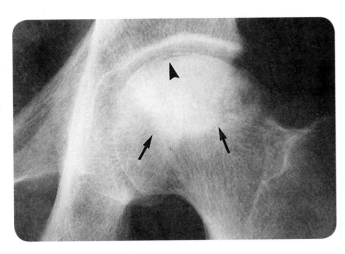

Figure 7.12 Avascular necrosis: bite and crescent signs. AP hip. Note the homogeneous increase in density (*snow cap sign*) involving the upper aspect of the head with a curvilinear inferior border (*bite sign*) (*arrows*). Beneath the articular cortex a subchondral fracture (*crescent sign*) can be seen (*arrowhead*). (With permission from Yochum TR, Rowe LJ. *Yochum and Rowe's Essentials of Skeletal Radiology*, 3rd ed. Philadelphia, PA: Lippincott Williams & Wilkins; 2004.)

arthroplasty. In particular, surgical techniques such as periacetabular osteotomy, safe surgical dislocation of the hip, and hip arthroscopy provide safe and effective tools to correct anatomical problems. The treatment outcome in many mechanically compromised hips is limited by the degree of cartilage damage that occurred prior to treatment. The caveat is detection of early stages of the joint disease, which can be difficult with plain radiographs alone. Thus, MRI can help identify diagnoses such as femoroacetabular impingement, acetabular dysplasia, and labral injury, which are felt to be precursors to premature OA. Evaluation of the articular cartilage of the hip joint is challenging because of the thin cartilage and spherical geometry of the femoral head and acetabulum. Thus, the input of an experienced radiologist is important in choosing the most appropriate protocol for the MRI. MR arthrography has higher diagnostic performance than MRI for detecting labral tears but has lower diagnostic performance for evaluation of the articular cartilage. MRI technology is continuing to evolve, and advances that provide higher spatial resolution and improved tissue contrast will help identify those patients for whom early intervention with arthroscopy will be beneficial.

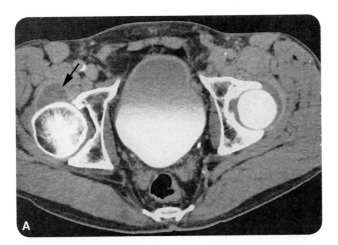

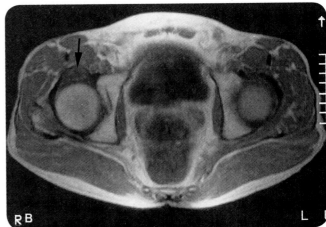

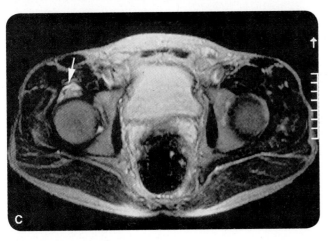

Figure 7.13 Inguinal mass: history of right hip pain. A: Soft tissue window computed tomographic (CT), axial pelvis. Note the cystic, low attenuation mass immediately anterior to the right femoral head (*arrow*). **B:** Proton density–weighted magnetic resonance imaging (MRI), axial pelvis. The area of decreased attenuation on the CT study displays a homogeneous low signal intensity on MRI (*arrow*). **C:** T2-weighted MRI, axial pelvis. Observe the homogeneous hyperintense signal intensity in this localized fluid collection (*arrow*). These findings are consistent with iliopsoas bursitis. **Comment:** This patient's history includes an inguinal hernia and the recent onset of right hip pain. At physical examination, a slightly pulsatile soft tissue mass was noted on deep palpation. (With permission from Yochum TR, Rowe LJ. *Yochum and Rowe's Essentials of Skeletal Radiology*, 3rd ed. Philadelphia: Lippincott Williams & Wilkins; 2004.)

SECTION 2 Regional Pain Syndromes

WHEN TO REFER

- Risk factors for AVN and hip pain
- Acute joint effusion with or without fever
- Fractures
- History of developmental or childhood hip pathology

Treatment and Clinical Course

Current treatments for **OA** of the hip entail a combination of nonpharmacologic, pharmacologic, and surgical therapies. Nonpharmacologic therapies, such as weight loss, land-based and water exercise, PT, and self-management education programs are generally supported by satisfactory or good, but not excellent, evidence. The pharmacologic therapies to reduce symptoms include acetaminophen, NSAIDs, COX 2 inhibitors, hyaluronic acid and glucosamine, all of which are of modest benefit. The risks associated with long-term use of NSAIDS and COX 2 inhibitors are a source of legitimate concern. Current studies are focused on discovery and development of disease modifying osteoarthritis drugs with hopes of modifying the progression of structural changes in OA and reducing the prevalence of the disease (9).

Given the developments in surgical management, early referral for advanced imaging such as MRI and specialized evaluation by orthopedists are reasonable steps to obviate progression to advanced OA.

Trochanteric bursitis is typically self-limited and responds to nonoperative management including rest, ice, NSAIDS, and PT. The PT involves stretching, flexibility, strengthening, and improving gait mechanics. Intrabursal injection of corticosteroids and local anesthetics are often effective when conservative strategies are unsuccessful. For intractable symptoms that fail injections and are felt not to be due to another cause, bursectomy can be effective.

ICD9

727.3 **Bursitis** *NEC*
   726.5 hip
   726.5 trochanteric area
924.9 **Contusion** *(skin surface intact)*
   924.01 hip
     924.00 with thigh
Derangement
   718.95 hip (joint) (internal) (old)
     835.00 current injury
     718.35 recurrent
   718.90 joint (internal)
     718.95 hip
   718.30 recurrent
     718.35 hip
Disorder
   733.90 cartilage NEC
     718.05 hip
829.0 **Fracture** *(abduction) (adduction) (avulsion) (compression) (crush) (dislocation) (oblique) (separation) (closed)*
   733.14 hip
716.60 **Monoarthritis**
   716.65 pelvic region (hip) (thigh)
715.95 **Osteoarthrosis/Osteoarthritis hip** *(degenerative) (hypertrophic)*
780.96 **Pain(s)**
   719.40 joint
     719.45 hip
848.9 **Sprain, strain** *(joint) (ligament) (muscle) (tendon)*
   843.9 hip
     843.9 and thigh
726.90 **Tendinitis, tendonitis**
   726.5 trochanteric

References

1. Zacher J, Gursche A. 'Hip' pain. *Best Pract and Res Clin Rheum* 2003;17:71–85.
2. Ganz R, Leunig M, Leuni-Ganz K, Harris WH. The etiology of osteoarthritis of the hip: an integrated mechanical concept. *Clin Orthop Relat Res.* 2008 Feb;466(2):264–72.
3. Tibor LM, Sekiya JK. Differential diagnosis of pain around the hip joint. *Arthroscopy* 2008;24:1407–1421.
4. Strauss E, Nho S, Kelly B. *Greater Trochanteric Pain Syndrome. Sprots Med Arthrosc Rev.* 2010;18:11.
5. Schapira D, Nahir M, Scharf Y. Trochanteric bursitis: a common clinical problem. *Arch Phys Med Rehabil.* 1986;67:815–7.
6. Martin HD, Shears SA, Palmer IJ. Evaluation of the hip. *Sports Med Arthrosc Rev* 2010;18:63–75.
7. Young-Jo K, Bixby S, Mamish TC. Imaging structural abnormalities in the hip joint: instability and impingement as a cause of osteoarthritis. *Semin Musculoskelet Rad* 2008;12:334–345.
8. Kijowski R. Clinical cartilage imaging of the knee and hip joints. *Am J Rad* 2010;195: 618–628.
9. Hunter DJ Pharmacologic therapy for osteoarthritis–the era of disease modification. *Nature Rev Rheum.* 2010;7(1):13–22.
10. Cush JJ, Lipsky PE. Approach to articular and musculoskeletal disorders. In: Fauci AS, Braunwald E, Kasper DL, et al. *Harrison's Principles and Practice of Internal Medicine*, 17th ed: http://www.accessmedicine.com/content.aspx?aID=2869993.

CHAPTER 8 Sports-Related Conditions and Injuries

Lisa L. Willett

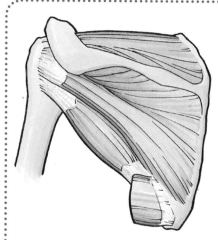

A 52 year old male with type 2 diabetes mellitus began an exercise program to improve his diabetic control. He has been playing tennis three times a week for the past month. He presents to his physician complaining of right shoulder pain. The pain is worse in certain positions.

Sporting activities are an important component of a healthy lifestyle. Patients of all ages are encouraged by physicians to exercise for health benefits. However, sports activities can lead to injuries. As our adult population ages and a larger proportion of the population embraces healthier lifestyle, sports-related conditions and injuries are predicted to increase.

There are many types of sports-related injuries, ranging from chronic overuse to traumatic injuries. Lower extremity overuse injuries occur from jogging, walking, jumping, or cycling. Examples of chronic overuse injuries include patellofemoral pain syndrome and Achilles tendinitis. Of the overuse injuries of the upper extremity, both rotator cuff tendinitis and lateral epicondylitis are the most common. Injuries related to trauma can result from high-impact sporting activities, and include ligament tears (such as an anterior cruciate ligament tear), ligament sprains (lateral ankle sprain), fractures, joint dislocations, or head injuries. The epidemiology of sporting injuries is limited. In studies (1), lower extremity injuries are more common than upper extremity, with the most common sites being the knee and ankle.

Injuries of the Rotator Cuff

CLINICAL PRESENTATION

Rotator cuff tendinitis is common in athletes who participate in repetitive overhead activities, such as softball, baseball, tennis, or golf. The rotator cuff is comprised of four muscles, the supraspinatus, infraspinatus, teres minor, and subscapularis, whose tendons attach to the proximal humerus (Fig. 8.1). Impingement of the tendons between the head of the humerus and the acromion can lead to inflammation and subsequent tears of one or more of the tendons. The supraspinatus is the most frequently involved. Symptoms include "ache-like" shoulder pain, often worse at night, exacerbated by abduction or flexion of the arm as well as activities that involve overhead movement of the arm. If the tear is complete, patients may note weakness and decreased range of motion (2).

EXAMINATION

The physical exam findings vary depending on which of the four tendons are involved, and the degree of injury. If there is only inflammation, the patient will experience pain; partial or full-thickness tears results in weakness and decreased range of motion. Although over 20 maneuvers have been described to test rotator cuff tears, the 3 maneuvers most useful for predicting a rotator cuff

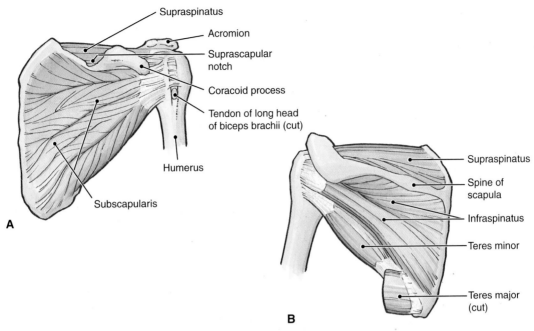

Figure 8.1 Rotator cuff muscles. **A**, anterior; **B**, posterior. The supraspinatus (**A** and **B**), infraspinatus (**B**), teres minor (**B**), and subscapularis (**A**) canvas the perimeter of the glenohumeral joint capsule. (From Moore KL, Agur AMR. Essential Clinical Anatomy, 2nd ed. Baltimore: Lippincott Williams & Wilkins, 2002. Figure 7.12, p. 425.)

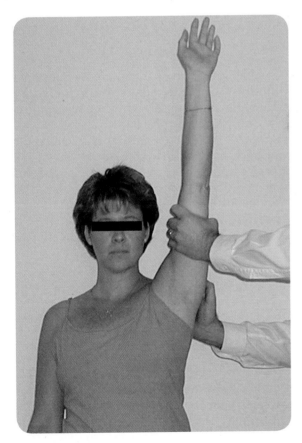

Figure 8.2 Impingement sign. Impingement of the greater tuberosity on the coracoacromial ligament occurs when the shoulder is forward flexed to 90 degrees and internally rotated, reproducing the patient's pain. From Koval KJ, MD and Zuckerman JD, MD. Atlas of Orthopaedic Surgery: A Multimeidal Reference. Philadelphia: Lippincott Williams & Wilkins, 2004.

tear are: supraspinatus weakness, weakness in external rotation, and a positive impingement sign (3,4). The test to elicit supraspinatus weakness ("empty can sign") involves having the patient abduct his arm to 90 degrees, with 30 degrees forward adduction. With the patient's thumb pointing down toward the floor, the examiner pushes down on the arm at the distal humerus as the patient resists. To elicit weakness in external rotation, a finding consistent with infraspinatus compromise, the patient holds his arms against his torso, flexes his elbows at 90 degrees with the thumbs turned up and the arm rotated internally 20 degrees. The patient is then asked to externally rotate the arm against the examiner's resistance. A positive impingement sign (Fig. 8.2) is elicited with the arm down, externally rotated and then passively elevated to an overhead position. The patient will experience pain with internal rotation of the arm. Another maneuver, the painful arc sign (Fig. 8.3) can be helpful to exclude a rotator cuff tear; a positive is interpreted when pain is elicited with active range of motion between 60 and 100 degrees of abduction and it has a high sensitivity (97.5%) for rotator cuff tear. Therefore, if this sign is absent, the patient is unlikely to have a tear.

STUDIES

If the exam and history are consistent with rotator cuff tendinitis, further studies are not necessary. However, if the pain persists, plain radiographs are indicated. Superior migration of the humeral head can be seen if a large rotator cuff tear is present. Magnetic resonance imaging (MRI) is the preferred test for diagnosing rotator cuff disorders, although ultrasonography is emerging as a cost-effective alternative with similar sensitivity and specificity.

SECTION 2 Regional Pain Syndromes

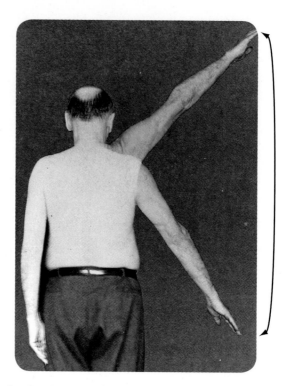

Figure 8.3 Painful arc sign. From Moore KL, PhD, FRSM, FIAC & Dalley AF II, PhD. Clinical Oriented Anatomy (4th ed.). Baltimore: Lippincott Williams & Wilkins, 1999.

TREATMENT

Multiple therapies are available to treat rotator cuff injuries. Nonoperative therapy consists of 6 weeks to 3 months of nonsteroidal anti-inflammatory agents (NSAIDS), intra-articular steroid injections, passive and active exercises with physical therapy, plus heat, cold, or ultrasonography therapy. Patients who fail nonoperative treatment can be referred to orthopedics for surgical repair with open, mini-open, or arthroscopic techniques. In a systematic review of 137 studies of nonoperative and operative treatments (5), evidence was not conclusive to recommend one therapy over another. Older age, increased size of the tear, and greater preoperative symptoms were associated with recurrent tears. Duration of symptoms was not associated with poorer outcomes.

CLINICAL COURSE

Regardless of the treatment approach, the majority of patients with rotator cuff injuries improve.

Patellofemoral Pain Syndrome

CLINICAL PRESENTATION

Patellofemoral pain syndrome (PFPS) is one of the most common sports injuries, and the most common cause of knee pain (1). It is seen in sports involving running, jumping, quick stops, and turning. The cause of patellofemoral pain is due to malalignment of the patella as it tracks in the trochlear groove of the femur. Symptoms of PFPS include unilateral or bilateral anterior knee pain, described as a dull ache in the peri- or retro-patellar region of the knee. It is initiated by the sporting activity, but can progress to become constant. Pain is exacerbated by squatting, walking up or down stairs, and prolonged sitting. It is also known as chondromalacia patellae or patellofemoral joint syndrome (2).

CLINICAL POINTS

- Overuse injuries are common when patients begin exercise programs.

- Lower extremity injuries are more common than upper extremity, with the most common sites being the knee and ankle.

- The most common cause of knee pain amongst patients exercising is patellofemoral pain syndrome.

- Conservative management with rest, ice, physical therapy, and nonsteroidal anti-inflammatory agents is effective first line therapy.

PHYSICAL EXAMINATION

Several exam maneuvers have been described, but evidence to support their diagnostic utility is limited. The physical exam is often normal in patients with PFPS, and the diagnosis is made from the patient's clinical history, and excluding other causes of knee pain. One may find atrophy of the vastus medialis muscle, tight hamstrings, and patellar instability. To assess for the presence of patellar instability, the patient's knee is flexed to 20 degrees. Manual pressure is applied both medially and laterally to the patellar. Displacement of the patella more than 75% of its width suggests an increased risk for subluxation.

STUDIES

Further diagnostic testing is not warranted once a clinical diagnosis of PFPS is made, and when trauma, effusion, or other concerning symptoms are absent. Plain radiographs may demonstrate evidence of patellofemoral malalignment. Lateral views can demonstrate patella alta (a high-riding patella, which increases risk for subluxation), patellar tilt, and trochlear depth. An infrapatellar, or "sunrise view," demonstrates patellofemoral articulation and may be a further clue of malalignment.

TREATMENT

Treatment of PFPS is primarily conservative and includes NSAIDs, rest, and ice. Physical therapy is important to provide dynamic stabilization of the patella. This includes exercises to strengthen the vastus medialis muscle, and therapy to stretch the iliotibial band and hamstring muscles. Patellar taping and stabilization braces with a hole for patellar tracking are recommended. Published data also support acupuncture and ultrasound therapy.

CLINICAL COURSE

It can take several months to achieve symptomatic relief. If there is no improvement after 9 months of conservative therapy, surgical realignment of the patellofemoral joint can be considered.

Iliotibial Band Syndrome

CLINICAL MANIFESTATIONS

The iliotibial band constitutes connective tissue that connects the ilium to the fibula. Trauma due to overuse, most commonly seen in long distance runners, can manifest itself as a dull ache underneath the lateral aspect of the knee as the band traverses next to the lateral femoral condyle on its way to insert on the fibula. On occasions the pain radiates up the thigh following the course of the band up to its insertion in the ilium. While this syndrome is almost exclusively seen on runners, specific risk factors include running longer distances than the patient is accustomed to run, running on uneven surfaces, or having uneven contact with the surface as it happens when wearing worn shoes.

EXAMINATION

While clinical symptoms are highly characteristic of this syndrome, especially in the right subset of patients, there is one maneuver that can help confirm the diagnosis. Placing the patient on the lateral decubitus position, with the affected limb upward, the examiner moves the affected limb forward and downward in an attempt to reproduce the symptoms in the affected area; on occasions pain is not reproduced but tightness can be felt along the iliotibial band. For comparison the maneuver is repeated by testing the opposite ilial-band with the patient now in the lateral decubitus position with the affected side downward.

TREATMENT

Management for this condition is mostly supportive, including rest. Use of NSAIDS is indicated for relief of pain. The use of local corticosteroids injection should be limited to patients not responding to more conservative measures; patients should restrain from running at least for 2 to 3 weeks after the injection. Running on even surfaces and wearing appropriate running shoes can also help alleviate this problem.

CLINICAL COURSE

Most patients improved dramatically with rest and the use of NSAIDS. Occasional patients require the use of local corticosteroids injections. Rarely surgical release of the band might prove curative for patients.

Achilles Tendinopathy

CLINICAL PRESENTATION

The Achilles tendon is one of the most commonly involved sites of overuse injuries. It occurs in men participating in running and repetitive jumping activities. Achilles tendinopathy refers to pain, swelling, and impaired performance of the tendon; tendinitis or tendinosis is when inflammation or degeneration has been confirmed. There are two types of Achilles tendinopathy, based on the location of the injury. Insertional tendinitis occurs within 2 cm of the insertion on the posterior aspect of the calcaneous. Non-insertional, or mid-substance, injuries occur 2 to 6 cm proximal to the insertion, where the vascular distribution is limited. Achilles tendon injuries progress through a series of stages. The initial injury is limited to the surrounding tendon sheath, and can progress to affect the tendon itself, ultimately leading to scar, degeneration, and partial or complete rupture. Rupture should be considered when patients describe a "pop" or notes a change in chronic pain, or experiences weakness with standing on their toes.

Symptoms of Achilles tendinitis are ankle pain, initially following exercise. The pain is localized over the Achilles tendon, at the inferior aspect of the posterior calf. With chronic inflammation, the pain will become constant, associated with weakness and morning stiffness in the affected ankle.

PHYSICAL EXAMINATION

The physical exam findings vary with the extent of injury. Pain on palpation is common, with swelling and limited range of motion with foot dorsiflexion. A tender nodule on the tendon that moves with ankle flexion can be palpated. If the patient has an Achilles rupture, a palpable gap may be noted at the rupture site, followed by swelling, edema, and bruising. The Thompson (Fig. 8.4) test reliably predicts a complete rupture. The patient is placed prone on the examination table, with the ankles suspended off the table; the examiner then squeezes the posterior calf to elicit a normal plantar flexion response. If there is absence of plantar flexion, considered a positive Thompson test, then the patient likely has a tendon rupture and imaging should be pursued. Ultrasound and MRI are both useful for the diagnosis of and to determine the extent of the Achilles tendon injury. If a tear is suspected clinically, an MRI is the test of choice.

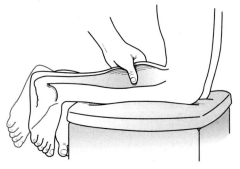

Figure 8.4 The Thompson Test demonstrates a rupture of the Achilles tendon. Adapted from Browner B, Jupiter J, Levine A. *Skeletal Trauma: Fractures, Dislocations, and Ligamentous Injuries,* 2nd ed. Philadelphia: WB Saunders, 1997.

TREATMENT

Treatment of Achilles tendinitis is conservative, and includes NSAIDs, rest, and ice. Physical therapy exercises have been shown to be effective. Eccentric exercises, which involve heel drops from a step surface, significantly improve pain by 16 weeks and should be part of a physical therapy program. Extracorporeal shockwave therapy (ESWT), splints, and insoles are also effective. Local steroid injection has no proven efficacy and risks tendon rupture. Treatment of Achilles tendon rupture is early surgical repair (6).

CLINICAL COURSE

Most patients with Achilles tendonitis recover fully with conservative treatment; risk of recurrence is unfortunately common once overuse activity is reinitiated. Appropriate orthotics devices, gradual reengagement with activities, and appropriate warming up maneuvers are of help. Patients with a ruptured Achilles tendon managed in a nonsurgical fashion have poor prognosis with high rate of re-rupture and long term functional morbidity.

Ankle Sprain
CLINICAL PRESENTATION

Ankle injuries are among the most common of all musculoskeletal injuries. The most common mechanism of injury results from a lateral ankle inversion where the ankle joint is in plantar flexion, causing the ankle to "roll" (7) Sporting activities such as basketball, soccer, and ice skating are high risk activities for ankle injury, as is a history of a prior ankle sprain. The lateral collateral ankle ligaments are most easily injured, and include the anterior and posterior talofibular ligaments (ATFL and PTFL) and the calcaneofibular ligament (CFL) (Fig. 8.5). High ankle sprains, or syndesmotic sprains, are caused by dorsiflexion and eversion of the ankle with internal rotation of the tibia, with injury to the posterior and anterior tibiofibular ligaments. Ankle

Right foot — Lateral view

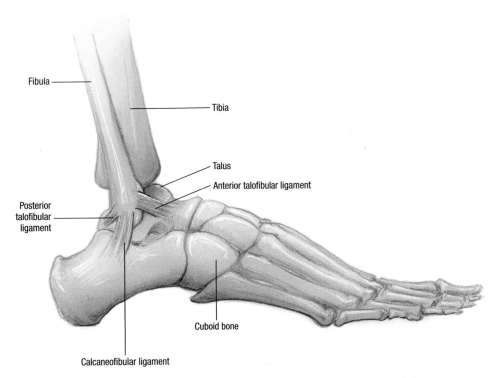

Fibula
Tibia
Talus
Anterior talofibular ligament
Posterior talofibular ligament
Cuboid bone
Calcaneofibular ligament

Figure 8.5 Ankle ligaments, right foot, lateral view. Asset provided by Anatomical Chart Co.

sprains are classified as Grade 1 through 3 depending on the severity of injury (presence of a tear, functional status, pain and swelling, ecchymosis, and weight-bearing ability).

PHYSICAL EXAMINATION

On physical examination, the ankle should be inspected for swelling, ecchymosis, and the location and degree of pain on palpation. Maneuvers, such as the anterior drawer test and the talar tilt test evaluate for joint stability (Fig. 8.6). The anterior drawer test evaluates for an ATFL tear. The examiner stabilizes the affected lower leg with one hand while cupping the heel with the other hand. Anterior force is applied to the heel in an attempt to move the talus anteriorly. The amount of displacement is then compared to the unaffected ankle. The talar tilt test evaluates a calcaneofibular ligament tear. Instead of anterior force, an inversion stress is applied to the talus. Patients with ankle injuries should also be evaluated with the Ottawa Ankle Rules (8). These clinical prediction rules have almost 100% sensitivity for ankle fracture and if negative, effectively rules out a fracture. If positive, radiographic imaging should be obtained.

TREATMENT

Treatment of lateral ankle sprains is controversial and limited by lack of clinical trials (9). Acutely, patients should apply rest, ice, compression, and elevation, and protect the ankle from further injury for 72 hours. The evidence

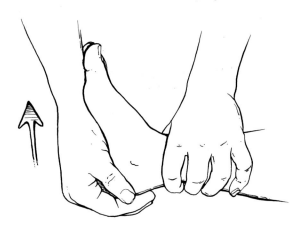

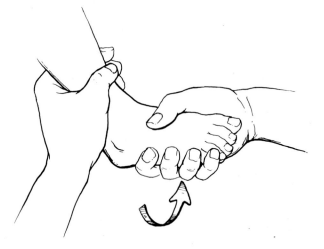

PATIENT ASSESSMENT

- Exam maneuvers can determine whether a ligament tear is present.

- Some highly sensitive maneuvers (Ottowa rules) are effective at decreasing the likelihood of a significant tear or fracture.

- Imaging is indicated when a ligament or tendon tear is suspected.

- Ultrasound and MRI can determine the degree of tendon injury.

Figure 8.6 Evaluation of ankle joint stability. The anterior drawer test (*top*) and the talar tilt test (*bottom*).

supports NSAIDs for pain control and improvements in swelling. Functional treatment with taping, bandages, or wraps has more favorable outcomes than immobilization with a cast. Although data is lacking on appropriate timing of surgery, patients with an unstable joint should be referred to an orthopedic surgeon for further evaluation.

NOT TO BE MISSED

1. Weakness of the muscles of the rotator cuff or a positive impingment sign can imply a rotator cuff tear.

2. Achilles tendon rupture presents with a palpable gap at the rupture site, swelling, edema, and bruising. This requires imaging and surgical referral.

3. Unstable joints should be referred to orthopedic surgery for further evaluation.

ICD9

726.71 **Achilles bursitis or tendinitis**
717.7 **Chondromalacia of patella**
727.61 **Complete rupture of rotator cuff**
844.2 **Cruciate ligament of knee**
726.10 **Disorders of bursae and tendons in shoulder region, unspecified**
829.0 **Fracture** *(abduction) (adduction) (avulsion) (compression) (crush) (dislocation) (oblique) (separation) (closed)*
  733.16 ankle
  733.14 femur (neck)
  733.15 specified NEC
  733.16 fibula
  733.14 hip
  733.11 humerus
  733.12 radius (distal)
  733.19 specified site NEC
  733.16 tibia
  733.12 ulna
  733.12 wrist
780.96 **Pain(s)**
  719.40 joint
    719.46 knee
726.1 **Rotator cuff syndrome of shoulder and allied disorders**
840.4 **Rotator cuff (capsule)**
726.32 **Lateral epicondylitis**
717.83 **Old disruption of anterior cruciate ligament**
Sprain, strain *(joint) (ligament) (muscle)*
  848.9 (tendon)
  845.00 ankle
    845.00 and foot
  841.9 elbow
  845.10 foot
  842.10 hand
  843.9 hip
    843.9 and thigh
  844.9 knee
    844.9 and leg
    717.5 old
  844.9 leg
  844.9 and knee
  846.9 low back
  846.0 lumbosacral
    724.6 chronic or old

WHEN TO REFER

- Physical therapy referral is important for treating rotator cuff injuries, patellofemoral pain syndrome, and Achilles tendinitis.

- Patients who fail nonoperative physical therapy after 6 to 9 months may benefit from orthopedic intervention.

- Unstable joints should be referred for orthopedic evaluation.

SECTION 2 Regional Pain Syndromes

References

1. Murray IR, Murray SA, MacKenzie K, Coleman S. How evidence based is the management of two common sports injuries in a sports injury clinic? *Br J Sports Med* 2005;39:912–916.
2. Barry NN, McGuire JL. Overuse syndromes in adult athletes. *Rheum Dis Clin North Am* 1996;22(3):515–530.

3. Ebell MH. Diagnosing rotator cuff tears. *Am Fam Physician* 2005;71(8):1587–1588.

4. Burbank KM, Stevenson JH, Czarnecki GR, et al. Chronic shoulder pain: Part I. *Evaluation and Diagnosis, Am Fam Physician* 2008;77(4):493–497.

5. Seida JC, LeBlanc C, Schouten JR, et al. Systematic Review: Nonoperative and operative treatments for rotator cuff tears. *Ann Intern Med* 2010;153(4):246–255.

6. Magnussen RA, Dunn WR, Thomson AB. Nonoperative treatment of midportion Achilles tendinopathy: A systematic review. *Clin J Sport Med* 2009;19:54–64.

7. Ivins D. Acute ankle sprain: An update. *Am Fam Physician* 2006;74:1714–1726.

8. Michael JA, Stiell IG. Ankle Injuries. In Tintinalli JE, Kelen GD, Stapczynski JS, eds. *Emergency Medicine: A Comprehensive Study Guide*, 6th ed, McGraw Hill, 2004.

9. Kerkhoffs GMMJ, Rowe BH, Assendelft WJJ, et al. Immobilisation and functional treatment for acute lateral ankle ligament injuries in adults. *Cochrane Database of Systematic Reviews* 2002;(3):CD003762.

Specific Rheumatic Diseases: Diagnosis and Treatment

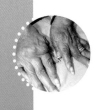

Chapter 9 **Rheumatoid Arthritis, Including Sjögren's Syndrome**

Zachary M. Pruhs, James R. O'Dell, and Ted R. Mikuls

Chapter 10 **The Seronegative Spondyloarthropathies**

Dennis W. Boulware

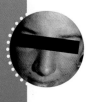

Chapter 11 **Systemic Lupus Erythematosus**

Michelle A. Petri

Chapter 12 **Raynaud's Phenomenon and Systemic Sclerosis**

Laura B. Hughes and Barri Fessler

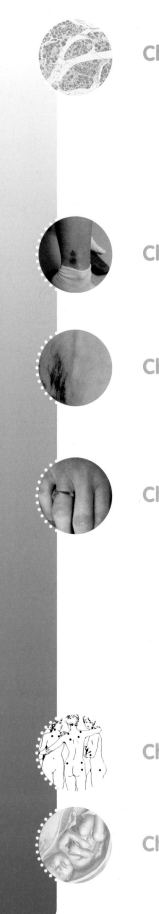

Chapter 13 **Inflammatory Myopathies: Polymyositis, Dermatomyositis, and Related Conditions**

Irene Z. Whitt and Frederick W. Miller

Chapter 14 **Vasculitis**

Bao Quynh N. Huynh and S. Louis Bridges, Jr

Chapter 15 **Giant Cell Arteritis and Polymyalgia Rheumatica**

Angelo Gaffo

Chapter 16 **Overlap Syndromes and Unclassified or Undifferentiated Connective Tissue Disease**

Iris Navarro-Millán and Graciela S. Alarcón

Chapter 17 **Fibromyalgia**

Graciela S. Alarcón

Chapter 18 **Pregnancy and Rheumatic Diseases**

Michael Lockshin

9 Rheumatoid Arthritis, Including Sjögren's Syndrome

Zachary M. Pruhs, James R. O'Dell, and Ted R. Mikuls

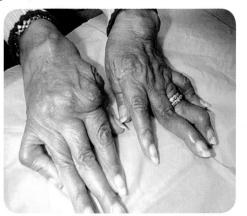

A 45-year-old woman presents with 4 months of worsening pain and stiffness in her finger joints, wrists, and balls of the feet bilaterally. Her symptoms are worse in the morning, improve with activity, and are associated with occasional warmth and swelling of the hands. Hand radiographs show periarticular erosions and osteopenia (Fig. 9.1).

Introduction

Rheumatoid arthritis (RA) is a systemic inflammatory disease with its primary manifestation in the synovium. The hallmark of the disease is a chronic, symmetric polyarthritis (synovitis) that typically affects the hands, wrists, and feet initially and later may involve any synovial joint. Although RA primarily involves the synovium, features of systemic disease are present in almost all patients and range in severity from fatigue to severe multisystem vasculitis. In recent years, significant advances in therapy have occurred, however, RA continues to result in substantial morbidity for most patients. RA patients have a higher mortality rate than the general population that is primarily related to increased cardiovascular disease burden.

Epidemiology

RA affects all racial groups worldwide and while it is seen more commonly in some populations, the prevalence in most cohorts is estimated to be 0.5% to 1%. In the developed world there appears to be a trend toward decreasing RA incidence and prevalence since the 1960s. Overall, RA is two to three times more prevalent in women than in men. A study in Minnesota reported an incidence of 50/100,000 person-years in men and 98/100,000 person-years in women (1). The preponderance of women with new onset RA was most striking in the younger age groups, but nearly equal for patients >75 years of age. The incidence of

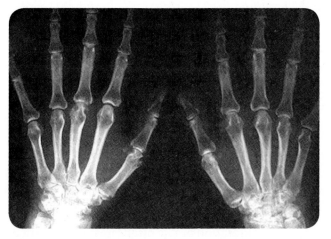

Figure 9.1 Radiograph of hands and wrists in a patient with rheumatoid arthritis; findings demonstrate periarticular osteopenia and erosions.

RA increases with age, with female excess in each age range found in most studies.

GENDER AND HORMONAL INFLUENCES

The greatest differences in incidence rates between men and women are seen in patients below 50 years of age, where RA is relatively uncommon in men. Therefore, hormonal mechanisms are felt to play a part in RA risk. In the past, the use of oral contraceptive pills were thought to be protective in the development of RA and postpartum flares of RA are also well documented in addition to an ameliorating impact on disease during late-term pregnancy. More recent studies suggest that while longer periods of breastfeeding may protect from RA, neither parity nor use of oral contraceptive pills appears to decrease risk of disease. In a recent large cohort study, use of postmenopausal hormone therapy showed no significant improvements in either risk or severity of RA (2). Some have suggested that men with RA may have mild testosterone deficiencies, and replacement may result in some decrease in symptoms.

GENETIC AND ENVIRONMENTAL RISK FACTORS

First-degree relatives of those with RA are at increased risk of developing the condition, with siblings of severely affected patients at highest risk. Monozygotic twins have a concordance rate of about 12% to 21%, whereas dizygotic twins have a rate about one quarter of this. Genetic predisposition varies widely with ethnicity and geography. While worldwide prevalence is estimated at ~0.5% to 1%, Native Americans of the Pima and Chippewa tribes have an RA prevalence of 5.3% and 6.8% respectively, an increased disease burden thought to be mediated by increased genetic risk among these populations.

Select human leukocyte antigens (HLA) class II molecules represent the most important genetic risk factor in RA and the relationship extends across ethnic groups. There is extensive evidence linking a host of HLA-DRB1 variants (often called "shared epitope" or SE alleles) with increased susceptibility to anti-cyclic citrullinated peptide (anti-CCP) antibody positive RA. Although not as strongly associated with disease risk as HLA-DRB1 SE containing alleles, several non-HLA genetic risk factors for disease susceptibility have now been defined including polymorphisms in PTPN22, STAT4, CTLA4, PADI4, and C-rel. However, genetic testing in RA (for either diagnostic or prognostic purposes) remains largely confined to research without widespread clinical application.

Of the many environmental factors linked to RA risk, cigarette smoking is perhaps the best documented. Smoking has been associated with a 50% to 70% increased risk of RA, a risk that is greatest among those carrying HLA-DRB1 SE containing alleles (a gene-environment interaction). Other factors reported to influence RA risk include occupational exposures (related to silica inhalation) and alcohol use, the latter reported to exert a protective effect.

Clinical Presentation

The hallmark symptoms of RA include:

1. Stiffness—typically greater in the morning and relieved with activity.
2. Pain—often a chief complaint of the patients and frequently difficult to quantify.
3. Tenderness—palpation with a lateral joint squeeze will elicit pain in patients with active synovitis.
4. Swelling—results from synovial proliferation and is often most prominent at the small joints of the hands and feet.
5. Deformity—develops due to stretching of tendons and ligaments along with bony erosion and is typically irreversible.

CLINICAL POINTS

- Rheumatoid arthritis (RA) is a clinical diagnosis based primarily on a thorough history and physical exam aided by the select use of laboratory tests and imaging.

- Patients with RA suffer from increased morbidity and mortality, the latter primarily due to an excess of cardiovascular disease.

- The cornerstone of RA treatment is early aggressive therapy treating to a goal of low disease activity or remission to prevent permanent damage.

- The ultimate goal of RA treatment is to achieve and maintain complete remission.

- Long-term goals of RA treatment also include the prevention of disability and improved survival.

- Immediate RA treatment goals include: decreasing pain, preventing joint damage and maintaining function, and controlling other symptoms of inflammation.

Table 9.1 Extra-articular Manifestations of Rheumatoid Arthritis

SYSTEM	MANIFESTATIONS
Mucocutaneous	Subcutaneous nodules, pyoderma gangrenosum, Sjögren's syndrome
Cardiopulmonary	Pleuritis, pulmonary fibrosis, interstitial lung disease, bronchiectasis, coronary artery disease/atherosclerosis, pericarditis (can be constrictive)
Vascular	Vasculitis
Renal	Glomerulonephritis (rare)
Ophthalmologic	Retinal vasculitis, scleritis, episcleritis
Hematologic	Anemia of chronic disease, thrombocytosis, Felty's syndrome (triad of leucopenia, splenomegaly, and RA), large granular lymphocyte (LGL) syndrome
Neurologic	Neuropathy
Musculoskeletal	Osteoporosis

The diagnosis of RA should be considered in any patient with inflammatory arthritis, especially if the hands and feet are involved. The patient's response to the question, "What is the worst time of day for your joints?" is often telling. Patients with inflammatory arthritis such as RA usually report significant morning stiffness (often lasting >1 hour), whereas patients with osteoarthritis (OA) and other mechanical syndromes are usually worse later in the day after activity. In addition, significant fatigue may be present even in early RA.

EXTRA-ARTICULAR MANIFESTATIONS OF RA

Extra-articular manifestations of RA (ExRA) range in severity from nodular skin lesions to systemic vasculitis (Table 9.1). In a large cohort study over a 30-year time span, more than 40% of RA patients had extra-articular involvement with nearly 13% of those categorized as severe (3). The most frequent manifestations of ExRA were subcutaneous nodules found in 34% of patients. The most frequent severe manifestation of ExRA was pericarditis (5%). Predictors of severe ExRA include smoking at time of diagnosis, anti-CCP and RF positivity. Importantly, patients with ExRA have significantly increased morbidity and patients with severe ExRA have a markedly increased mortality.

SJÖGREN'S SYNDROME

Sjögren's syndrome is well recognized as an extra-articular manifestation of RA. Sjögren's is a connective tissue disease affecting the exocrine glands characterized by dry eyes and mouth that is frequently associated with other connective tissue diseases including RA (4). Sjögren's syndrome is often classified by whether it is primary (occurring in isolation) or secondary (occurring concomitantly with another rheumatic condition) with signs and symptoms that can be mimicked in select viral infections (e.g., Hepatitis C, HIV), lymphoproliferative malignancy, and sarcoidosis. The relationship between RA and Sjögren's was first noted in 1933 by Henrik Sjögren himself. Patients suffering from Sjögren's will often present with parotid and lacrimal gland swelling in addition to their symptomatic complaints.

PATIENT ASSESSMENT

- Bilateral polyarticular inflammatory arthritis often confined to the hands and feet may be characteristic early in the disease course.

- Inflammatory markers (ESR and CRP) may be normal at the time of presentation in one third to half of the patients.

- Rheumatoid factor (RF) is positive in ~70% of patients but is not specific; anti-CCP antibody has a similar sensitivity to RF but is highly specific (>95%) for RA.

SECTION 3 Specific Rheumatic Diseases

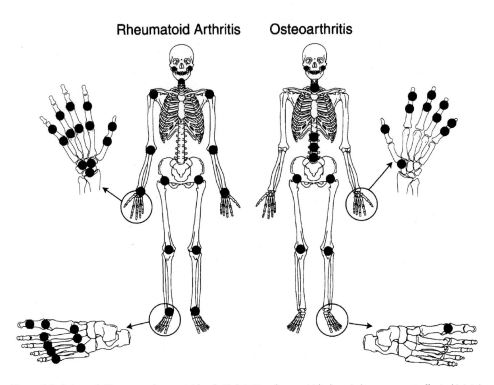

Figure 9.2 Osteoarthritis versus rheumatoid arthritis joint involvement (darker circles represent affected joints). From O'Dell JR. Rheumatoid arthritis: the clinical picture. In: Koopman WJ, ed. *Arthritis and Allied Conditions: A Textbook of Rheumatology,* 14th ed. Philadelphia: Lippincott Williams & Wilkins, 2001:1153–1186, with permission.

Diagnosis may be aided by the Schirmer's (assessing for ocular dryness) and Rose Bengal tests as well as salivary gland or lip biopsy; positive serologies for ANA, anti-SSA/SSB, and RF are characteristic of Sjögren's syndrome. Sjögren's may exhibit extraglandular involvement including visceral (heart, lungs, kidney, gastrointestinal tract, central/peripheral nervous system) and non-visceral (skin, muscles, joints) manifestations. Classification of the disease is guided by the revised rules for classification from the American–European Consensus Group (Table 9.2).

Examination

Joint distribution is critical in the diagnosis of RA. Initially, RA is often limited to the hands and feet. In the hands, the proximal interphalangeal joints (PIPs) and metacarpal phalangeal joints (MCPs) are most likely to be involved early in the disease course. Figure 9.2 compares and contrasts the joints most commonly involved in RA and OA. In the hand, the distal interphalangeal joints (DIPs) are characteristically involved in OA (Heberden nodes) but seldom involved in RA, the PIPs may be involved with either, whereas MCP involvement is the rule in RA and seldom occurs in OA. The wrist is frequently involved in RA, whereas only the first carpal–metacarpal joint is commonly involved in OA. A remarkable feature of RA is the symmetry of involvement.

If inflammation persists over time, permanent damage, including tendon, ligament, cartilage, and subchondral bone destruction can occur, with resultant joint deformity and disability. Although inflammation and deformity are most often seen initially in the hands and feet, the disease may later affect larger joints. Involvement of the knees, hips, and shoulders accounts for significant morbidity including work disability in a large percentage of patients. With early and effective treatments, deformity and severe disability are occurring less frequently.

Table 9.2 Revised International Classification Criteria for Sjögren's

1. Ocular symptoms: a positive response to at least one of the following questions:
   Have you had daily, persistent, troublesome dry eyes for more than 3 months?
   Do you have a recurrent sensation of sand or gravel in the eyes?
   Do you use tear substitutes more than three times a day?

2. Oral symptoms: a positive response to at least one of the following questions:
   Have you had a daily feeling of dry mouth for more than 3 months?
   Have you had recurrently or persistently swollen salivary glands as an adult?
   Do you frequently drink liquids to aid in swallowing dry food?

3. Ocular signs: objective evidence of ocular involvement defined as a positive result for at least one of the following two tests:
   Schirmer's I test, performed without anesthesia (5 mm in 5 minutes)
   Rose Bengal score or other ocular dye score (4 or more according to van Bijsterveld's scoring system)

4. Histopathology: in minor salivary glands (obtained through normal-appearing mucosa) focal lymphocytic sialoadenitis, evaluated by an expert histopathologist, with a focus score of 1 or more, defined as a number of lymphocytic foci (which are adjacent to normal-appearing mucous acini and contain more than 50 lymphocytes) per 4 mm^2 of glandular tissue

5. Salivary gland involvement: objective evidence of salivary gland involvement defined by a positive result for at least one of the following diagnostic tests:
   Unstimulated whole salivary flow ($<$1.5 mL in 15 minutes)
   Parotid sialography showing the presence of diffuse sialectasias (punctate, cavitary, or destructive pattern), without evidence of obstruction in the major ducts
   Salivary scintigraphy showing delayed uptake, reduced concentration, or delayed excretion of tracer

6. Autoantibodies: presence in the serum of one or both of the following autoantibodies:
   Antibodies to Ro (Sjögren's syndrome A) antigens
   Antibodies to La (Sjögren's syndrome B) antigens

Revised rules for classification

For primary Sjögren's syndrome:

In patients without any potentially associated disease, primary Sjögren's syndrome may be defined as follows:

The presence of any four of the six items is indicative of primary Sjögren's syndrome, as long as either histopathology or serology is positive

The presence of any three of the four objective criteria items (i.e., items 3, 4, 5, and 6)

For secondary Sjögren's syndrome:

In patients with a potentially associated disease (e.g., another well-defined connective tissue disease), the presence of item 1 or item 2 plus any two from among items 3, 4, and 5 may be considered as indicative of secondary Sjögren's syndrome

Exclusion criteria:
   Past head and neck radiation treatment
   Hepatitis C infection
   AIDS
   Preexisting lymphoma
   Sarcoidosis
   Graft versus host disease
   Use of anticholinergic drugs (since a time shorter than fourfold the half-life of the drug)

Adapted from Vitali C, Bombardieri S, Jonsson R, et al. Classification criteria for Sjögren's syndrome: a revised version of the European criteria proposed by the American-European Consensus Group. *Ann Rheum Dis* 2002;61(6):557.

SECTION 3 Specific Rheumatic Diseases

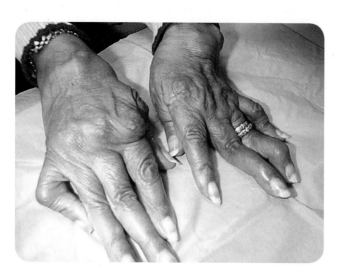

Figure 9.3 Swan neck and boutonniere deformities (fifth digits) in a patient with long-standing RA.

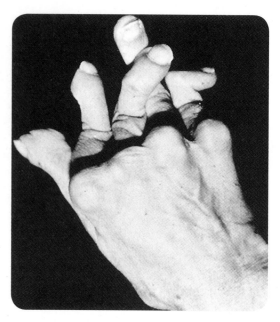

Figure 9.4 Arthritis mutilans. From Koopman WJ, Moreland LW, eds. *Arthritis and Allied Conditions: A Textbook of Rheumatology*, 15th ed. Philadelphia: Lippincott Williams & Wilkins, 2005.

FINGERS

Non-reducible flexion contractures of the proximal interphalangeal (PIP) joint with concomitant hyperextension of the distal interphalangeal (DIP) joint of the finger known as "boutonniere" deformity may occur with progressive disease. Hyperextension at the proximal interphalangeal joint with flexion of the distal interphalangeal joint or "swan-neck" deformity is also seen in RA (Fig. 9.3). Although similar deformities can be seen in systemic lupus erythematosus (SLE), these are typically reducible (the so-called Jaccoud's arthropathy). "Triggering" of the finger occurs when thickening or nodule formation of the tendon interacts with the concomitant tenosynovial proliferation, trapping the tendon (stenosing tenosynovitis). Tendon rupture may occur due to infiltrative synovitis in the digit or bony erosions that produce surfaces that cut the tendon at the wrist (especially the flexor pollicis longus). Arthritis mutilans ("opera glass hands") results if destruction is severe and extensive, with dissolution of bone (Fig. 9.4).

METACARPOPHALANGEAL JOINTS

Two typical deformities may occur at the metacarpophalangeal (MCP) joints—volar or palmar subluxation of the fingers relative to the metacarpal bones and ulnar deviation (Fig. 9.5). Most cases of ulnar deviation are accompanied by radial deviation of the wrist, roughly proportional to the degree of ulnar deviation of the fingers. Although RA is the most common cause of ulnar deviation, other arthritides, as well as certain neurologic deficiencies, may result in ulnar deviation as well.

WRISTS

The wrist is the site of multiple potential problems in patients with RA. The combination of ulnar drift of the

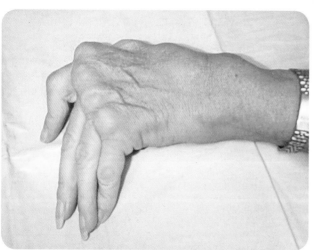

Figure 9.5 Ulnar deviation and subluxation of digits with boutonniere deformity of second digit.

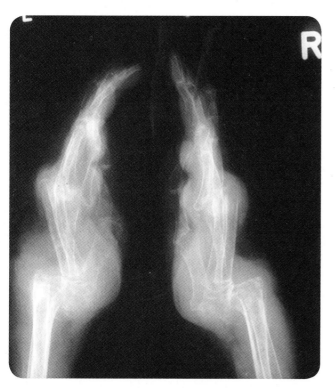

Figure 9.6 Radiograph showing wrist destruction and subluxation in a patient with RA. William J. Koopman, Larry W. *Moreland, Arthritis and Allied Conditions: A Textbook of Rheumatology*, 15th ed. Philadelphia: Lippincott Williams & Wilkins, 2005.

fingers and radial deviation of the wrist is known as a "zig-zag" deformity. Wrist subluxation may lead to rupture of the extensor tendons of the little, ring, and long fingers (Fig. 9.6), as the end of the distal ulna may be roughened secondary to erosion of bone and may abrade the tendons as they move back and forth during normal hand function. Entrapment of the median nerve as it passes through the carpal tunnel (carpal tunnel syndrome) leads to numbness and decreased sensation on the palmar aspect of the thumb, index, long, and radial aspect of the ring fingers, and later to weakness and atrophy of the muscles in the thenar eminence (Fig. 9.7).

ELBOW

Elbow involvement is often detected by palpable synovial proliferation at the radiohumeral joint and is commonly accompanied by a flexion deformity. If synovitis or effusion is present in the elbow, complete extension will not occur; therefore, complete extension is an excellent sign that significant synovitis or effusion is absent. Olecranon bursal involvement is common, as are rheumatoid nodules in the bursa and along the extensor surface of the ulna (Fig. 9.8). Ulnar nerve entrapment and corresponding neuropathy can occur with significant elbow involvement.

SHOULDERS

Shoulders are commonly involved, with nocturnal pain being particularly troubling, as it is often difficult for patients with shoulder problems to find a comfortable position for sleep. Swelling occurs initially anteriorly but may be difficult to detect and is present on examination in a minority of patients at any point in time.

FEET AND ANKLES

Ankle joint involvement is seldom seen in the absence of midfoot or metatarsophalangeal involvement. Major structural changes occur in the midfoot and foot due to the combination of chronic synovitis and weight bearing. Posterior

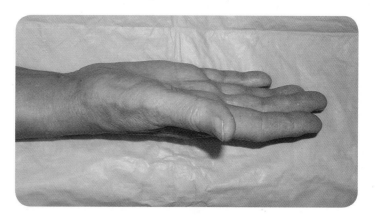

Figure 9.7 Thenar atrophy in a patient with RA and severe carpal tunnel syndrome.

SECTION 3 Specific Rheumatic Diseases

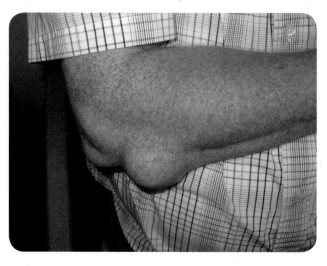

Figure 9.8 Subcutaneous nodule in a patient with RA.

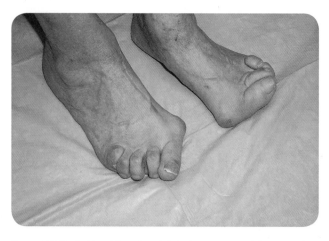

Figure 9.9 Feet with subluxation of digits in a patient with long-standing RA.

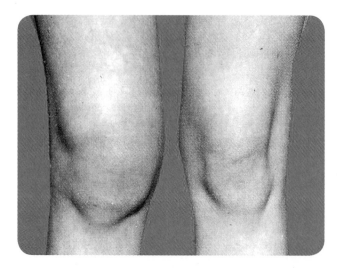

Figure 9.10 Patient with RA and a large right knee effusion. From Koopman WJ, Moreland LW, eds. *Arthritis and Allied Conditions: A Textbook of Rheumatology*, 15th ed. Philadelphia: Lippincott Williams & Wilkins, 2005.

tibialis tendon involvement or rupture may lead to subtalar subluxation, which results in eversion and migration of the talus laterally. Midfoot disease leads to loss of normal arch contour with flattening of the feet. Metatarsophalangeal (MTP) joint inflammation occurs in most patients and is often one of the earliest disease manifestations. The great toe typically develops hallux valgus (bunion). Subluxation of the phalanx at the metatarsophalangeal joint of the other toes predominantly occurs dorsally (Fig. 9.9). The toes may exhibit compensatory flexion due to a fixed length of the flexor tendons, resulting in "hammer toes" (named because they resemble piano key hammers). When dorsal subluxation occurs, the soft-tissue pad on the plantar surface of the metatarsal heads is displaced, allowing the metatarsal heads to protrude and become the primary weight-bearing surface. This is painful and calluses develop. This can result in patient reports of feeling like they are "walking around with pebbles" in their shoes.

KNEES

Large knee effusions may develop in RA with abundant proliferation of synovium (Fig. 9.10). Persistent effusions may lead to inhibition of quadriceps function by spinal reflexes with subsequent muscular atrophy. With chronic effusions the knee is more comfortable in the flexed position, and flexion deformities occur that greatly increase the work expended to walk. Baker or popliteal cysts are common and may be responsive to intra-articular corticosteroid injection.

HIPS

Limited motion or pain with internal and/or external rotation is the hallmark of hip involvement whereas localized lateral hip pain is more often due to trochanteric bursitis. Patients with true hip joint pathology characteristically report pain in the mid-groin with rotation or with weight bearing.

CERVICAL SPINE

Neck pain on motion and occipital headache are common manifestations of cervical spine involvement and occur in a proportion of patients with long-standing disease. The atlantoaxial (C1–C2) joint is a synovium-lined joint and is susceptible to the same proliferative synovitis and subsequent instability that are seen in the peripheral joints. The possibility of significant C1–C2 instability should be considered before a patient with RA undergoes surgical procedures to avoid compromise to the cervical cord or brainstem during intubation or as the patient is transferred while asleep. Patients with severe destruction in the hands (arthritis mutilans) are very likely to have symptomatic cervical spine abnormalities, as are those taking significant amounts of corticosteroids.

CRICOARYTENOID JOINT

Since synovial tissue is present around the cricoarytenoid joint, involvement of this joint may occur in up to one fourth of RA patients. A sense of "fullness" that is aggravated by speaking or swallowing is usually the initial symptom. Hoarseness and inspiratory symptoms may develop. Severe involvement may rarely produce enough restriction of joint motion to cause acute, life-threatening dyspnea and emergent tracheotomy may be required.

Studies

Select laboratory and imaging studies may be helpful in the diagnosis of RA. Both rheumatoid factor (RF) and anti-CCP antibody are positive in ~70% of patients. However, RF has only modest disease specificity, whereas anti-CCP antibody is seen almost exclusively in RA. Often relatively unremarkable early in the disease course, radiographs of involved joints may show soft tissue swelling, periarticular osteopenia, and periarticular erosions with disease progression. Acute phase reactants (erythrocyte sedimentation rate and C-reactive protein) are elevated in ~50% of patients at presentation and may be valuable in assessing response to therapy. Other laboratory abnormalities may include anemia of chronic disease and reactive thrombocytosis. Although not universally employed, MRI and ultrasound may be sensitive in detecting early changes in RA.

Diagnosis of Rheumatoid Arthritis

The importance of making an accurate diagnosis of RA as early as possible cannot be overemphasized. All modern treatment paradigms stress early aggressive disease-modifying antirheumatic drug (DMARD) therapy. It is critical to ensure that effective treatments are begun when they have the maximum chance of making the biggest differences, while at the same time protecting patients who do not have RA from the potential toxicities of unnecessary therapies.

CLASSIFICATION CRITERIA OF RHEUMATOID ARTHRITIS

In 2010 the American College of Rheumatology (ACR) and the European League Against Rheumatism (EULAR) collaboratively issued new RA classification criteria (Table 9.3). The new criteria were developed to augment the 1987 ACR RA classification criteria (Table 9.4) which have been criticized for a lack of sensitivity for the detection of early disease. Under the 2010 criteria, a definitive diagnosis of RA is ascribed to patients with a score of six or more (of a possible ten points) from four scoring domains including number and location of involved joints, serologic abnormality, acute phase reactant elevation, and duration of symptoms. While the 2010 criteria will assist in identifying homogeneous groups of patients for trials of early intervention, the utility of the new ACR/EULAR criteria in "real-life" practice is yet to be established.

Other Conditions that Can Resemble Rheumatoid Arthritis

When presented with a patient who has joint pain, the first challenge is to discern if the problem is due to mechanical derangements, OA, or inflammation. Stiffness, swelling, tenderness, warmth, and pain with motion are hallmarks of

---

NOT TO BE MISSED

- The differential diagnosis for RA is broad and includes viral infections (e.g., Hepatitis C and parvovirus), paraneoplastic syndromes, and other rheumatic diseases (lupus, osteoarthritis, etc.).

- RA is associated with extra-articular manifestations including subcutaneous nodules, serositis, lung disease, vasculitis, Sjögren's syndrome, inflammatory eye disease, and osteoporosis leading to fractures.

- Patients with RA should be evaluated for cervical spine involvement especially as part of any preoperative assessment.

- Although uncommon, cricoarytenoid joint involvement may lead to airway obstruction.

- RA is characterized by a higher risk for malignancy including lymphoma (non-Hodgkin) and lung cancer.

SECTION 3 Specific Rheumatic Diseases

Table 9.3 2010 American College of Rheumatology/European League Against Rheumatism Classification Criteria for Rheumatoid Arthritis

Target population (Who should be tested?): Patients	Score
1) who have at least one joint with definite clinical synovitis (swelling)	
2) with the synovitis not better explained by another disease	
Classification criteria for RA (score-based algorithm: add score of categories A–D; a score of ≥6/10 is needed for classification of a patient as having definite RA)[a]	
A. Joint involvement[b]	
1 large joint	0
2–10 large joints	1
1–3 small joints (with or without involvement of large joints)[c]	2
4–10 small joints (with or without involvement of large joints)	3
>10 small joints (with at least 1 small joint)	5
B. Serology (at least one test result is needed for classification)	
Negative RF and negative ACPA	0
Low-positive RF or low-positive ACPA (positive but <3x upper limit of normal)	1
High-positive RF or high-positive ACPA (positive, >3x upper limit of normal)	2
C. Acute phase reactants (at least one test result is needed for classification)	
Normal CRP and normal ESR	0
Abnormal CRP or abnormal ESR	1
D. Duration of symptoms	
<6 weeks	0
≥6 weeks	1

[a]Although patients with a score of <6/10 are not classifiable as having RA, their status can be reassessed and the criteria might be fulfilled cumulatively over time.

[b]Joint involvement refers to any *swollen* or *tender* joint on examination, which may be confirmed by imaging evidence of synovitis. "Large joints" refers to shoulders, elbows, hips, knees, and ankles.

[c]"Small joints" refers to the metacarpophalangeal joints, proximal interphalangeal joints, second through fifth metatarsophalangeal joints, thumb interphalangeal joints, and wrists.

Adapted from Aletaha, et al. 2010. Rheumatoid arthritis classification criteria: An American College of Rheumatology/European League Against Rheumatism collaborative initiative. *Arthritis Rheum* 2010; 62(9):2569–2581.

active articular inflammation. The presence of severe morning stiffness is indicative of an inflammatory process, while "gelling" of the joints for merely a few minutes in the morning and after rest is more consistent with OA and mechanical derangements. The diagnosis of RA is most difficult early in the disease course or when relatively few joints are involved; unfortunately, diagnosis is often delayed several months after the onset of symptoms, precluding the initiation of early treatment.

Signs and symptoms of inflammatory arthritis may be associated with many syndromes other than RA. A history directed at eliciting the associated features of other arthritides is essential. For instance, the presence of photosensitivity or nephritis suggests the possibility of SLE, while conjunctivitis and dactylitis may suggest reactive arthritis. Systemic vasculitis, such as polyarteritis nodosa or

Table 9.4 The 1987 Revised Criteria for the Classification of Rheumatoid Arthritis

CRITERION	DEFINITION
1. Morning stiffness	Morning stiffness in and around the joints lasting at least 1 hour before maximal improvement
2. Arthritis of three or more joint areas	At least three joint areas simultaneously have had soft tissue swelling or fluid (not bony overgrowth alone) observed by a physician. The 14 possible areas are right or left PIP, MCP, wrist, elbow, knee, ankle, and MTP joints
3. Arthritis of hand joints	At least one area swollen (as defined above) in a wrist, MCP, or PIP joint
4. Symmetric arthritis	Simultaneous involvement of the same joint areas (as defined in 2) on both sides of the body (bilateral involvement of PIPs, MCPs, or MTPs is acceptable without absolute symmetry)
5. Rheumatoid nodules	Subcutaneous nodules, over bony prominences, or extensor surfaces or in juxta-articular regions, observed by a physician
6. Serum rheumatoid factor	Demonstration of abnormal amounts of serum rheumatoid factor by any method for which the result has been positive in <5% of normal control subjects
7. Radiographic changes	Radiographic changes typical of rheumatoid arthritis on posteroanterior hand and wrist radiographs, which must include erosions or unequivocal bony decalcification localized in or most marked adjacent to the involved joints (osteoarthritis changes alone do not qualify)

For classification purposes, a patient shall be said to have rheumatoid arthritis if he/she has satisfied at least 4 of these 7 criteria. Criteria 1 through 4 must have been present for at least 6 weeks. Patients with two clinical diagnoses are not excluded. Designation as classic, definite, or probable rheumatoid arthritis is not to be made.

Adapted from Arnett et al. The American Rheumatism Association 1987 Revised Criteria for the Classification of Rheumatoid Arthritis. *Arthritis Rheum* 1988;31(3):315–324.

Wegener granulomatosis, may be associated with disabling joint pain, although objective signs of arthritis are infrequent. Hypothyroidism can produce rheumatic symptoms, and is seen in increased association with RA. Finally, the crystalline arthropathies including gout and calcium pyrophosphate deposition disease frequently present as inflammatory arthritis and may mimic RA.

CRYSTALLINE ARTHROPATHIES

Patients with gout develop uric acid crystal deposition in the joints and may present with symptoms similar to RA. Classically, gout presents with podagra (inflammation and pain in the great toe) or pauciarticular joint swelling with exquisite pain. In contrast to RA, there is a male preponderance and typically male patients develop symptoms in the third and fourth decades of life (with women developing initial flares much later, well after menopause). High serum uric acid is suggestive but not diagnostic of gout, however, uric acid levels may be normal or even low during acute gout attacks. Definitive diagnosis is made through aspiration of intracellular negatively birefringent uric acid crystals from the synovial fluid, examined under polarized microscopy. In select cases chronic gout can present in a "pseudo-rheumatoid" fashion. Thus, gout should be considered, particularly in patients with hyperuricemia who are seronegative for RF and anti-CCP antibody.

Patients with calcium pyrophosphate crystal deposition (CPPD) or pseudogout may also present with pauciarticular pain and inflammation, especially in the wrists and knees. Patients with pseudogout may have a history of trauma to the affected joints. Pseudogout typically presents after the fifth decade of life and has a slight female preponderance. Definitive diagnosis is made through aspiration of weakly positive birefringent crystals from the synovial fluid (polarized microscopy). Importantly, pseudogout may be associated with other underlying metabolic illnesses including hyperparathyroidism, hypothyroidism, and hemochromatosis. Further workup should be considered in patients diagnosed with pseudogout. Like chronic gout, CPPD can closely mimic RA in select circumstances.

SLE

Patients with SLE may present with polyarticular arthritis and arthralgias similar to RA with a similar joint distribution. However, patients with SLE frequently have other disease manifestations including skin and internal organ involvement. The presence of photosensitive skin rash, serositis, renal disease, or hematologic abnormality (e.g., cytopenias) in a patient with inflammatory arthritis is suggestive of SLE. Additionally, >95% of patients with SLE will have a positive antinuclear antibody (ANA) titer as opposed to 30% to 40% of RA patients. The presence of anti-double stranded DNA or anti-Smith antibody is highly specific to SLE.

SPONDYLOARTHROPATHIES

The spondyloarthropathies (reactive arthritis, psoriatic arthritis, and inflammatory bowel disease) may appear similar to RA at presentation. The spondyloarthropathies often present with inflammation found at enthesis or site of tendon insertions (Achilles tendon insertion, plantar fascia, shafts of fingers or toes) known as enthesitis. Asymmetric oligoarthritis (fewer than four joints), usually of the weight-bearing joints, is more common in these disorders than in RA. The presence of conjunctivitis/iritis, urethritis, and mucocutaneous or intestinal manifestations in the spondyloarthropathies also differentiate these conditions from RA. In addition, inflammatory symptoms of the axial skeleton strongly suggest the diagnosis of one of the spondyloarthropathies, recognizing that RA can affect the cervical spine.

PALINDROMIC RHEUMATISM

Palindromic rheumatism is a remitting, recurring, nondestructive, inflammatory arthritis with recurrences over at least 6 months. Attacks rarely last more than 1 week and generally involve only a few joints, with the joints ultimately involved being similar to those involved in typical RA. The disease eventually evolves into typical RA over time in one quarter to half of the patients. Women with RF and/or anti-CCP antibody with early hand involvement are more likely to develop RA than patients without these features.

REMITTING SERONEGATIVE SYMMETRIC SYNOVITIS WITH PITTING EDEMA

Remitting seronegative symmetric synovitis with pitting edema (RS3PE) is characterized by a very abrupt onset of marked dorsal swelling of the hands with pitting edema, wrist synovitis, and flexor tendinitis of the fingers. Similar swelling and synovitis may also be seen in the feet and ankles. Patients can often precisely pinpoint the time of onset. In general, the prognosis is excellent, although RS3PE occurring with an underlying malignancy as part of a paraneoplastic syndrome has been reported. For the most part, patients respond dramatically to low-dose corticosteroids. RF and anti-CCP antibody are not generally present and radiographic joint destruction does not typically occur.

POLYMYALGIA RHEUMATICA

Polymyalgia rheumatica (PMR) generally presents with an abrupt to subacute onset of pain and stiffness in the shoulder and hip girdles of patients >50 years of age. Fever, weight loss, and lethargy can occur and may be severe. Restriction of shoulder movement secondary to pain and soft-tissue contracture is common. The stiffness and restricted mobility are exquisitely sensitive to treatment with modest dose prednisone, with marked clinical responses typically observed with doses as low as 10 to 15 mg/day. Persistent small joint synovitis of the hands and feet distinguishes RA from PMR, although morning stiffness may otherwise be identical. RA of acute onset with PMR symptoms in the elderly often has an excellent prognosis.

VIRAL ARTHRITIS

Polyarthritis may be the presenting feature of viral infections. Clues leading to the etiologic agent may be evident in the history and examination. In contrast to RA, viral associated arthritis is more often self-limited. Fever and cutaneous manifestations may suggest an infectious process. Viral infections that can closely mimic RA include rubella, parvovirus B19, and viral hepatitis (particularly hepatitis C which can lead to chronic arthralgias and low-titer positive RF).

Treatment

GOALS

The status of the individual patient at any point in time should always be assessed relative to treatment goals. Specific treatment goals are well accepted and easy to understand in such conditions as hypertension, hyperlipidemia, or diabetes. In RA, goals are more difficult to quantify but no less important. With improving therapies, remission is becoming a more realistic, although still elusive, goal. No one single measure adequately describes the status of a patient with RA. Rather, combinations of abnormalities detected by laboratory testing, physical examination, radiologic examination, and assessment of pain and functional status are used.

The American College of Rheumatology (ACR) has recommended a core set of composite criteria (Table 9.5) for the ongoing evaluation of therapies in patients with RA. The components of this core set are excellent parameters to follow in individual patients in clinical practice, as well as in clinical research situations. Frequently used composite measures of disease activity include the Disease Activity Score (DAS), the Routine Assessment of Patient Index Data 3 (RAPID-3), and the Clinical Disease Activity Index (CDAI). The latter measures can be calculated in "real-time" with suggested thresholds defined corresponding to low disease activity and remission.

Medications

There are four main classes of medications used in the treatment of RA: nonsteroidal anti-inflammatory drugs (NSAIDs), corticosteroids, synthetic DMARDs,

Table 9.5 American College of Rheumatology Disease Activity Measures for Rheumatoid Arthritis Core Set

DISEASE ACTIVITY MEASURES

1. Tender joint count
2. Swollen joint count
3. Patient's assessment of pain
4. Patient's global assessment of disease activity
5. Physician's global assessment of disease activity
6. Patient's assessment of physical function
7. Acute-phase reactant value

and biologic DMARDs. As control of RA symptoms and prevention of long-term disability from the disease depends on stopping the inflammatory process, there is a trend toward earlier, more aggressive utilization of both synthetic and biologic DMARDs (5).

NSAIDs

NSAIDs may be useful early on in the course of RA, particularly when the diagnosis is still in question. NSAIDs may relieve pain, swelling, and stiffness in the short term while the diagnostic workup is completed. NSAID use carries risk of significant side effects including gastrointestinal ulcers and increased risk of bleeding. It is important to recognize that the long term use of NSAIDs has not been shown to slow disease progression in RA, therefore their use as monotherapy is not recommended.

CORTICOSTEROIDS

While corticosteroids are potent inhibitors of inflammation and may prevent disease progression in RA, their use is associated with a host of side effects including weight gain, hypertension, glucose intolerance, hyperlipidemia, osteoporosis, and cataracts among others. Patients on corticosteroids have higher rates of infection and a recent study reports a dose dependent increase in risk of pneumonia for patients on long-term corticosteroid therapy for RA (6). Ideally, corticosteroids should be used as a bridge to DMARD therapy and should generally not be employed as monotherapy in RA.

SYNTHETIC DMARDs

Given the long-term goal of suppression of inflammation in RA, synthetic DMARDs have become a cornerstone of therapy. Methotrexate in particular has demonstrated utility in preventing disease progression as well as reducing mortality in RA patients (7). With an established track record, acceptable risk of toxicity, and low cost, methotrexate now constitutes first-line therapy for RA in the absence of contraindications to its use. Other synthetic DMARDs include leflunomide, sulfasalazine, minocycline, azathioprine, cyclosporine, and hydroxychloroquine. In 2008 the ACR issued recommendations for the use of synthetic DMARDs in RA patients who had not previously received DMARDs based on disease duration and activity (8). Each medication has unique side effect profiles and monitoring requirements (Table 9.6). Synthetic DMARDs are frequently used in combination as well as concomitantly with the biologic DMARDs to achieve optimal control of RA disease activity.

Table 9.6 Guidelines for Monitoring the Treatment of Rheumatoid Arthritis

DRUG	POTENTIAL TOXIC EFFECTS	BASELINE EVALUATION	SYSTEM REVIEW OR EXAMINATION	LABORATORY TESTS	COMMENTS
Hydroxychloro quine	Macular changes	None unless patient >40 years old or previous eye problems	Visual changes, fundoscopic and visual field exam yearly	None	Best tolerated DMARD
Leflunomide	Myelosuppression, hepatic fibrosis	CBC, ALT, albumin, hepatitis B and C serologies	Diarrhea, weight loss, elevated blood pressure	CBC, ALT, albumin every 4–8 weeks	Long half-life; pregnancy contraindicated; patients should limit alcohol intake
Sulfasalazine	Neutorpenia, myelosuppression	CBC; consider G6PD and ALT assessment for patients at risk	Fever, bruising, pallor	CBC every 2–4 weeks for 3 months, then every 3 months	Enteric coated tablets may be better tolerated
Minocycline	Hyperpigmentation, nausea, dizziness	None	Hyperpigmentation	None	May interfere with efficacy of oral contraceptives
Azathioprine	Myelosuppression	CBC, creatinine, ALT	Fever, bruising, pallor	CBC every 2 weeks until stable dose, then every 1–3 months	Works well in combinations
Cyclosporine	Renal insufficiency, anemia, hypertension	CBC, creatinine, blood pressure	Edema; check blood pressure monthly	Creatinine every 2 weeks until stable dose, then every month; CBC every three months	Poor long-term continuation rate
Methotrexate	Myelosuppression, hepatic fibrosis, pneumonitis	CBC, recent chest radiograph, ALT, creatinine and albumin, hepatitis B and C serologies	Mouth ulcers, shortness of breath, new-onset cough, nausea	CBC, ALT, albumin every 4–8 weeks	Pregnancy contraindicated; patients must avoid alcohol, initiate folic acid supplementation concurrent with medication
TNF-α inhibitors: (Etanercept, Infliximab, Adalimumab, Golimumab, Certolizumab)	Infections	Screen for latent tuberculosis	Infections; symptoms of CHF or demyelinating disease	None unless also on DMARDs	Discontinue during infections
Anakinra	Pneumonia, neutropenia	Screen for asthma	Infections	CBC monthly for 3 months then every 3 months	Discontinue during infections
Abatacept	Infections	Screen for latent tuberculosis; hepatitis B and C serologies	Infections	None unless also on DMARDs	Discontinue during infections
Rituximab	Infections	Screen for hepatitis B and C serologies in at risk patients, CBC, creatinine	Infections, abdominal pain, mucocutaneous reactions	CBC every 2–4 months	Discontinue during infections; may increase risk of progressive multifocal leukoencephalopathy
Tocilizumab	Infections	Screen for latent tuberculosis, CBC AST/ALT, lipid panel	Infections, abdominal pain, symptoms of demyelinating disease	CBC and AST/ALT every 1–2 months, lipid panel at 1–2 months and then every 6 months	Discontinue during infections

Modified from O'Dell. Therapeutic Strategies for Rheumatoid Arthritis. *N Engl J Med* 2004;350(2):591–602.

BIOLOGIC DMARDs

Biologic DMARDs represent a relatively new class of agents designed to inhibit the inflammatory process by selectively targeting cytokines and other cellular ligands. There are currently nine biologic DMARDs approved in the treatment of RA. Similar to synthetic DMARDs, the ACR has issued recommendations for the use of biologic DMARDs including etanercept, infliximab, adalimumab, anakinra, abatacept, and rituximab (8). Biologic agents are typically employed as second-line therapy and are often used in conjunction with a synthetic DMARD, particularly methotrexate. Use of multiple biologics concurrently is not recommended due to higher rates of adverse events, particularly serious infection and lack of additive effect. Increased risk of serious infections is a concern with the use of biologic DMARDs, and screening for latent tuberculosis prior to initiation of treatment is recommended. The biologic DMARDs should be administered under the direction of a rheumatologist.

TREATMENT OF SJÖGREN'S SYNDROME

Treatment of Sjögren's syndrome is geared toward symptomatic relief and prevention of disease complications. Treatments for xerostomia and xerophthalmia include topical agents (artificial saliva and tears) and muscarinic agonists. Good oral hygiene and regular dental care are paramount to prevent tooth loss. Systemic involvement and refractory cases may require immunosuppressive therapies. Arthralgias and myalgias may respond well to NSAIDs and/or hydroxychloroquine. Visceral involvement may require corticosteroids which should be used cautiously as steroids may accelerate periodontal disease and oral candidiasis in Sjögren's patients. In cases of life threatening visceral involvement, mycophenolate mofetil, azathioprine, or cyclophosphamide therapy may be required. Investigations into the possible role of biologic agents (rituximab, abatacept) in treating Sjögren's are ongoing.

Clinical Course

NATURAL HISTORY

The natural history of RA, if not optimally managed, includes progressive joint inflammation, bony erosion, and deformity with resultant functional disability as well as increased mortality. In the period from the 1950s to the 1980s, RA was thought to have a "good" overall prognosis with symptomatic use of aspirin and NSAIDs. By the mid-1980s, clinicians began to recognize that patients with longer duration of RA symptoms had much worse outcomes and called for therapies and strategies to gain improved long-term disease control. The early, aggressive use of DMARDs and biologic agents has led to much tighter control of RA disease activity and in the developed world in particular, RA outcomes have improved significantly since the mid-1980s (9).

LONG TERM OUTCOMES

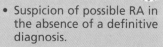

WHEN TO REFER

- Suspicion of possible RA in the absence of a definitive diagnosis.
- Known RA with questions regarding optimal treatment.

Outcomes for RA patients have been improving in the past few decades. A recent article comparing similar cohorts of RA patients receiving standard care from 1985 and 2000, respectively, found patients in 2000 had significant improvements in number of swollen joints as well as in measures of physical functioning and disease activity scores. The cohort from 2000 also demonstrated improvement in objective findings, including both laboratory and radiographic scores. Compared to the older cohort, more contemporary patients are also far more likely to be on DMARD therapy (66% vs. 13%) and methotrexate in particular (76% vs. 10%) (10).

Once the diagnosis of RA has been established and appropriate care is initiated, patients typically have improved outcomes compared to years past. While only a minority of RA patients is followed in published studies, outcomes in terms of radiographic change, joint replacement, work disability, and overall clinical and functional status appear to be improving.

ICD9

716.9 **Arthritis, arthritic** *(acute) (chronic) (subacute)•*
  crystals (see also Gout)
    275.49 [712.1] dicalcium phosphate•
    275.49 [712.2] pyrophosphate•
    275.49 [712.8] specified NEC•
  079.99 [711.5] due to or associated with viral disease NEC•
  274.00 gouty
    274.01 acute
  714.30 juvenile rheumatoid (chronic) (polyarticular)
    714.31 acute
    714.33 monoarticular
    714.32 pauciarticular
  714.4 postrheumatic, chronic (Jaccoud's)
  696.0 psoriatic
  714.0 rheumatic
    acute or subacute – see Fever, rheumatic
    714.0 chronic
    720.9 spine
  714.0 rheumatoid (nodular)
    714.1 with splenoadenomegaly and leukopenia
    714.2 visceral or systemic involvement
    714.30 juvenile (chronic) (polyarticular)
    714.31 acute
    714.33 monoarticular
    714.32 pauciarticular
716.9 **Arthropathy**
  136.1 [711.2]Behçet's •
    714.4 postrheumatic, chronic (Jaccoud's)
729.0 **Fibrositis** *(periarticular) (rheumatoid)*
274.9 **Gout,** *gouty*
  274.00 arthritis
  274.01 acute
  274.00 arthropathy
  274.01 acute
  274.02 chronic (without mention of tophus (tophi))
    274.03 with tophus (tophi)
  274.03 tophi
  274.81 ear
  274.82 specified site NEC
710.0 **Lupus**
  695.4 erythematosus (discoid) (local)
    710.0 disseminated
    710.0 systemic
719.3 **Palindromic, arthritis•**
725 **Polymyalgia**
  725 rheumatica

References

1. Gabriel SE, Crowson CS, O'Fallon WM. The epidemiology of rheumatoid arthritis in Rochester, Minnesota, 1955–1985. *Arthritis Rheum.* 1999;42(3):415–420.

2. Walitt B, Pettinger M, Weinstein A, et al. Effects of postmenopausal hormone therapy on rheumatoid arthritis: the women's health initiative randomized controlled trials. *Arthritis Rheum.* 2008;59(3):302–310.

3. Turesson C, O'Fallon WM, Crowson CS, et al. Extra-articular disease manifestations in rheumatoid arthritis: incidence trends and risk factors over 46 years. *Ann Rheum Dis.* 2003;62(8):722–727.

4. Theander E, Jacobsson LT. Relationship of Sjogren's syndrome to other connective tissue and autoimmune disorders. *Rheum Dis Clin North Am.* 2008;34(4):935–47, viii–ix. http://www.ncbi.nlm.nih.gov/entrez/query.fcgi?cmd=Retrieve&db=PubMed&dopt=Citation&list_uids=18984413.

5. O'Dell JR. Therapeutic strategies for rheumatoid arthritis. *N Engl J Med.* 2004;350(25):2591–2602. http://www.ncbi.nlm.nih.gov/entrez/query.fcgi?cmd=Retrieve&db=PubMed&dopt=Citation&list_uids=15201416.

6. Wolfe F, Caplan L, Michaud K. Treatment for rheumatoid arthritis and the risk of hospitalization for pneumonia: associations with prednisone, disease-modifying antirheumatic drugs, and anti-tumor necrosis factor therapy. *Arthritis Rheum.* 2006;54(2):628–634. http://www.ncbi.nlm.nih.gov/entrez/query.fcgi?cmd=Retrieve&db=PubMed&dopt=Citation&list_uids=16447241.

7. Choi HK, Hernan MA, Seeger JD, et al. Methotrexate and mortality in patients with rheumatoid arthritis: a prospective study. *Lancet.* 2002;359(9313):1173–1177. http://www.ncbi.nlm.nih.gov/entrez/query.fcgi?cmd=Retrieve&db=PubMed&dopt=Citation&list_uids=11955534.

8. Saag KG, Teng GG, Patkar NM, et al. American College of Rheumatology 2008 recommendations for the use of nonbiologic and biologic disease-modifying antirheumatic drugs in rheumatoid arthritis. *Arthritis Rheum.* 2008;59(6):762–784. http://www.ncbi.nlm.nih.gov/entrez/query.fcgi?cmd=Retrieve&db=PubMed&dopt=Citation&list_uids=18512708.

9. Sokka T. Long-term outcomes of rheumatoid arthritis. *Curr Opin Rheumatol.* 2009;21(3):284–290. http://www.ncbi.nlm.nih.gov/entrez/query.fcgi?cmd=Retrieve&db=PubMed&dopt=Citation&list_uids=19342954.

10. Pincus T, Sokka T, Kautiainen H. Patients seen for standard rheumatoid arthritis care have significantly better articular, radiographic, laboratory, and functional status in 2000 than in 1985. *Arthritis Rheum.* 2005;52(4):1009–1019. http://www.ncbi.nlm.nih.gov/entrez/query.fcgi?cmd=Retrieve&db=PubMed&dopt=Citation&list_uids=15818706.

10 The Seronegative Spondyloarthropathies

Dennis W. Boulware

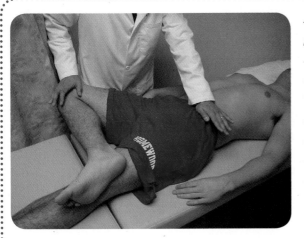

A 22-year-old man presents with a 3-month history of low back stiffness when he first arises in the morning. He finds that changing his exercise habits and going to the gym early in the morning helps reduce the duration of stiffness. His father and paternal grandfather have experienced a lifetime of back problems with fixed stooped postures and he is concerned he will have a similar outcome.

Clinical Presentation

For many years the seronegative spondyloarthropathies were confused understandably with rheumatoid arthritis due to common features of significant morning gel and inflammatory peripheral arthritis. This led to confusion in terminology with names such as rheumatoid spondylitis, rheumatoid variants, and so on. With better understanding of the histocompatibility genes, though, they are known now to be a clinically and etiologically distinct cluster of diseases with shared common features and clinical characteristics that distinguish them from each other. This chapter discusses the four main types of seronegative spondyloarthropathies: ankylosing spondylitis, reactive arthritis or Reiter's disease, psoriatic arthritis, and enteropathic arthritis associated with inflammatory bowel disease (IBD). As a group, they are rheumatoid factor negative, hence the name seronegative, and have radiographic and/or clinical sacroiliitis, typical vertebral abnormalities, inflammatory peripheral arthritis, enthesopathy, uveal tract involvement, familial clustering, and the frequent presence of human leukocyte antigen B27 (HLA-B27).

All of these conditions are a form of an inflammatory arthritis and significant morning gel phenomenon is expected during times of active inflammation. Stiffness requiring over an hour to resolve after prolonged periods of inactivity, such as immediately after awakening in the morning, is a common feature and the duration required for resolution often correlates with the severity of the condition. Morning gel or morning stiffness is a common feature with all inflammatory arthritides and likely led to the early confusion with rheumatoid arthritis. Similarly, activity helps to improve the sensation of stiffness and patients with any inflammatory arthritis will report improvement with activity as opposed to worsening with activity, as is common in mechanical disorders and osteoarthritis. The pattern of peripheral joint

CLINICAL POINTS

- More common in men than women.
- Onset usually in early adulthood.
- As an inflammatory arthritis, morning gel usually lasts several hours.
- Sacroiliitis usually causes buttock pain and stiffness.
- The extra-articular features (skin, mucous membranes, eyes, and bowel) help identify the specific diagnosis.

involvement in the seronegative spondyloarthropathies is asymmetric and oligoarticular, or may have no peripheral joint involvement with only axial involvement as often happens in ankylosing spondylitis, unlike the symmetrical distal small joint involvement seen in rheumatoid arthritis.

A seronegative spondyloarthropathy should be considered in a person with significant morning gel phenomenon of over an hour in duration, who does not have symmetrical small joint polyarthritis, but may have low back pain or asymmetric oligoarthritis, especially with inflammatory hip or shoulder involvement. Enthesopathies such as tendinitis or bursitis are common in all the seronegative spondyloarthropathies. At this point, nonarticular features can help make the correct diagnosis. In ankylosing spondylitis and reactive arthritis, the male-to-female ratio is strongly male dominant, hence female sex makes those conditions possible, but statistically less likely. The presence of certain extra-articular manifestations can assist the clinician in narrowing the differential diagnosis and lead to the correct diagnosis. Skin lesions that are papulosquamous in morphology, well demarcated, erythematous, and scaly suggestive of psoriasis will make psoriatic arthritis the most likely diagnosis, although it can reflect keratoderma blenorrhagicum seen in reactive arthritis. Mucous membrane lesions that may be painless such as urethritis and oral ulcers make reactive arthritis most likely, but can be seen in ankylosing spondylitis and enteropathic arthritis. Mucosal ulcers seen in the rectum or colon strongly suggest an enteropathic arthritis, but are also seen in reactive arthritis and ankylosing spondylitis. The overlap in clinical presentation of these diseases reflects that these conditions represent a spectrum of diseases that differ phenotypically, but have a common, albeit complex, genotypic pathogenic basis. When the clinician suspects the diagnosis of one of the seronegative spondyloarthropathies, closer examination of the extra-articular features will be more fruitful in identifying the specific disease.

Ankylosing Spondylitis

The classic patient with ankylosing spondylitis will be a male with an onset in his late teens or early twenties with morning stiffness, low back pain, and radiographic bilateral sacroiliitis. The duration of stiffness will be over an hour and usually 3 to 4 hours, varying directly with the severity of the disease. Physical activity will improve his stiffness and back pain unlike the pain and stiffness from a mechanical back disorder or osteoarthritis that worsens with activity. Nonsteroidal anti-inflammatory drugs, even over-the-counter products will provide relief although it may be incomplete relief of pain and stiffness.

Pain and stiffness reflect the inflammatory nature of the condition and an onset of pain or stiffness after the age of 40 years is very unusual. While the disease is more common in men, women are not immune from developing ankylosing spondylitis and often have less back symptoms and more peripheral asymmetric oligoarthritis. The pain from sacroiliitis is commonly reported as low back pain by the patient, but may be felt as buttock or gluteal pain, or pain in the anterior and/or lateral thighs. Extra-articular features are less common in ankylosing spondylitis than the other seronegative spondyloarthropathies, but do occur in a minority of patients. Iritis or anterior uveitis, occurring in up to 20% patients, is one of the more common extra-articular features often predating the development of the musculoskeletal manifestation. Oral mucosal ulcerations and shallow rectal or colonic ulcerations can be seen less frequently than iritis and uveitis. Finally, an IgA nephritis and leukocytoclastic cutaneous vasculitis resembling Henoch–Schönlein purpura has been reported.

Reactive Arthritis

Although commonly associated with Reiter's syndrome and the classic triad of arthritis, urethritis, and uveitis, reactive arthritis includes many more extra-articular manifestations than the classic triad, especially involving the skin and the mucosal membranes. The arthritis is usually an acute, additive, and asymmetric one with enthesitis and/or axial arthritis commonly seen and combined with keratoderma blenorrhagicum, diarrhea, cervicitis, urethritis, conjunctivitis, painless oral ulcers, and/or circinate balanitis. Identifying a prior recent infectious event is not always possible, but reactive arthritis is known to occur after dysenteric type illness or genitourinary infections. Typically, reactive arthritis follows the infection within 1 to 4 weeks, with fever being common and arthritis being the last clinical feature to present. Reactive arthritis is the most common musculoskeletal condition seen in active HIV infection and HIV should be considered in any new diagnosis of reactive arthritis, or worsening reactive arthritis. Finally, reactive arthritis is reported to occur after treatment of infections or immunization.

Psoriatic Arthritis

Psoriasis is a chronic autoimmune skin condition that has a higher prevalence of a coexisting chronic inflammatory arthritis than is seen in the general population. The skin disease usually predates the onset of arthritis, although the converse relationship is seen and the concurrent onset of psoriasis and arthritis is the least common mode of presentation. The pattern of joint involvement is variable but typically follows five different patterns: symmetric polyarthritis, distal interphalangeal joint involvement, oligoarthritis, arthritis mutilans, and axial involvement.

Enteropathic Arthritis Associated with Inflammatory Bowel Disease

The inclusion of IBD in this group of diseases emphasizes the relationship between gut inflammation and joint inflammation. Other gastrointestinal conditions, such as celiac disease, and intestinal bypass surgery are occasionally accompanied by joint inflammation, but these are not considered as spondyloarthropathies. Crohn's disease and ulcerative colitis are discussed together since the musculoskeletal and gastrointestinal features cannot be easily differentiated. Musculoskeletal issues are the most common extraintestinal manifestations of IBD and appear in 2% to 20% of patients with either ulcerative colitis or Crohn's disease, with peripheral arthritis seen more frequently in patients with colonic involvement and more extensive bowel disease. The frequency of peripheral arthritis in IBD ranges up to 20% of patients, with a higher prevalence in Crohn's disease. In both Crohn's disease and ulcerative colitis, the arthritis generally is pauciarticular, asymmetric, frequently transient or migratory, and typically nondestructive with common recurrences. Infrequently, the peripheral arthritis becomes chronic and destructive. Enthesopathies can cause sausage digit deformities, Achilles tendinitis, and plantar fasciitis. Axial involvement involving the sacroiliac joints or spine occurs in both diseases with prevalence rates of 10% to 20% for sacroiliitis and 7% to 12% for spondylitis reported, although the actual figures are probably higher because of the existence of subclinical axial involvement.

In most cases of Crohn's disease, intestinal symptoms antedate or coincide with the joint manifestations, with the articular symptoms preceding the intestinal symptoms by years. In ulcerative colitis, there is a more distinct temporal relationship between attacks of arthritis and flares of bowel disease.

Extraintestinal and extra-articular manifestations are similar to those seen in IBD, including erythema nodosum, pyoderma gangrenosum, anterior uveitis, episcleritis, and aphthous oral ulcers.

Examination

Physical examination of the affected painful or dysfunctional peripheral joints should assess the presence of inflammatory synovitis, which is the hallmark of an inflammatory arthropathy. These findings include soft tissue swelling that could mask palpation of bony landmarks in mild cases to impeding full passive range of motion and cause visible bulging in severe cases. Examination must include axial joints including the sacroiliac joints and spine.

There are several methods for examination of the sacroiliac joints, none of which are very sensitive or specific when done alone. The sacroiliac joints lie inferior to the posterior superior iliac spine, and direct palpation of this area (Fig. 10.1) usually detects gluteal muscle tenderness as opposed to sacroiliac joint tenderness, since the joint lies deep beneath the gluteal muscles and traverses obliquely from the surface making palpation of the joint directly impossible. Indirect compression of the sacroiliac joint can be done by several methods. With the patient supine, compression and loading of the anterior superior iliac spines with the examiner's upper body weight will compress the sacroiliac joint with tenderness felt in the sacral area (Fig. 10.2). The patient can also be positioned on their side with compression and loading of the iliac crest with the examiner's upper body weight; with sacroiliitis, tenderness may be felt in the sacral area (Fig. 10.3). Gaenslen's test is another test for sacroiliitis where one hip joint is flexed maximally on one side and the contralateral hip joint is extended. Gaenslen's test can be done with the patient supine, passively flexing one hip by approximating the knee to the patient's chest and allowing the other leg to fall over the side of an examination table, causing that hip to hyperextend. The test can also be performed with the patient in the lateral recumbent position with both hips flexed and with both knees approximating the chest, then taking the upper leg into full extension of that the knee and hip while hyperextending the hip (Fig. 10.4). The patient's position can be reversed and the other leg tested. The presence of sacroiliitis may cause the patient to experience tenderness

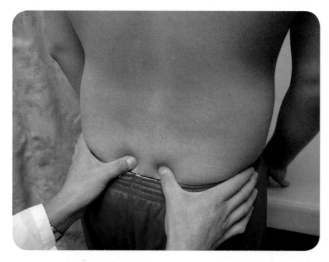

Figure 10.1 Examiner attempting to palpate directly the sacroiliac joints, which lie inferior to the posterior superior iliac spines. The sacral dimples mark the posterior superior iliac spine, which is the superior end of the sacroiliac joint.

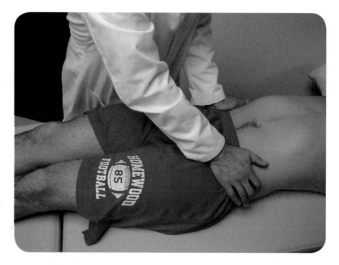

Figure 10.2 Testing for sacroiliitis by anterior loading of pelvis, with weight on the anterior superior iliac spines of the pelvis.

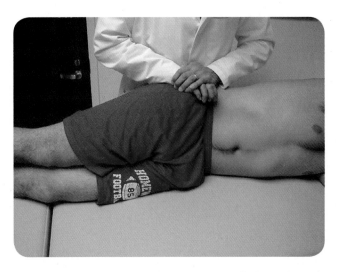

Figure 10.3 Testing for sacroiliitis by lateral loading of pelvis, with weight on the iliac wings of the pelvis.

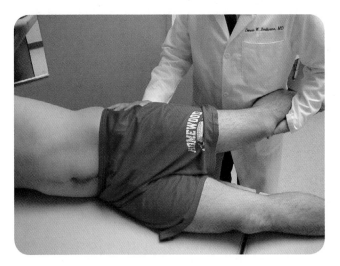

Figure 10.4 Testing for sacroiliitis using Gaenslen's maneuver placing leg in hypertension and loading the pelvis by torque.

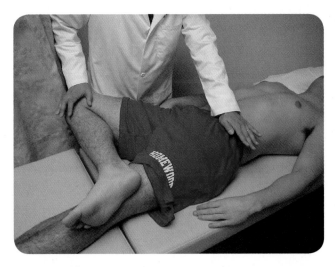

Figure 10.5 Testing for sacroiliitis using Patrick's test and loading the pelvis by torque.

in the sacral area. Finally, Patrick's maneuver can be done by placing the patient in a supine position and flexing one knee and hip to 90 degrees, then placing the flexed leg's foot on the contralateral knee. The flexed leg should be relaxed and using one hand on the flexed knee and the other hand on the contralateral anterior superior iliac spine to stabilize the pelvis, the examiner will push the flexed knee toward the examination table (Fig. 10.5). Both legs can be tested as the maneuver compresses one sacroiliac joint while distracting the other side. Sacroiliitis can cause discomfort felt in the sacral area during the test. Obviously, the patient must have stable hips as the maneuver places great stress on the ipsilateral hip joint. None of these tests individually is reliable and the clinician should pursue imaging studies if sacroiliitis is suspected or a concern.

Spinal involvement typically starts in the lumbar region and ascends up the spine. Loss of lumbar flexion is an early event and can be detected by use of the modified Schöber's test (Fig. 10.6A, B). With the patient standing erect, the clinician will place one mark between the posterior superior iliac spines and use a tape measure, placing the 0 end 10 cm above the original mark. The clinician will hold the 0 end of the tape measure in place and ask the patient to bend forward attempting to touch their toes and fully flexing the lumbar spine. The clinician will measure the distance of displacement when the lumbar spine is fully flexed from the 0 end of the tape measure to the original mark between the posterior superior iliac spines. A normal lumbar spine will increase the distance from 10 to at least 15 cm. Examination of the thoracic and cervical spine should also be performed with particular emphasis for limited motion in chest excursion by measuring chest circumference between full inspiration and expiration. Flexion contractures of the cervical spine can be detected by measuring the cervical fleche or distance from the occiput to the wall when the patient stands with their back to the wall with their heels, knees, buttock, and shoulders pressed against the wall. A normal cervical fleche is 0 cm.

An examination for extra-articular manifestations, particularly of the skin and mucous membranes is essential. The peripheral and axial articular involvement will not differentiate between the seronegative spondyloarthropathies and only the presence or absence of the extra-articular features will help in identifying the correct diagnosis.

Studies

The laboratory is of little help in evaluating the patient with a suspected seronegative spondyloarthropathy except to confirm the presence of systemic

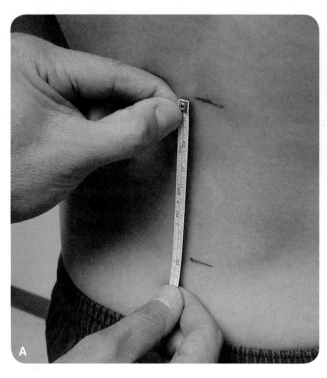 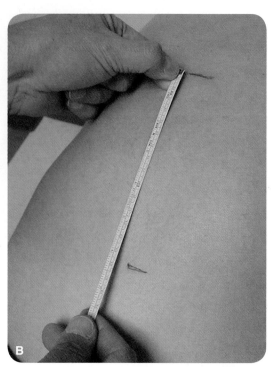

Figure 10.6 A. Start of the modified Schöber's test measuring 10 cm above the midline between the sacral dimples or posterior superior iliac spine with the patient erect. **B.** End of the modified Schöber's test measuring the additional distance above the midline between the sacral dimples or posterior superior iliac spine with the patient maximally flexed attempting to touch their toes.

inflammation through an abnormal C-reactive protein or erythrocyte sedimentation rate. The use of HLA-B27 is debatable as it is not always found in the seronegative spondyloarthropathies and can be found in certain populations without an inflammatory arthropathy. Since low back pain is a very common ailment, the presence of HLA-B27 can result in erroneous diagnoses of a seronegative spondyloarthropathy.

Imaging studies can be helpful in several of the seronegative spondyloarthropathies. In suspected sacroiliitis, plain x-ray will identify sacroiliitis or spondylitis with more precision than physical examination. In ankylosing spondylitis, the sacroiliac involvement is bilateral and starts early with erosions along the sacroiliac joint, followed later by sclerosis and eventual fusion. In psoriatic arthritis, reactive arthritis, and enteropathic arthritis, the sacroiliac involvement can be unilateral and involve more exuberant sclerosis than seen in ankylosing spondylitis. When there is spinal involvement, syndesmophytes will be seen and tend to be more exuberant and proliferative in psoriatic arthritis and reactive arthritis as opposed to ankylosing spondylitis. Early syndesmophytes commonly occur in the thoracolumbar area and are best viewed on lateral views as calcification of the annulus fibrosis or anterior longitudinal ligament shows first on this view.

Radiographic appearance of peripheral joints is similar to that of rheumatoid arthritis except in the case of psoriatic arthritis, which causes an erosive pattern that creates a pencil-in-cup appearance of the joint. In these cases, the proximal component of the joint is whittled to a point and the distal convex surface broadens to take on the appearance of a cup.

Treatment

The major aims of management include patient education regarding the natural history of the condition, reasonable reassurance of the patient's expectations, the

NOT TO BE MISSED

- Psoriasis
- Enthesitis
- Keratoderma blenorrhagicum
- Circinate balanitis
- Uveitis or anterior iritis
- Mucous membrane involvement with oral ulcers, rectal ulcers, and so on
- Inflammatory bowel disease, both ulcerative colitis and Crohn's disease

use of anti-inflammatory medications, physical therapy and lifestyle modifications aimed at retarding spinal and joint deformities, and the appropriate use of disease modifying anti-rheumatic drugs for destructive peripheral arthropathies.

Nonsteroidal anti-inflammatory drugs (NSAIDs) are effective for the pain and stiffness associated in axial and peripheral joint involvement, but should be used judiciously with appropriate caution for gastrointestinal ulceration and renal insufficiency. Anecdotally, use of NSAIDs can exacerbate psoriasis and IBD.

Use of disease modifying anti-rheumatic drugs are indicated when there is evidence of destructive peripheral disease or axial disease refractory to NSAIDs alone. Referral to a rheumatologist is advisable at this point.

Despite the relationship of infections preceding reactive arthritis, there are no conclusive studies that the use of antibiotics is of any significant value.

Clinical Course

The clinical course for the seronegative spondyloarthropathies varies considerably for each condition and within each condition. In ankylosing spondylitis, sacroiliitis is seen in virtually all cases, but peripheral arthritis is less common. Ankylosing spondylitis is more common in young men who have typical low back pain and stiffness, but when it occurs in women and children, they can have an atypical presentation with more peripheral arthritis, enthesitis, and cervical involvement. The prognosis in ankylosing spondylitis is good in most patients where only 10% become significantly disabled and 90% are able to pursue full-time employment. A predictable pattern of disease usually emerges after the first 10 years with destructive hip involvement being an indicator of a poor functional outcome.

In reactive arthritis, the prognosis and course of individual patients with Reiter syndrome are varied and unpredictable, regardless of whether they present with the classic triad, ACR criteria, or incomplete Reiter syndrome. Most patients demonstrate an initial episode of acute arthritis with a mean duration of 2 to 3 months, but which may last up to a year. Some patients develop recurrent attacks with disease-free intervals. A minority of patients demonstrates a chronic course of peripheral arthritis and they have a greater potential for progressive spondylitis. Predicting which patients will develop recurrent attacks or chronic reactive arthritis is difficult and inexact. Factors that may predict a poorer or more chronic outcome include hip arthritis, ESR >30 mm/hour, poor response to NSAIDs, lumbar spine involvement, sausage digits, and/or an onset before 16 years of age. Yet despite the potential for chronic disease, studies have shown that patients with reactive arthritis typically maintain a higher level of continued employment than individuals with other inflammatory arthritides. Severe disability is uncommon and is frequently secondary to aggressive, destructive lower-extremity involvement, aggressive axial involvement, or blindness.

In psoriatic arthritis, there can be several patterns of joint involvement, with the polyarticular pattern resembling rheumatoid arthritis, the most common form. The polyarticular pattern responds well to disease modifying anti-rheumatic drugs and clinically has a good outcome allowing full functioning and continued employment. More aggressive disease responds well to more aggressive disease modifying anti-rheumatic drugs such as methotrexate and the TNF inhibitors that are used for treating psoriasis as well.

In both psoriatic arthritis and enteropathic arthritis associated with IBD, aggressive treatment of the psoriasis and IBD is highly recommended, as in some cases the severity of the arthritis parallels the severity of the skin or bowel disease.

WHEN TO REFER

- When in doubt of the exact diagnosis.
- When the peripheral arthritis is deforming, erosive, and/or destructive.
- When disease modifying anti-rheumatic drugs are needed.

SECTION 3 Specific Rheumatic Diseases

ICD9

716.9 **Arthritis, arthritic** *(acute) (chronic) (subacute)*
   569.9 [713.1] due to or associated with gastrointestinal condition NEC
      099.3 [711.1] Reiter's disease/Reactive arthritis
      696.0 psoriatic
720.9 **Spondylitis**
   720.0 ankylosing (chronic)

Additional Reading

1. Davis JC. Ankylosing spondylitis. In Koopman WJ, Moreland LW, eds. *Arthritis and Allied Conditions.* 15th ed. Philadelphia: Lippincott Williams and Wilkins, 2005;1319–1334.
2. Khan MA, Sieper J. Reactive arthritis. In Koopman WJ, Moreland LW, eds. *Arthritis and Allied Conditions.* 15th ed. Philadelphia: Lippincott Williams and Wilkins, 2005;1335–1356.
3. Bennett RM. Psoriatic arthritis. In Koopman WJ, Moreland LW, eds. *Arthritis and Allied Conditions.* 15th ed. Philadelphia: Lippincott Williams and Wilkins, 2005;1357–1374.
4. Mielants H, Baeten D, De Keyser F, Veys EM. Enteropathic arthritis. In Koopman WJ, Moreland LW, eds. *Arthritis and Allied Conditions.* 15th ed. Philadelphia: Lippincott Williams and Wilkins, 2005;1375–1400.
5. Boulware DW, Arnett FC, Cush JJ, Lipsky PE, Bennett RM, Mielants H, De Keyser F, Veys EM. The seronegative spondyloarthropathies. In Koopman WJ, Boulware DW, Heudebert GR, eds. *Clinical Primer of Rheumatology.* Philadelphia: Lippincott Williams and Wilkins, 2003;127–163.

CHAPTER 11

Systemic Lupus Erythematosus

Michelle A. Petri

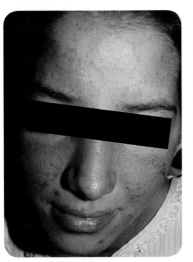

A 23-year-old Caucasian woman presents to her primary care doctor with complaints of 9 months of fatigue, pain in muscles including the neck and shoulder area, and red cheeks after sun exposure, lasting for an hour or so. On the physical examination, the cheeks have several pustules. Laboratory data are ordered and show a positive ANA 1:80 (homogeneous pattern), normal complete blood count, normal chemistries, and normal urinalysis. Does she have systemic lupus erythematosus?

Clinical Presentation

EPIDEMIOLOGY

Systemic lupus erythematosus (SLE) is a multisystem autoimmune disease. It occurs predominantly in women, but 10% of patients are men. The onset is predominantly in the 20s and 30s, but it can present in older patients (it is rare before puberty). It is both more common and more severe in African–Americans and Hispanic–Americans than in Caucasians. It is estimated that about 300,000 Americans have SLE.

PATHOGENESIS

Lupus autoantibodies are present for 5 to 7 years before the clinical onset of SLE occurs. There is a polygenic genetic predisposition, with as many as 100 genes, many affecting inflammatory pathways, such as HLA DR and DQ alleles, interferon, interleukin-6, and the glucocorticoid receptor pathway. Female hormones are another factor in pathogenesis. Men with SLE tend to be hypoandrogenic. Abnormal responses to common viruses, such as Epstein Barr virus, may play an inciting role (1). Environmental precipitants include ultraviolet light, trimethoprim/sulfa, infections, silica, and mercury.

ORGAN MANIFESTATIONS

Because SLE is a multisystem disease, multiple presentations are possible. The most common organs involved at presentation are cutaneous and musculoskeletal.

Cutaneous Lupus

In SLE, there can be acute, subacute, and chronic subtypes of cutaneous lupus. Acute cutaneous lupus is a photosensitive maculopapular inflammatory rash. Classically it is called a "malar rash" if on the bridge of the nose and cheeks, but it can also be on the "V" area of the chest or on the forearms. It is usually raised and lasts for days to months. It must be differentiated from flushes/ blushes, acne rosacea (with pustules), seborrhea, solar urticaria (with pruritus), and polymorphous light eruption. In the case presentation, there were pustules and a history of transient rash: both would argue against lupus.

Subacute cutaneous lupus erythematosus (SCLE) can occur in an annular form (that may be mistaken for a fungal rash or Lyme disease) or a psoriaform rash. SCLE can occur without SLE, and in many cases is caused or aggravated by commonly used medications, including hydrochlorothiazide, terbinafine, statins, calcium-channel blockers, ACE-inhibitors, interferon alpha and beta, and TNF inhibitors (2).

The most common chronic cutaneous lupus is discoid lupus. It can occur without SLE. Only about 5% of patients with discoid lupus progress to SLE. Discoid lupus is a scarring rash, usually on the scalp, ears, face, and arms. It can be disfiguring, leading to scarring alopecia, and hypo- and hyperpigmentation.

SLE can also cause cutaneous vasculitis, presenting as palpable purpura or digital gangrene, but this is rare.

MUSCULOSKELETAL LUPUS

The majority of SLE patients will have inflammatory arthralgias, meaning joint pain with morning stiffness, in the distribution of the small joints of the hands (PIPs and MCPs) and wrists, and, less commonly, large joints. There can be true synovitis of these joints. Erosions are unusual. Instead, SLE patients can develop Jaccoud's arthropathy, with reducible joint deformation due to tendon and ligament laxity. Myositis can occur in SLE, but it is rare. When a patient with SLE has muscle pain, the usual cause is fibromyalgia.

LUPUS NEPHRITIS

Lupus nephritis presents as proteinuria, hematuria, and sometimes red blood cell casts. It is subdivided into mesangial, mesangial proliferative, focal, diffuse proliferative, membranous, and end-stage sclerosis. A renal biopsy is necessary to determine the International Society of Nephrology (ISN) class, which leads to important information on prognosis and treatment. Diffuse proliferative glomerulonephritis (Class IV) is the most likely class to lead to renal failure.

HEMATOLOGIC LUPUS

SLE can affect all cell lines. The most common finding is leukopenia and lymphopenia. Prednisone can cause or worsen lymphopenia. Usually cytopenias from lupus are mild and do not require treatment. Autoimmune hemolytic anemia is usually Coombs positive. The most frequent anemias found in SLE patients, however, are iron-deficiency anemia and the anemia of chronic disease (also called the anemia of chronic inflammation). Thrombocytopenia can occur due to SLE, as well as due to antiphospholipid antibodies.

SEROSITIS

SLE can cause pleurisy, pleural effusions, pericarditis, pericardial effusion, and rarely, ascites.

NEUROLOGIC LUPUS

SLE can lead to psychosis, seizures, stroke, coma, encephalopathy, cranial neuropathy, peripheral neuropathy, myelitis, and mononeuritis multiplex (3). The most common neurologic complaint, though, is cognitive impairment, that can occur in 80% patients, 10 years after diagnosis (4).

CONSTITUTIONAL

Active SLE can lead to fever, weight loss, lymphadenopathy, and splenomegaly. Although fatigue can be part of an acute SLE flare, most chronic fatigue in SLE is not associated with active lupus, but rather with fibromyalgia, deconditioning, depression, hypothyroidism, anemia, and other comorbidity.

Examination

SKIN

Acute cutaneous lupus is an erythematosus maculopapular rash on the face, "V" area of the chest, and forearms (i.e., sun exposed areas). Discoid lupus (a deeper rash that can cause scarring) can be found on the scalp, just above the eyebrows, in the ears, and on the palate.

Oral ulcers can be found on the buccal mucosa and the tongue. They can be painful or painless. Nasal ulcers can also occur.

The hair in lupus is both thin and fragile. It tends to break off around the frame of the face (lupus "frizzies"). Circumscribed areas of total hair loss are more likely due to discoid lupus (causing scarring alopecia) or alopecia areata.

SLE patients can have livedo reticularis, a violaceous mottling of the extremities. This can also occur from antiphospholipid antibodies.

HEAD

SLE patients with secondary Sjögren's may have parotid enlargement or eye or mouth dryness.

NECK

SLE can cause cervical lymphadenopathy, usually small in size. Thyroid enlargement can occur from autoimmune thyroid disease.

CHEST

SLE can cause restrictive lung disease. This can lead to basilar crackles. Lupus pleurisy may cause a pleural rub or pleural effusion.

HEART

Pericarditis can cause a pericardial rub or distant heart sounds, if there is large pericardial effusion. Pulmonary hypertension can cause an accentuated P2. Active lupus causes tachycardia. Heart murmurs are very common in SLE.

ABDOMEN

Abdominal serositis can cause ascites. Budd-Chiari (from antiphospholipid antibodies) also causes ascites. SLE can cause hepatosplenomegaly.

EXTREMITIES

Pedal edema can be a sign of lupus nephritis or pulmonary hypertension. Raynaud's phenomenon is common in SLE.

MUSCULOSKELETAL

Lupus can cause tenderness or true swelling of the PIPs, MCPs, wrists, knees, and ankles (but not the DIP joints). Tenderness in muscles is usually fibromyalgia, not lupus myositis. A proximal myopathy can occur from corticosteroids.

Table 11.1 ACR Classification Criteria

Malar rash	Hematologic disorder
Discoid rash	Immunologic disorder:
Photosensitivity	Anti-dsDNA
Oral ulcers	Anti-Sm
Arthritis	Lupus anticoagulant
Serositis	Anticardiolipin
Renal disorder	False–positive test for syphilis
Neurologic disorder	Antinuclear antibody

NEUROLOGIC

SLE can cause cranial and peripheral neuropathy, and longitudinal myelitis. Antiphospholipid antibodies can cause stroke.

Studies

LABORATORY ASSESSMENT

The laboratory assessment to diagnose SLE includes the tests necessary to assess organ involvement (complete blood count with differential, serum creatinine, urinalysis, urine protein/creatinine ratio) but also a battery of serologic tests of lupus autoantibodies, including ANA, anti-dsDNA, anti-Ro, anti-La, anti-Smith, anti-RNP, direct Coombs, antiphospholipid antibodies (lupus anticoagulant and anticardiolipin), C3, and C4.

Diagnosis of SLE

The diagnosis of lupus is still an art. There are classification criteria for SLE, which can be helpful. The ACR Classification Criteria requires the presence of four of the eleven criteria to classify a patient as having SLE. Although not perfect, they do emphasize the multisystem nature of the disease. ANA is not sufficient to diagnose lupus – most people with a positive ANA are normal. A patient with ANA and muscle pain, for example, likely has fibromyalgia (not lupus) – as in the case presentation (Table 11.1).

Clinical Course

SLE is about equally divided into the "flare pattern", in which patients have exacerbations followed by improvement, and "chronic activity", in which there is always some activity. Remission, not requiring prednisone or immunosuppressive treatment, is very rare.

Survival in SLE has improved since the 1950s, but plateaued in the 1980s. Early in SLE, the major causes of death are active disease and infection, whereas, later in SLE, the major cause of death is cardiovascular disease (5).

Treatment

GENERAL MEASURES

SLE patients should practice sun protection and use sunscreen as ultraviolet light increases SLE flares. Because of the high risk of cardiovascular disease, a low fat, low cholesterol diet is recommended.

SLE increases the risk of infection. Vaccinations for influenza yearly and pneumococcus every 5 years are recommended. Only inactivated vaccines

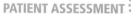

PATIENT ASSESSMENT

• A true photosensitive rash should be raised and should last for days to weeks after sun exposure.

• Fibromyalgia is much more common than lupus. Are fibromyalgia tender points present? Is there prolonged morning stiffness in the small joints of the hands and wrists to suggest inflammatory polyarthralgia?

should be used if the SLE patient is on prednisone and/or immunosuppressive drugs.

SLE increases the risk of malignancy. General guidelines should be followed in terms of PAP smears, mammograms, and colonoscopy.

SLE itself, but also sun avoidance, increases the risk of vitamin D deficiency. 25-hydroxyvitamin D levels should be checked, and replacement prescribed.

Osteopenia and osteoporosis are common, due to SLE itself, but especially due to corticosteroid use. DEXA scans are recommended every 2 years, especially in SLE patients on corticosteroids.

HYDROXYCHLOROQUINE

Hydroxychloroquine should be prescribed to all SLE patients. The dose is 400 mg (200 mg twice daily) in an average person, but the dose should not exceed 6.5 mg/kg, and should be reduced in renal insufficiency or renal failure. Hydroxychloroquine helps cutaneous lupus and lupus arthritis. It prevents 50% of SLE flares (6), helps to prevent renal and neurologic lupus, improves survival, and improves hyperlipidemia. The risk of retinopathy is one out of 5,000 after 5 years of use.

NSAIDs

NSAIDs are helpful for lupus arthritis and serositis. However, they should not be used in patients with lupus nephritis. Long-term use may increase the risk of cardiovascular disease. Ibuprofen may block the therapeutic effect of aspirin.

PREDNISONE/CORTICOSTEROIDS

Prednisone leads to 80% of permanent organ damage after the diagnosis of SLE (7). Its use should be minimized. A chronic need for prednisone should lead to a referral to a rheumatologist, who can consider the addition of steroid-sparing regimens. Mild/moderate lupus flares may be treated with a "burst" of steroids (medrol dosepack or one time intramuscular triamcinolone 100 mg) instead of chronic oral steroids. Severe flares may require "pulse" therapy with intravenous methylprednisolone 1000 mg for 3 days, followed by oral prednisone. The risk of osteonecrosis goes up dramatically with doses of oral prednisone of 20 mg or higher.

IMMUNOSUPPRESSIVE DRUGS

Methotrexate

Methotrexate is helpful for lupus arthritis and cutaneous lupus. Doses are usually between 7.5 and 25 mg weekly, with daily folic acid. Monitoring of the complete blood count and liver function tests is necessary. It cannot be used in pregnancy.

Leflunomide

Leflunomide is used for lupus arthritis and has shown benefit for lupus nephritis as well. Doses vary from 10 to 20 mg daily. Monitoring of the complete blood count and liver function tests is necessary. Mild hair loss can occur. It cannot be used in pregnancy.

Azathioprine

Azathioprine is an immunosuppressive drug with broad applicability in SLE. Doses of 1 mg to 2 mg/kg are usually used. Thiopurine methyltransferase (TPMT) testing is recommended to identify patients at greater risk of toxicity (cytopenias, liver function test elevation). It can be used in pregnancy when needed to control lupus activity.

Mycophenolate Mofetil

Mycophenolate mofetil has been widely studied in lupus nephritis (8, 9), where it is equivalent to cyclophosphamide in induction therapy (although superior in non-Caucasians) (10) and superior to azathioprine for maintenance therapy. Monitoring of complete blood count and liver function tests is needed. It cannot be used in pregnancy.

Cyclophosphamide

Cyclophosphamide was widely used for lupus nephritis, but with a high price in terms of toxicity (premature ovarian failure, infections, and later malignancy). Mycophenolate mofetil is now the first choice for lupus nephritis, with some possible exceptions (such as rapidly progressive glomerulonephritis). Cyclophosphamide is still used for refractory lupus nephritis and for CNS-lupus. It is usually given as an intravenous "pulse" monthly (750 mg/m^2 BSA) as an induction therapy for 6 months, and sometimes continued as a maintenance therapy quarterly for up to 2 more years.

High Dose Cyclophosphamide

High dose cyclophosphamide (200 mg/kg over 4 days) was not superior to the usual monthly intravenous cyclophosphamide regimen in a clinical trial (11). It is used as a salvage therapy for SLE patients failing all other therapies, with or without autologous stem cell transplantation (12).

BIOLOGICS

Rituximab

Rituximab, a monoclonal antibody directed against CD20 on B cells, was not superior to standard of care for nonrenal lupus or to mycophenolate mofetil for renal lupus. However, it has been effective in studies of patients with hematologic lupus, CNS-lupus, and catastrophic antiphospholipid antibody syndrome.

Belimumab

Belimumab is the first FDA-approved treatment for SLE in 50 years. It targets the B lymphocyte stimulator protein (BLyS), a growth factor for B cells. In Phase 3 clinical trials, it led to a 10% to 14% improvement over standard of care in the Systemic Lupus Responder Index, reduced flares, led to a greater reduction in prednisone (and less need for increased prednisone), reduced anti-dsDNA, and increased complement (13).

ANTIPHOSPHOLIPID ANTIBODIES

About 50% of SLE patients may have an antiphospholipid antibody (lupus anticoagulant, anticardiolipin, or anti-beta 2 glycoprotein I). These antibodies cause hypercoagulability and increase pregnancy loss. Prophylactic therapy with aspirin (81 mg) and hydroxychloroquine is recommended. Use of estrogen, SERMs, and thalidomide should be avoided, as they increase the risk of thrombosis. If an SLE patient with antiphospholipid antibodies has a thrombotic event, then anticoagulation (with a target INR of 2 to 3) is recommended lifelong (14).

SJÖGREN'S SYNDROME

Ten percent of SLE patients will develop Sjögren's syndrome. Only about half of patients with secondary Sjögren's will have Sjögren's autoantibodies (anti-Ro

WHEN TO REFER

- To confirm diagnosis
- Before instituting corticosteroids
- If the patient requires more than 7.5 mg of prednisone
- To evaluate proteinuria
- For a rash not responsive to hydroxychloroquine
- For CNS symptomatology
- For dyspnea

or anti-La). The diagnosis can be confirmed with the Schirmer's test or equivalent documentation. For eye dryness, Restasis (cyclosporine) eye drops are recommended. For eye and mouth dryness, Evoxac (cevimeline) 30 mg three times a day can be helpful.

CARDIOVASCULAR RISK FACTORS

Because the major late cause of death in SLE is cardiovascular disease, it is essential to control traditional cardiovascular risk factors. Lupus itself can increase hypertension and hyperlipidemia, due to lupus nephritis. Prednisone increases hypertension, hyperlipidemia, diabetes mellitus, and obesity (15).

ICD9

710.0 **Lupus**
   695.4 discoid (local)
   695.4 erythematodes (discoid) (local)
   695.4 erythematosus (discoid) (local)
    710.0 disseminated
    710.0 systemic
  710.0 [583.81] nephritis
    710.0 [580.81] acute
    710.0 [582.81] chronic
583.9 **Nephritis, nephritic** *(albuminuric) (azotemic) (congenital) (degenerative) (diffuse) (disseminated) (epithelial) (familial) (focal) (granulomatous) (hemorrhagic) (infantile) (nonsuppurative, excretory) (uremic)*
  710.0 [583.81] lupus
    710.0 [580.81] acute
    710.0 [582.81] chronic
  714.4 postrheumatic, chronic (Jaccoud's)

References

1. Harley JB, James JA. Epstein-Barr virus infection may be an environmental risk factor for systemic lupus erythematosus in children and teenagers [letter]. *Arthritis Rheum* 1999;42(8):1782–1783.
2. Callen JP. Drug-induced subacute cutaneous lupus erythematosus. *Lupus* 19(9):1107–1011.
3. Hanly JG, Urowitz MB, Su L, , et al. Prospective analysis of neuropsychiatric events in an international disease inception cohort of SLE patients. *Ann Rheum Dis* 2010;69(3):529–535.
4. Brey RL, Holliday SL, Saklad AR, et al. Neuropsychiatric syndromes in SLE: Prevalence using standardized definitions in the San Antonio Study of Neuropsychiatric Disease Cohort. *Neurology* 2002;58:1214–1220.
5. Urowitz MB, Gladman DD, Abu-Shakra M, et al. Mortality studies in systemic lupus erythematosus. Results from a single center. III. Improved survival over 24 years. *J Rheumatol* 1997;24(6):1061–1065.
6. Canadian Hydroxychloroquine Study Group. A randomized study of the effect of withdrawing hydroxychloroquine sulfate in systemic lupus erythematosus. *N Engl J Med.* 1991;324:150–154.
7. Gladman DD, Urowitz MB, Rahman P, et al. Accrual of organ damage over time in patients with systemic lupus erythematosus. *J Rheumatol* 2003;30(9):1955–1959.
8. Ginzler EM, Dooley MA, Aranow C, et al. Mycophenolate mofetil or intravenous cyclophosphamide for lupus nephritis. *N Engl J Med* 2005;353(21):2219–2228.
9. Contreras G, Pardo V, Leclercq B, et al. Sequential therapies for proliferative lupus nephritis. *N Engl J Med* 2004;350(10):971–980.
10. Appel GB, Contreras G, Dooley MA, et al. Mycophenolate mofetil versus cyclophosphamide for induction treatment of lupus nephritis. *J Am Soc Nephrol* 2009;20(5):1103–1112.
11. Petri M, Brodsky RA, Jones RJ, Gladstone D, Fillius M, Magder LS. High dose Cyclophosphamide versus Monthly Intravenous Cyclophosphamide for Systemic Lupus Erythematosus: A prospective Randomized Trial. *Arthritis Rheum* 2010;62:1487–1493.

12. Burt RK, Traynor A, Statkute L, et al. Nonmyeloablative hematopoietic stem cell transplantation for systemic lupus erythematosus. *J Amer Med Assoc* 2006;295:527–535.

13. Navarra SV, Guzmán RM, Gallacher AE, et al. Efficacy and safety of belimumab in patients with active systemic lupus erythematosus: a randomised, placebo-controlled, phase 3 trial. *Lancet* 2011; 377(9767):721–731.

14. Crowther MA, Ginsberg JS, Julian J, et al. A comparison of two intensities of warfarin for the prevention of recurrent thrombosis in patients with the antiphospholipid antibody syndrome. *N Engl J Med* 2003; 349(12):1133–1138.

15. Petri M, Lakatta C, Magder L, et al. Effect of prednisone and hydroxychloroquine on coronary artery disease risk factors in systemic lupus erythematosus: a longitudinal data analysis. *Am J Med* 1994;96: 254–259.

12 Raynaud's Phenomenon and Systemic Sclerosis

Laura B. Hughes and Barri Fessler

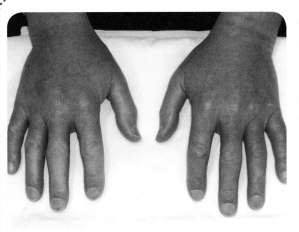

A 42-year-old man presents complaining of swollen hands. His fingers turn blue and white, and are associated with pain when exposed to cold temperatures. He notes heartburn and the sensation of food sticking in his esophagus.

Examination reveals diffusely edematous hands with skin thickening affecting the fingers. Nail-fold microscopy shows dilated loops with areas of dropout (Fig. 12.1).

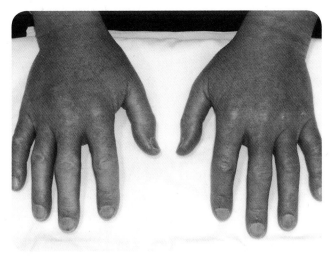

Figure 12.1 Skin thickening of both hands. Pallor of the 2nd, 3rd, and 4th digits of the right hand.

Raynaud's Phenomenon

INTRODUCTION

Raynaud's phenomenon (RP) is an exaggerated vasospastic response to cold temperature or emotional stress. First described by Maurice Raynaud in 1862 it is characterized by intermittent acral bleaching, followed by cyanosis and erythroderma. The typical tricolor sequence is driven by vasoconstriction of digital arteries (white phase), decreased blood flow in capillaries and venules (blue phase), followed by reactive hyperemia (red phase). Population-based surveys estimate the prevalence of RP in women between 6% and 20% and men between 3% and 12.5% (1).

CLINICAL PRESENTATION AND EXAMINATION

Raynaud's phenomenon occurs as a primary (not associated with an underlying disease) or secondary syndrome (associated with an underlying disease) (2). The distinction between primary and secondary RP is important as their pathophysiology differs, and the prognosis, severity, and treatment may also differ (3). Primary RP is characterized by the following diagnostic criteria: a definite history of symmetric episodic attacks of acral pallor or cyanosis; absence of peripheral vascular disease; absence of tissue necrosis; normal nail-fold capillary examination; a negative antinuclear antibody (ANA) test; and a normal erythrocyte sedimentation rate (4). Patients with primary RP often are younger and have minimal pain with attacks. In patients with secondary RP, the course is often more severe and frequently results in ischemic changes and digital ulceration (4). Many connective tissue diseases are associated with secondary RP, most notably systemic sclerosis (SSc), where it is often the initial manifestation. It may also occur in systemic lupus erythematosus (SLE), myositis, Sjögren's syndrome, rheumatoid arthritis, mixed connective tissue disease, vasculitis, and undifferentiated connective tissue disease. Secondary RP can also occur in noninflammatory conditions including hand–arm vibration syndrome, thoracic outlet syndrome, occlusive vascular diseases (e.g., arteriosclerosis, atheroemboli, thromboangiitis obliterans), hematologic diseases (e.g., paraproteinemia, cryoglobulinemia, cryofibrinogenemia, cold agglutinin disease, polycythemia), and from medications (e.g., amphetamines, beta-blockers, cocaine, nicotine, antineoplastic agents) (5).

Clinical clues to suggest secondary RP include later age of onset, asymmetric finger involvement, intense pain, tissue necrosis, signs or symptoms of another disease (e.g., alopecia, rash, sicca symptoms, oral ulcers, photosensitivity, skin thickening, arthralgias, dyspnea, gastroesophageal reflux disease (GERD), muscle weakness), and abnormal nail-fold capillaroscopy (5). Nail-fold capillaries can be examined through a drop of oil using an ophthalmoscope set at 40 diopters. The presence of enlarged or tortuous capillary loops suggests an underlying connective tissue disease, whereas these findings in association with capillary dropout are more suggestive of SSc.

If a thorough history and physical examination, including nail-fold capillaroscopy, reveals little evidence for an underlying disease, a clinical diagnosis of primary RP can be made. If there is clinical suspicion of a secondary cause, or an abnormal nail-fold capillary pattern is observed, serologic testing should be performed, including an ANA and erythrocyte sedimentation rate. An abnormal nail-fold capillary pattern in a patient with RP has been found to be the best predictor of an eventual disease transition to secondary RP. Elevated titers of ANA antibodies including anticentromere, antinucleolar, or anti-ScL70 antibodies, in a patient with RP, suggest the presence of—or eventual development of—an underlying connective tissue disease.

STUDIES

Raynaud's phenomenon is a clinical diagnosis. If secondary causes are suspected, an evaluation to asses for atherosclerotic disease is indicated as well as for an underlying connective tissue disorder, including serologies for SLE, Sjögren's syndrome, and an autoimmune myositis.

TREATMENT

Treatment choices for RP depend on the severity of the condition and the presence of an underlying disease. The goals of therapy are to improve quality of life and prevent tissue injury. In patients with primary RP, a conservative, nonpharmacologic approach is most important, although medications may be necessary. General education regarding the disease itself as well as the use of nonpharmacologic lifestyle modifications is recommended. Avoiding unnecessary cold exposure or sudden temperature changes such as moving from a hot environment to an air-conditioned room is essential. Patients should understand that the entire body and not just the digits should be kept warm. Strategies such as wearing thermal underwear, hats, scarves, and insulated footwear help keep the body warm. The digits should be protected from cold with gloves and/or hand warmers. Patients should avoid medications that promote vasoconstriction, such as decongestants, amphetamines, beta-blockers, and caffeine. Similarly, smoking cessation is also recommended because nicotine is vasoconstrictive. Physical maneuvers that promote vasodilation in the digits can also be taught to lessen the severity of an attack, including rotating the arms in a windmill pattern and placing the hands in warm water or in a warm body fold (such as the axilla). If these measures fail to improve the quantity and/or severity of attacks, there are a number of pharmacologic therapies that can be initiated. Calcium channel blockers are the most widely used class of drugs for the treatment of RP. Among the different classes of calcium channel blockers, the dihydropyridine group has been the most effective, with doses of nifedipine ranging from 30 to 180 mg daily or amlodipine from 5 to 20 mg daily. The long-acting or slow-release preparations are generally preferred as they are better tolerated and achieve a more sustained response. If a patient has a suboptimal response to maximum-dose calcium channel blockers, the addition of a direct vasodilator—such as topical nitroglycerin—can be used. Indirect vasodilators have also been evaluated, including angiotensin converting enzyme (ACE) inhibitors (e.g., enalapril, captopril), angiotensin II receptor antagonists (e.g., losartan), and selective serotonin reuptake inhibitors (e.g., fluoxetine). More recently, phosphodiesterase type 5 inhibitors (e.g., sildenafil, tadalafil, vardenafil) have been used for patients with severe RP with digital ischemia. Bosentan, an endothelin 1 receptor antagonist, has demonstrated success in treating digital ulcers in patients with scleroderma and secondary RP. Prazosin, a sympatholytic agent, and pentoxyphilline, a phosphodiesterase inhibitor, have also been reported to improve RP symptoms. Digital or thoracic sympathectomy or intravenous prostaglandin infusions (e.g., iloprost, epoprostenol) can be utilized in patients with RP who are refractory to oral medical therapy, typically in the acute setting where there is critical digital ischemia. Low-dose aspirin has also been recommended in patients with digital ischemia.

CLINICAL COURSE

Patients with primary RP are unlikely to develop progression of their disease or damage digital ischemia. Education about the nature of RP and instruction in nonpharmacologic measures can often reduce the frequency and severity of attacks and improve quality of life. Patients with secondary RP, especially those with SSc, are more likely to develop digital ulcers and tissue ischemia. Referral to a rheumatologist is recommended for patients with secondary RP or difficult-to-treat primary RP.

Systemic Sclerosis

INTRODUCTION

Scleroderma is a general term that refers to cutaneous fibrosis. It may be subdivided into two major categories: systemic sclerosis (SSc, also referred to as systemic scleroderma) and localized scleroderma. The most common forms of SSc are *limited scleroderma* and *diffuse scleroderma*, which are differentiated by the extent of skin thickening. Limited scleroderma (previously referred to as "CREST" syndrome) is defined as skin thickening that affects only the extremities distal to the elbows and/or knees. Diffuse scleroderma is defined as skin thickening proximal to the elbows and/or knees in addition to distal extremity involvement and truncal involvement. The face may be involved in both limited and diffuse scleroderma. In addition to skin, systemic involvement affecting the vasculature, gastrointestinal (GI) tract, lungs, heart, joints, and kidneys is frequently seen in both the forms of scleroderma. Cutaneous fibrosis may also occur in a *localized* form of scleroderma (not to be confused with the *limited* form), which includes morphea (one or more patches of thickened skin), linear scleroderma (a line of thickened skin usually affecting an extremity), and scleroderma *en coup de sabre* (linear scleroderma affecting the forehead and face). There is usually no visceral organ involvement in patients with localized scleroderma. Finally, patients may develop internal organ fibrosis along with scleroderma-specific antibodies but in the absence of skin thickening; this syndrome is referred to as *scleroderma sine scleroderma* and is very rare.

The etiology of SSc is unknown, but believed to be multifactorial, involving genetic predisposition and environmental exposures. Monozygotic and dizygotic twin studies have shown a low rate of disease concordance. Only 1.6% of patients with SSc have a first-degree relative with the disease, suggesting a small genetic contribution to disease susceptibility. The risk of other autoimmune diseases—such as SLE and rheumatoid arthritis—is increased in first-degree relatives of patients with SSc. There is some evidence that links SSc with exposures to silica, vinyl chloride, and organic solvents; however, an environmental exposure is not apparent in the majority of patients.

The typical age of onset of SSc is 30 to 50 years. It is more common in women than men (3–5:1). The incidence of SSc in the United States ranges from 9 to 19 cases per million. Prevalence estimates range from 28 to 286 cases per million population.

There are three fundamental pathological processes that explain the majority of clinical and laboratory manifestations seen in SSc. *Excessive deposition of collagen* in the skin and internal organs results in skin thickening, pulmonary fibrosis, and GI dysmotility. A noninflammatory *vasculopathy* contributes to Raynaud's phenomenon (RP), pulmonary arterial hypertension (PAH), scleroderma renal crisis (SRC), and gastric antral vascular ectasia (GAVE). Finally, *alterations in cellular* and *humoral immunity* are manifested by production of autoantibodies including anticentromere, anti-SCL70 (anti-DNA topoisomerase 1), and anti-RNA polymerase III antibodies.

CLINICAL PRESENTATION AND EXAMINATION

The tempo of disease expression differs between the two major forms of SSc: limited SSc typically develops over many decades, whereas diffuse SSc rapidly evolves over 1 to 2 years. Raynaud's phenomenon, discussed above, is usually the first manifestation of SSc, preceding the development of other clinical features by months to years. In patients with limited SSc, RP may be present for 20 to 30 years before the onset of skin thickening. In patients with diffuse SSc, RP usually develops concomitantly with the skin thickening or within a year of the cutaneous changes. The hallmark of SSc is skin involvement. Initially the skin becomes pruritic and the extremities become diffusely swollen and erythematous. As collagen is deposited, the skin becomes indurated and thickened. The fingers begin to taper as they fibrose (called "sclerodactyly") and digital flexion contractures may develop as the skin becomes progressively taut. The skin thickening starts distally affecting the hands and feet and progresses proximally. The face, chest, abdomen, and back may also be affected. Areas of spotty hypopigmentation and hyperpigmentation ("salt and pepper" appearance) may develop in patients with dark skin. Telangiectasias are more commonly seen on the hands and face of patients with limited SSc. Calcium deposits (calcinosis cutis) may occur in the hands, elbows, knees, and legs, and are usually a late manifestation of SSc, seen more frequently in limited disease. The subcutaneous calcium deposits may erupt through the skin, leading to drainage that can be mistaken for infection. Tendon friction rubs may be palpated in the wrists, elbows, knees, and ankles. Ulcerations over the fingertips, knuckles, or elbows because of skin thickening, vascular insufficiency, and trauma may develop, causing significant morbidity.

Gastrointestinal involvement is present in up to 90% of patients and is the second most common organ affected following skin involvement. Esophageal hypomotility and incompetence of the lower esophageal sphincter causing dysphagia and GERD is common, and may result in the development of strictures, Barrett's esophagus, and/or aspiration. Gastroparesis and dysmotility, which may occur throughout the GI tract, are due to atrophy of smooth muscle

PATIENT ASSESSMENT

- Nail-fold capillaroscopy is helpful in distinguishing primary RP from secondary RP.

- If there is clinical suspicion for secondary cause of RP on the basis of history and/or physical examination, serologic testing should be performed.

- Skin biopsies are not mandatory for diagnosis of SSc, but they may help rule out other diagnoses.

- If one of the SSc-associated autoantibodies is present (e.g., anticentromere, anti-SCL70, anti-RNA polymerase III), it is helpful in confirming the diagnosis, but *not* all patients with SSc have one of these antibodies.

and fibrosis in the gut wall. Bacterial overgrowth in the small bowel, malabsorption, pseudo-obstruction, and GAVE (watermelon stomach) are frequent complications. Primary biliary cirrhosis occurs in 2% to 8% of patients with SSc with limited disease.

Pulmonary disease is now the major cause of mortality in patients with SSc. The two major clinical manifestations are pulmonary fibrosis and pulmonary arterial hypertension, the former typically occurring in 75% of patients with diffuse disease and the latter in approximately 50% of patients with limited disease. However, these conditions are not mutually exclusive. Patients with extensive pulmonary fibrosis can develop PAH, and patients with PAH can develop mild pulmonary fibrosis. Dyspnea on exertion may be acute or insidious. Aspiration pneumonia and pulmonary hemorrhage may also be seen. Cardiac disease consisting of arrhythmias, pericardial effusions, or heart failure may occur and is associated with a poor prognosis. (9)

Scleroderma renal crisis used to be the most common cause of death in patients with SSc prior to the introduction of ACE inhibitors. It typically occurs in the setting of rapidly progressive skin thickening in a patient with diffuse disease; it is also associated with anti-RNA polymerase III antibodies and a history of antecedent high-dose corticosteroid usage. The manifestations include malignant hypertension present in 90% of patients, along with a rising creatinine and microangiopathic hemolytic anemia and thrombocytopenia. Normotensive SRC occurs in 10% of patients.

Musculoskeletal involvement includes arthralgias, nonerosive arthritis, joint contractures because of restriction of motion from skin thickening, tendon friction rubs, myopathy, and compression neuropathies. Bone resorption of the digital tufts (called acro-osteolysis) develops because of chronic vascular insufficiency and ischemia. Carpal tunnel syndrome or ulnar neuropathy may be seen because of compression from cutaneous fibrosis.

STUDIES

There are several autoantibodies that can be observed in patients with SSc; however, 40% to 50% of patients do *not* have one of these antibodies. Therefore if an antibody is present, it is helpful in establishing the diagnosis and predicting the prognosis, but it is not essential for the diagnosis. The centromere pattern on ANA testing (also called anticentromere antibodies) is associated with limited SSc, PAH, and severe RP with ischemia. The nucleolar pattern on ANA testing is also associated with SSc. Anti-DNA topoisomerase 1 (also known as anti-ScL70) antibodies are associated with diffuse SSc and pulmonary fibrosis. Antibodies to RNA polymerase III are associated with an increased risk of SRC and decreased incidence of lung disease (6,10).

In contrast to many other autoimmune diseases, acute-phase reactants (e.g., erythrocyte sedimentation rate, C-reactive protein) are not elevated in SSc. If they are elevated, a search for a concomitant condition—such as infection, malignancy, or another inflammatory disease—is warranted. Anemia of chronic disease is frequently seen in SSc; if iron-deficiency anemia is noted, GI evaluation for blood loss is indicated.

The diagnosis of SSc is established on the basis of a combination of characteristic symptoms, physical findings, specific serologies, and sometimes skin biopsies. The published classification criteria (used for enrolling patients into clinical trials in the past) consist of a major criterion (proximal scleroderma) and two or more minor criteria (sclerodactyly, digital pitting scars or loss of substance from the finger pad, and bibasilar pulmonary fibrosis). These criteria are inadequate because they omit the majority of patients with limited SSc and do not incorporate SSc-associated antibodies; therefore, they are currently being revised (7). Cutaneous fibrosis is not specific to SSc; there are several other fibrosing disorders that have been described, including nephrogenic fibrosing dermopathy, eosinophilic fasciitis, scleredema, and scleromyxedema, and should always be considered in the differential diagnosis. History (e.g., a patient with renal failure who was exposed to gadolinium during magnetic resonance imaging), physical examination findings (e.g., absence of skin thickening on the hands, absence of RP), and laboratory testing (e.g., elevated thyroid-stimulating hormone, monoclonal gammopathy on serum protein electrophoresis) may help to elucidate other etiologies for skin thickening.

TREATMENT

The management of SSc is targeted to specific organ manifestations because there is no effective therapy that treats the underlying disease process. To date, no medication has been demonstrated to make a substantial, clinically significant impact on skin fibrosis; however, medications such as methotrexate and mycophenolate mofetil are used in select patients because of modest effects demonstrated in studies. Interestingly, skin thickening in patients with diffuse SSc will start to spontaneously regress after 2 to 5 years of disease; however, the internal manifestations do not spontaneously improve and actually may continue to worsen over time. Given the almost universal presence of GERD in patients with SSc, all patients should be treated with proton pump inhibitors (e.g., omeprazole, pantoprazole) as esophageal disease may be subclinical, and treatment may help to prevent strictures, development of Barrett's esophagus, and aspiration pneumonitis. Promotility agents (e.g., erythromycin, metoclopramide, or domperidone) may be helpful in patients with gastroparesis, and treatment with rotating antibiotics is useful in patients with bacterial overgrowth. Frequently, patients with SSc lose weight and may require supplemental oral or parenteral nutrition. In patients found to have active interstitial lung disease, cyclophosphamide is used; whether azathioprine or mycophenolate mofetil are useful in the treatment of SSc-associated interstitial lung disease (ILD) is currently under investigation. Scleroderma renal crisis is treated with ACE inhibition and blood pressure control. The role of ACE inhibitors for prophylaxis against SRC is unknown. There is a strong association of corticosteroid usage with subsequent development of SRC; therefore, steroid use in SSc should be minimized or avoided completely. Although PAH used to be uniformly fatal within 1 to 2 years, there are now numerous medications that help to prolong survival and improve quality of life, including endothelin receptor antagonists (e.g., bosentan, ambrisentan), phosphodiesterase inhibitors (e.g., sildenafil, tadalafil), and prostacyclin analogues (e.g., epoprostenol, treprostinil). Any patient with SSc with PAH should be followed by a pulmonary hypertension specialist for optimum assessment and treatment. Patients with SSc should be encouraged to exercise and/or participate in physical therapy to increase flexibility, strength, and exercise capacity. In addition, attention should be paid to the presence of mood disorders as depression is common because of the altered self-image, frustration because of loss of hand dexterity, muscle weakness, and chronic pain. Counseling and psychiatric treatment should be encouraged, if indicated. In addition, support groups can provide emotional support to patients and their families (8).

CLINICAL COURSE

Screening for restrictive lung disease and pulmonary vascular disease in patients with SSc—consisting of pulmonary function tests and an echocardiogram (with special attention to the right side of the heart and pulmonary artery pressure)—should be performed at diagnosis for baseline measurement and at least annually thereafter, more frequently (every 3–6 months) if the patient has rapidly progressive skin disease or is symptomatic. If the PFTs suggest an underlying restrictive lung disease, a high-resolution CT of the lungs should be

WHEN TO REFER

- If SSc is suspected, patients should be referred to a rheumatologist for confirmation of diagnosis, assessment of organ involvement, and treatment plan.

- Patients with SSc should be referred for annual PFT and echocardiography.

- If pulmonary hypertension is suspected then all patients should be referred to a pulmonary hypertension specialist for confirmation by right-heart catheterization.

performed to determine if there is evidence of parenchymal inflammation and/or fibrosis; the distinction is important because only inflammation is treatable and reversible. Pulmonary function tests can also suggest the presence of pulmonary vascular disease if there is an isolated reduction in diffusion capacity of the lung for carbon monoxide (DLCO) with preservation of lung volumes (Forced Vital Capacity (FVC)/DLCO ratio .1.6). If the echocardiogram and/or PFTs suggest pulmonary vascular disease, a right-heart catheterization should be performed to determine if PAH is present. Treatment for PAH should not be based on estimated pulmonary artery (PA) pressure on echocardiogram because there are significant false-negative rates (in early PAH) and false-positive rates (in pulmonary fibrosis). Serum creatinine and urinalysis should be monitored quarterly. Patients should be encouraged to check their blood pressure several times a week at home especially if they have rapidly progressive diffuse skin disease or are anti-RNA polymerase III positive.

ICD9
Raynaud's
   443.0 disease or syndrome (paroxysmal digital cyanosis)
Sclerosis, sclerotic
   710.1 systemic (progressive)
Scleroderma, sclerodermia *(acrosclerotic)*
   (diffuse) (generalized) (progressive)
   710.1 (pulmonary)
   701.0 circumscribed
   701.0 linear
   701.0 localized (linear)
   778.1 newborn

References

1. Fraenkel L. Raynaud's phenomenon: Epidemiology and risk factors. *Curr Rheumatol Rep* 2002;4(2): 123–128.
2. Richter JG, Sander O, Schneider M, et al. Diagnostic algorithm for Raynaud's phenomenon and vascular skin lesions in systemic lupus erythematosus. *Lupus* 2010;19(9):1087–1095.
3. Bakst R, Merola JF, Franks AGJ, et al. Raynaud's phenomenon: Pathogenesis and management. *J Am Acad Dermatol* 2008;59(4):633–653.
4. LeRoy EC, Medsger TA, Jr. Raynaud's phenomenon: A proposal for classification. *Clin Exp Rheumatol* 1992;10(5):485–488.
5. Block JA, Sequeira W. Raynaud's phenomenon. *Lancet* 2001;357(9273):2042–2048.
6. Perera A, Fertig N, Lucas M, Medsger TA, Jr. Clinical subsets, skin thickness progression rate and serum antibody levels in systemic sclerosis patients with anti-topoisomerase I antibody. *Arthritis Rheum* 2007;56:2740–2746.
7. Hudson M, Fritzler MJ, Baron M; Canadian Scleroderma Research Group. Systemic sclerosis; establishing diagnostic criteria. *Medicine (Baltimore)* 2010;89(3):159–165.
8. Khanna D, Denton CP. Evidence-based management of rapidly progressive systemic sclerosis. *Best Pract Res Clin Rheumatol* 2010;24(3):387–400.
9. Tyndall AJ, Bannert B, Vonk M, et al. Causes and risk factors for death in systemic sclerosis: A study from the EULAR Scleroderma Trials and Research (EUSTAR) database. *Ann Rheum Dis* 2010;69(10):1809–1815.
10. Gliddon AE, Dore CJ, Dunphy J, et al. Antinuclear antibodies and clinical associations in a British Cohort with limited cutaneous systemic sclerosis. *J Rheumatol*, 2011:38(4):702–705.

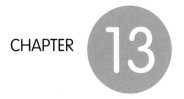

13 Inflammatory Myopathies: Polymyositis, Dermatomyositis, and Related Conditions

Irene Z. Whitt and Frederick W. Miller

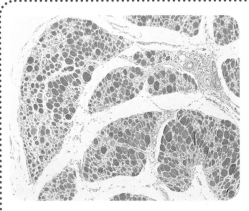

A previously healthy 54-year-old librarian comes to the clinic complaining of "tired and sore arms and legs" for the previous 7 weeks. This came on gradually after a cruise to the Caribbean, while playing golf in the sun all day, but she has continued to get weaker, to the point that she needs help getting in and out of her bathtub and has difficulty reaching high shelves at work. Despite avoiding the sun since the cruise ended, she has a faint, persistent "sunburn" on her hands and knees. She is fatigued and has difficulty with breathing while going upstairs. She has noticed more heartburn than usual, and sometimes solid food "comes back up." She denies taking any illicit drugs, has had no medication changes recently, and drinks wine only occasionally. Looking at her chart, you note that she has had a normal thyroid-stimulating hormone and electrolyte panel in the past 1 year, but she did not get the mammogram, Papanicolaou smear, or colonoscopy you had recommended.

Clinical Presentation

Inflammatory myopathies are diseases characterized by acquired muscle inflammation. This term encompasses a large number of disorders that include viral, fungal, and parasitic infections of muscle, toxic myopathies, and other causes of muscle damage. When the appropriate clinical, laboratory, and pathologic studies eliminate known causes of muscle inflammation, a diagnosis of idiopathic inflammatory myopathy (IIM) can be made (1). Idiopathic inflammatory myopathy is very rare, with an incidence of approximately 9 to 12 cases/million/year. It typically manifests either in young children or in adults in the fifth decade of life, though it can present at any age. Women are more affected than men (2).

The three most common forms of IIM are polymyositis (PM) and inclusion body myositis (IBM), where inflammation is found in multiple muscles, and dermatomyositis (DM), in which inflammatory changes occur in the skin as well as muscles. In PM and DM, inflammation is also frequently systemic, and occurs in other organs such as the joints, lungs, heart, or gastrointestinal (GI) tract. This inflammation manifests as direct organ infiltration by mononuclear cells, frequent immune abnormalities, and the production of autoantibodies. This, in addition to a

CLINICAL POINTS

- Idiopathic inflammatory myopathy is a diagnosis of exclusion, and the differential diagnosis can be challenging.

- Symmetric proximal muscle weakness predominates; a good functional assessment of the patient is required in order to distinguish true weakness from pain that limits function.

- Rashes in DM can be subtle, and most are not pathognomonic.

- Patients may have clinical weakness before or in the absence of elevated muscle enzymes; a muscle biopsy is required in most cases for definitive diagnosis, especially in patients without the pathognomonic rash of DM.

- Cancer has been associated with IIM, especially DM; age-appropriate cancer screening should be performed. Women with IIM should be evaluated for ovarian cancer.

NOT TO BE MISSED

A Differential Diagnosis of Muscle Weakness or Pain

Noninflammatory Myopathies

- Endocrine (hypo- and hyperthyroidism, acromegaly, diabetes, Cushing's syndrome, Addison's disease, hypo- and hyperparathyroidism, hypocalcemia, hypokalemia)

- Toxic (ethanol, corticosteroids, cocaine, statins, fibrates)

- Metabolic (acid maltase deficiency, carnitine deficiency, uremia)

- Congenital

- Mitochondrial

(Continued)

demonstrated response to therapies that decrease inflammation, has led to the classification of IIM as autoimmune diseases. Yet, the IIM themselves are a heterogeneous group of rare syndromes that differ considerably in their clinical presentations, pathologic findings, disease courses, and prognoses (3).

Most patients with DM present with characteristic rashes over the knuckles (Gottron's papules; see Fig. 13.1A) or around the eyes (heliotrope rash; Fig. 13.1B) and progressive, symmetric proximal muscle weakness, more pronounced in the legs than the arms, evolving over weeks to months. Patients with PM present with the weakness, but not the rash. They usually have hip muscle weakness, and notice increasing difficulty getting up from a chair or climbing stairs. The shoulder muscles often become symptomatic later, resulting in difficulty combing the hair or reaching objects on high shelves. Importantly, only one quarter of patients with DM or PM have significant muscle pain or tenderness. In the absence of objective weakness, hip or shoulder girdle pain as the only presenting complaint suggests an alternative diagnosis, such as polymyalgia rheumatica.

Other skeletal muscles can be affected, and 20% of patients have dysphagia (with nasal regurgitation of liquids signifying greater severity), while a smaller subset experiences respiratory insufficiency from respiratory muscle weakness. Subtle signs of extramuscular inflammation may also be present if carefully sought. Patients may have profound fatigue, persistent unexplained low-grade fevers, symmetric small-joint arthralgias or arthritis, abdominal pain, dyspnea on exertion from interstitial lung disease, or palpitations (from cardiac conduction abnormalities) and heart failure related to direct inflammation of the cardiac muscle.

DIFFERENTIAL DIAGNOSIS

The IIM are systemic connective tissue diseases, and many other organ systems can be involved, resulting in a wide range of possible presentations and symptoms that can mimic many other disorders. Thus, the differential diagnosis of IIM includes the many disorders associated with muscle complaints and is considerably challenging, not only because of the plethora of conditions to be considered, but also because IIM are so rare that few clinicians are thoroughly familiar with these diseases. One begins with clearly defining the patient's primary problems. Since patients may use "weakness" and "pain" interchangeably, questions should focus on (1) distinguishing myalgias from true weakness, which is often painless, by focusing on the patients' functional abilities (what they can and cannot do in their daily routine) (2); the location of weakness (proximal muscles in PM and DM vs. distal muscles in IBM and other disorders; symmetric weakness in PM and DM vs. asymmetric muscle involvement in IBM and other disorders) (3); the time frame and tempo of symptom progression and whether atrophy is present, signifying a chronic course most consistent with dystrophies (4); and any associated nonmuscular symptoms such as fatigue, low-grade fevers, rashes, breathing or swallowing difficulties, arthritis or arthralgias, which suggest a systemic disease, such as IIM.

Next, one needs to consider possible causes. Has the individual been exposed to any myotoxins, licit or illicit drugs, botanical or other over-the-counter preparations that could result in myopathy, or a metabolic abnormality such as hypokalemia? Has the patient had any recent unusual exposure, infection, or travel? Are there any symptoms or findings that suggest thyroid or parathyroid disease, diabetes, or an underlying malignancy? Is there a family history of a similar disorder that would suggest a dystrophy or inherited myopathy?

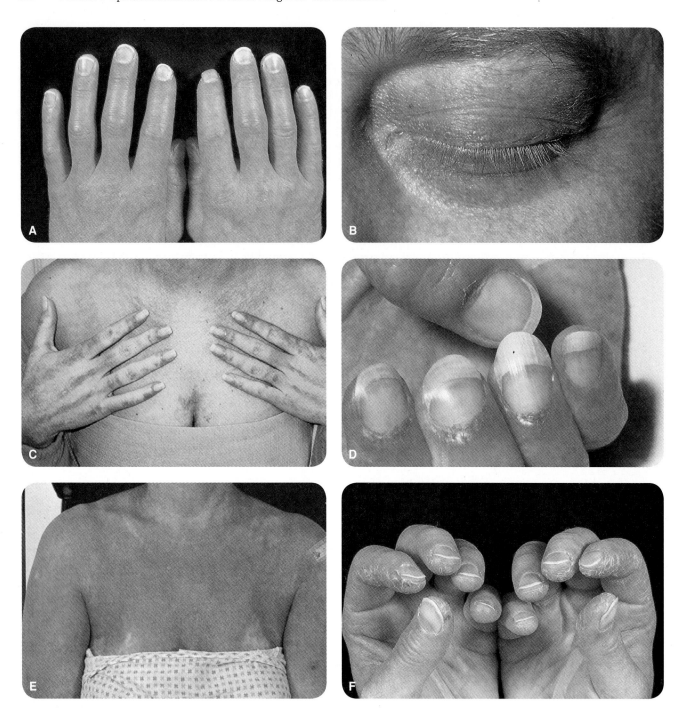

Figure 13.1 Skin changes seen in dermatomyositis. **A:** Gottron's papules are scaly papules overlying the extensor surfaces of the hands (over the meta-carpophalangeal and proximal interphalangeal joints in this case), elbows, knees, or malleoli. This patient also has sclerodactyly and arthritis of the metacarpophalangeal and proximal interphalangeal joints. **B:** The heliotrope rash is a purplish discoloration around the eyes, especially on the upper lids. **C:** Linear extensor erythema overlies the extensor surface of the hands beyond the usual location of Gottron's papules or sign. **D:** Periungual vas-culitic changes and cuticular overgrowth. **E:** Photosensitive diffuse erythroderma with accentuated erythema in the V of the neck (V sign) in a patient with cancer-associated dermatomyositis. **F:** Drying and cracking of the skin over the lateral and palmar surfaces of the fingers, known as "mechanic's hands," is seen frequently in patients with both DM and PM with one type of myositis-specific antibodies, the autoantibodies to aminoacyl-tRNA synthetases (the antisynthetase syndrome). With permission from Miller W. Frederick inflammatory myopathies: Polymyositis, dermatomyositis, and related conditions. In: Koopman WJ, Moreland LW, eds. *Arthritis and Allied Conditions: A Textbook of Rheumatology.* 15th ed. Baltimore: Lippincott Williams & Wilkins; 2005:6–7.

NOT TO BE MISSED (Continued)

Muscular Dystrophies

- Myotonia
- Neuropathies [amyotrophic lateral sclerosis (ALS), Guillain–Barre syndrome, diabetic plexopathy]
- Neuromuscular junction disorders (Eaton–Lambert syndrome and myasthenia gravis)
- Overuse syndromes
- Paraneoplastic (carcinomatous neuropathy, cachexia, myonecrosis)
- Rhabdomyolysis
- Tendonitis–fasciitis

Inflammatory Myopathies

Infectious

- Bacterial (*Staphylococcus*, *Streptococcus*, *Clostridia*, *Mycobacterium tuberculosis*)
- Viral (influenza, adenovirus, Epstein–Barr virus, coxsackievirus, hepatitis B and C, human immunodeficiency virus (HIV), human T-lymphotropic virus 1 (HTLV-1))
- Fungal (*Candida*, coccidiomycosis)
- Parasitic (trichinosis, toxocariasis, cysticercosis, trypanosomiasis, toxoplasmosis)
- Toxic (L-tryptophan, eosinophilia myalgia syndrome)
- Graft-versus-host disease
- Rheumatic conditions (giant cell arteritis, polyarteritis nodosum, overlap syndromes with lupus and scleroderma)
- Macrophagic or eosinophilic myofascitis
- Idiopathic Inflammatory Myopathies (see Table 13.1)

DIAGNOSTIC CRITERIA

Criteria to define the IIM syndromes and distinguish them from other myopathies were proposed more than 30 years ago (4) and remain useful today. Since these are diagnoses of exclusion, one must first do an evaluation directed by the history and physical examination findings to exclude the many other causes of myopathy. Once this has been accomplished, a diagnosis of IIM can be made using the findings of acute or subacute symmetric proximal muscle weakness, significant elevation of muscle enzymes, characteristic EMG abnormalities, and muscle biopsy findings or rashes consistent with IIM (Table 13.1). In unclear cases, additional clues that can assist in making the diagnosis of IIM include the presence of antinuclear antibodies (ANA) or myositis autoantibodies (5), a family history of autoimmune disease, detection of inflammatory changes in muscles by magnetic resonance imaging (MRI) (6), or a clinical response to immunosuppressive therapy (Table 13.2).

Inclusion body myositis is the most common IIM occurring in patients older than 50 years. Patients with IBM usually fulfill the IIM criteria, but in contrast, have more slowly progressive weakness of the quadriceps and distal muscles of the arms, in a somewhat asymmetric fashion; lower elevations of serum CK levels; and characteristic amyloid deposits and rimmed vacuoles within myocytes seen on light microscopy. Some inflammatory changes may be present, but amyloid deposition predominates. Although some patients may initially improve with immunosuppressive treatments, most have a gradual and relentless progression of muscle weakness.

Table 13.1 Bohan and Peter Criteria for the Diagnosis of Dermatomyositis (DM) and Polymyositis (PM)[a]

1. Symmetric weakness, usually progressive, of the proximal limb-girdle muscles
2. Elevation of serum levels of muscle-associated enzymes
   - CK, aldolase, LDH, AST/SGOT, ALT/SGPT
3. EMG triad of myopathy
   - Short, small, low-amplitude polyphasic motor unit potential
   - Fibrillation potentials, even at rest
   - Bizarre high-frequency repetitive discharges
4. Muscle biopsy evidence of chronic inflammation without other causes
   - Necrosis of type I or type II muscle fibers
   - Degeneration and regeneration of myofibers with variation in myofiber size
   - Focal collections of endomysial, perimysial, perivascular, or interstitial mononuclear cells
5. Characteristic rashes of dermatomyositis
   - Heliotrope rash, Gottron's papules, Gottron's sign

CK, creatine kinase; LDH, lactate dehydrogenase; AST/SGOT, aminotransferase/serum glutamic oxaloacetic transaminase; ALT/SGPT, alanine aminotransferase/serum glutamic pyruvic transaminase; EMG, electromyography.
[a]In patients in whom all known causes of myopathy have been excluded:
Definite IIM = For PM, all of the first four criteria
For DM, any three of the first four criteria plus the rash
Probable IIM = For PM, any three of the first four criteria
For DM, any two of the first four criteria plus the rash
Possible IIM = For PM, any two of the first four criteria
For DM, any one of the first four criteria plus the rash

Table 13.2 Useful Discriminators for Myositis in Confusing Cases of Myopathy

FEATURES LEADING TOWARD IIM	FEATURES LEADING AWAY FROM IIM
Family history of any autoimmune disease	Family history of muscular syndrome similar to the patient's (i.e., hereditary muscle disease)
Symmetric, chronic, proximal > distal weakness	Weakness related to exercise or involving the face
Muscle atrophy after chronic symptoms	Muscle atrophy early or hypertrophy at any point
Absence of neuropathy by examination or EMG	Presence of neuropathy
Lack of fasciculations and little muscle cramping	Fasciculations or prominent muscle cramping
Characteristic rash of DM	No rash or vasculitis
Features of CTD—fatigue, fevers, arthritis, ILD, etc.	No CTD symptoms
CK, AST, ALT, LDH, aldolase levels 2–100× normal	Enzymes <2× normal range or >100× normal
Positive ANA, ENA, or myositis antibodies[a]	Negative autoantibodies
Muscle biopsy evidence of myofiber degeneration/regeneration with inflammation, strong alkaline phosphatase staining in the interstitium	Myofiber vacuoles, ragged red fibers, parasites; no inflammation or alkaline phosphatase staining of the interstitium
MRI—spotty bright symmetric areas in muscle by STIR	MRI normal or only shows atrophy
Clinical response to immunosuppression	No clinical response to immunosuppression

EMG, electromyography; IIM, idiopathic inflammatory myopathy; DM, dermatomyositis; CK, creatine kinase; LDH, lactate dehydrogenase; AST, aminotransferase; ALT, alanine aminotransferase; MRI, magnetic resonance imaging; STIR, short tau inversion repeat; ANA, antinuclear antibody; ENA, antiextractable nuclear antigen antibody panel; CTD, connective tissue disease; ILD, interstitial lung disease; on specific testing, this includes the following antibodies: double-stranded DNA (dsDNA), SSA (anti-Ro), SSB (anti-La), anti-U1RNP, anti-Smith, and anti-scl70.

[a]Myositis autoantibodies. These include antisynthetase antibodies (the most common of which is anti-Jo-1), anti-SRP, anti-Mi-2, and others. Validated immunoprecipitation assays for these are available commercially.

PATIENT ASSESSMENT

- Subacute progressive proximal muscle weakness without other neurologic abnormality.
- Myalgias are not prominent.
- Systemic symptoms such as fatigue, arthritis, dysphagia, GI, lung, and cardiac abnormalities.
- Creatine kinase (CK) elevations >10 × upper limit of normal.
- Electromyography (EMG) showing fibrillations or positive sharp waves.
- Muscle biopsy and/or skin biopsy compatible with inflammation.
- Exclude the many other causes of muscle weakness.
- Serious complications: dysphagia from oropharyngeal muscle weakness can lead to aspiration; interstitial lung disease can be rapidly progressive and severe; and cardiac involvement can lead to conduction abnormalities necessitating pacemaker intervention.

Cancer-associated myositis is another IIM disorder, and on the basis of population studies (7), can be considered if both diagnoses are made within 2 years of one another. Treating the underlying cancer generally also treats the myositis. Although molecular genetic studies have identified genes responsible for many dystrophies, metabolic, and mitochondrial myopathies, some patients continue to defy diagnostic evaluations and remain enigmas.

Physical Findings

The physical examination begins with manual strength testing of proximal versus distal limb muscles and neck flexors. Carefully distinguish weakness from fatigability or pain that limits function by asking the patient to give a full effort on the examination. Note if a patient is able to rise from a squatting or sitting position without the use of his or her hands, how rapidly the patient is able to dress or undress, whether a waddling gait is present (demonstrating hip extensor weakness), and note what the patient can and cannot do compared to a previous time point. A simple activities-of-daily-living questionnaire that can be easily scored is often useful. The remainder of the neurologic examination, including sensory testing, should be normal; note that muscle tendon reflexes are preserved until the weakness is advanced. One should evaluate the function of other muscles and organs, including the heart (is the pulse irregular, suggesting conduction abnormalities, or are there signs of heart failure?); oropharynx (is swallowing normal?); respiratory muscles and lungs (note the patient's overall respiratory effort in addition to a careful lung examination listening for Velcro crackles that herald interstitial lung disease or coarse crackles signifying aspiration pneumonia). Any detected abnormalities should be pursued with appropriate tests, as indicated, such as an electrocardiogram (EKG), Holter monitoring, or echocardiogram, swallowing study, chest x-ray and/or computed tomographic (CT) scan of the chest, and pulmonary function tests with inspiratory and expiratory pressures (Table 13.3).

Many of the skin lesions described in patients with DM are subtle, and because they are often minimized by the patients themselves, they must be actively sought during the examination. None of them is pathognomonic, except Gottron's papules. These are palpable lesions overlying the extensor surfaces of the hand joints, elbows, knees, or malleoli with an erythematous base (Fig. 13.1A). Other rashes characteristic for DM include Gottron's sign, which is a scaling erythema without papules in the same distribution as Gottron's papules, and the heliotrope rash, a subtle, purplish discoloration around the eyes (Fig. 13.1B). In the absence of a prominent heliotrope rash, patients may have subtle periorbital edema. Other common rashes include a scaling scalp rash resembling psoriasis (pseudopsoriasis), sometimes associated with patchy alopecia if severe; linear extensor erythema (Fig. 13.1C); periungual vasculitic changes and cuticular overgrowth (Fig. 13.1D); photosensitive erythroderma; accentuated erythema in the V of the neck (V sign; Fig. 13.1E) or around the shoulders (shawl sign); and a drying and cracking of the skin over the lateral and palmar surfaces of the fingers, known as "mechanic's hands" (Fig. 13.1F). In patients with chronic or severe skin rashes and in children, subcutaneous calcium deposits, or calcinosis, develop over time.

Most importantly, if IIM (and DM in particular) is suspected, the clinical evaluation is not complete without a thorough age-appropriate cancer screening. Multiple population-based studies and registries have found an increased incidence of malignancies in patients with DM (standardized incidence ratio (SIR) 3.0:12.6) (7) and to a lesser degree in patients with PM (SIR 1.9) compared to the general population. Although the type of malignancy varies and is often age specific, the strongest associations were with ovarian, lung, pancreatic, GI, and non-Hodgkin lymphoma. Of special note, ovarian cancer was overrepresented in some series and should be specifically screened for in women with IIM, especially DM.

Pathogenesis

While the causes of the IIM are by definition unknown, evidence suggests that they likely result from one or more environmental stimuli acting on genetically susceptible individuals to induce chronic immune activation and subsequent myositis. Some environmental triggers are better understood than others. As with the case at the beginning of this chapter, excessive exposure to ultraviolet light has been shown to induce and exacerbate the rash of DM. In contrast, HIV and HTLV-1 infections have been associated with PM.

Many lines of indirect evidence suggest that inappropriate cellular immune activation is responsible for the pathologic effects seen in myositis and that the patterns of immune activation are distinct between the different IIMs, involving different cells and processes. In DM, a vasculopathy may be the primary

Table 13.3 Systemic Manifestations of IIM and Suggested Further Investigations

ORGAN SYSTEM	INVESTIGATIONS TO CONSIDER
General Fatigue Fevers Weight loss	*Differential diagnosis:* ESR, CRP, age-appropriate malignancy screening *Autoantibodies:* ANA, ENA, myositis autoantibodies
Musculoskeletal Muscle weakness, proximal > distal, upper and lower limbs, neck, rarely facial muscles	*Other causes:* fasting glucose, Ca, Phos, K, TSH, GGT (if alcohol) Laboratory tests of muscle enzymes (see text) Neurologic examination, EMG, muscle biopsy of the muscle most involved; consider MRI of muscle if unclear site for biopsy
Arthralgias or arthritis	X-rays of affected joints
Respiratory Dyspnea at rest and/or on exertion, dry cough, wheezing, rales	Chest x-ray
Pneumonia due to aspiration or immunosuppression	Chest x-ray, CT chest as needed
Interstitial lung disease	CT chest with prone positioning; pulmonary function tests
Cardiac Congestive heart failure Arrhythmias Myocarditis	Echocardiogram EKG, Holter monitoring Right ventricular heart biopsy; cardiac MRI
Gastrointestinal Dysarthria—poor tongue propulsions Dysphagia—upper and lower esophageal dysmotility	Formal swallowing evaluation
Reflux esophagitis	Empiric therapy; consider EGD if prolonged, severe dysphagia
Skin Dermatomyositis-specific rashes Dermatomyositis-associated rashes Panniculitis	Clinical photography (as baseline) and skin biopsy
Calcinosis cutis Periungual capillary changes	Can be seen on x-rays Examine with ophthalmoscope (on 40-diopter setting)
Raynaud's phenomenon	N/A
Association with malignancy	Age-appropriate cancer screening Ovarian cancer screening in women with IIM

ESR, erythrocyte sedimentation rate; CRP, c-reactive protein; ANA, antinuclear antibody; ENA, antiextractable nuclear antigen antibody panel; see Table 13.2 for specifics.

Ca, serum calcium level; Phos, serum phosphorus level; K, serum potassium level; TSH, thyroid-stimulating hormone; GGT, gamma-glutamyl transpeptidase, often helpful in distinguishing alcohol-related versus myositis-related transaminase elevation.

EMG, electromyography; CT, computed tomography; EKG, electrocardiogram, MRI, magnetic resonance imaging; EGD, esophagogastroduodenoscopy.

event responsible for the later muscle damage. Gene expression analysis has shown that interferon-alpha genes are overexpressed, producing an "interferon signature" that is more prominent when compared to PM/IBM or other autoimmune diseases. Thus, one model of pathogenesis (8) suggests that plasmacytoid dendritic cells, present in the perivascular space, become activated through an environment stimulus–genetic susceptibility interaction and secrete interferon-alpha. This in turn leads to specific protein expression, activation of CD4+ cells and B cells that secrete antibodies. The result is complement deposition, capillary injury, and pathologic changes of muscle infarction of the surrounding myocytes.

In contrast, it is immunoglobulin-related genes that are overexpressed in blood samples from patients with PM and IBM (8). This lead to a hypothesis that it is the myeloid dendritic cells, which are present in the endomysium surrounding the myocytes, that become activated through an unknown environmental trigger. They in turn activate CD8+ cytotoxic T cells, which directly destroy individual myocytes. Myeloid dendritic cells also stimulate plasma cells in muscle to overproduce immunoglobulins, which as yet have an ill-defined role in pathogenesis.

Studies (Laboratory, EMG, Muscle Biopsy, Imaging)

CLINICAL CHEMISTRY

One of the primary laboratory clues to a myopathy is the detection of elevated serum levels of enzymes originating from the cytoplasm of the muscle cell (sarcoplasm). The most frequently measured enzyme is CK because of its high sensitivity, muscle specificity, and relatively good correlation with disease activity and muscle strength. At the onset of illness, serum CK levels may be elevated as much as 10 to 100 times the upper limit of normal. Most of the elevation of serum CK levels in IIM is due to increases in the MM isoenzyme fraction, which is released from skeletal muscle. Elevation of the MB isoenzyme, found primarily in the myocardium, may also occur not only as a result of myocarditis but also as an indicator of skeletal muscle regeneration and myoblast activation. In patients with IIM, myoblast activation also results in elevation of other enzymes that correlate with CK levels, including lactate dehydrogenase (LDH), aldolase, serum glutamic oxaloacetic transaminase/aspartate aminotransferase (SGOT/AST), and serum glutamic pyruvic transaminase/alanine aminotransferase (SGPT/ALT). Elevations of the latter two have sometimes led to unnecessary liver biopsies.

Although the serum levels of CK and other muscle-derived enzymes are generally useful in following myositis activity and responses to therapy, they cannot substitute for a thorough evaluation of the patient, which includes functional assessment. First, there is a delay between the magnitude of the enzyme elevation and global disease activity; the CK levels tend to normalize 3 to 8 weeks before muscle strength improves and conversely may rise 5 to 6 weeks after a clinical relapse is detected. Therefore, clinical improvement or worsening in the patient must be correlated with CK levels, not the reverse. Second, a patient with IIM may have a normal CK level in the face of clinically active disease, as demonstrated by muscle weakness and accompanied by inflammation on muscle biopsy or MRI. This may be due to suppression of CK by corticosteroids, the presence of serum inhibitors of CK enzyme activity, or extensive muscle atrophy because of chronic disease. In addition, patients with systemic lupus erythematosus, rheumatoid arthritis, and other connective tissue diseases tend to have abnormally low CK levels; thus, a normal CK level in these patients may indicate active myositis. In contrast, racial and other differences not taken into account by the testing laboratory may result in falsely high CK levels. Because CK levels correlate with muscle mass, African Americans have significantly higher baseline CK levels than Caucasians, as do muscular athletes and marathon runners.

Abnormalities of nonspecific markers of inflammation—such as leukocytosis, elevated platelet counts, high C-reactive protein, and erythrocyte sedimentation rates—may be found in patients with myositis. These may be useful in assessing IIM activity, after being sure to exclude other coexisting processes such as infection or malignancy, which can also cause these abnormalities. Twenty-four-hour urinary creatinine excretion, which reflects muscle mass and damage, is elevated in many patients with muscle diseases. Additionally, abnormally low serum creatinine levels may be the result of loss of muscle mass and should alert one to the presence of chronic myositis.

IMMUNOLOGY

Immunologic abnormalities are sometimes the first clue that a patient has IIM. The most frequent abnormalities are hypergammaglobulinemia or the presence of an autoantibody. Antinuclear autoantibodies (ANAs) are the most common autoantibodies, but occur only in 25% of patients (9). The ANA usually displays a speckled pattern, although any other pattern can also be present. Other immune abnormalities include hypogammaglobulinemia, monoclonal gammopathy, cryoglobulinemia, and a variety of autoantibodies, some of which are strongly associated with myositis (myositis autoantibodies) (Table 13.2).

ELECTROMYOGRAPHY AND OTHER TESTS

Electromyography and nerve conduction velocity measurements are often performed to distinguish neuropathies from myopathies. They also can add to the probability that the patient has an inflammatory myopathy when characteristic abnormalities, such as fibrillations or positive sharp waves at rest and myopathic motor unit potentials, are present (Table 13.1). However, these findings are not pathognomonic for IIM and can also be seen in other cases, such as drug-induced myopathies. Thus, a muscle biopsy is usually needed to further narrow the differential.

In addition, radiographs, EKGs, and other laboratory studies should be performed on the basis of the nature of the symptoms and findings, and concern for the presence of cancer, which is associated with IIM (Table 13.3). This last issue is a difficult one, since there are no current guidelines on the number or specific tests for malignancy that should be performed. A prudent approach would be to start with the patient history and family history and pursue reasonable avenues in addition to age-appropriate screening. For example, a smoker should probably have a chest x-ray and CT chest to exclude malignancy; a 40-year-old with a family history of colon cancer should probably undergo a colonoscopy despite the young age; and a patient with recurrent high fevers should probably be investigated for lymphoma. In addition, all women with DM in particular should be carefully screened for ovarian cancer and followed up thoroughly if they have persistent vague abdominal pain. A screening pelvic and vaginal ultrasound is probably a good starting point, to be pursued by other testing.

MUSCLE BIOPSY

Although physicians may be reluctant to perform a muscle biopsy in what would appear to be straightforward cases of DM or PM, a biopsy should be included early in the evaluation of most patients, given the many other conditions that can closely mimic the IIM. The biopsy may reveal an unexpected disease, sometimes with important therapeutic, prognostic, or reproductive implications. It should be obtained in the muscle judged to be the weakest (usually the deltoid or quadriceps muscles), and on the side opposite from where the EMG was performed, to avoid a false-positive result. Nonetheless, the biopsy may not always be diagnostic. When a muscle cell dies for any reason, a secondary inflammatory process may occur. Therefore, muscle inflammation can be present in some dystrophies, especially facioscapulohumeral and dysferlin dystrophies, and in some toxic myopathies. In addition, inflammation in typical myositis may be missed because of its spotty nature or as a result of therapy. The yield can be improved by performing an MRI of the most clinically affected muscles, which can detect muscle inflammation and damage and thus direct the site of biopsy.

When it is detected, muscle inflammation in IIM consists of a preponderance of lymphocytes, which are often in direct contact with a dying myocyte (endomysial), as in the case of cytotoxic CD8+ T cells in PM (Fig. 13.2A); or

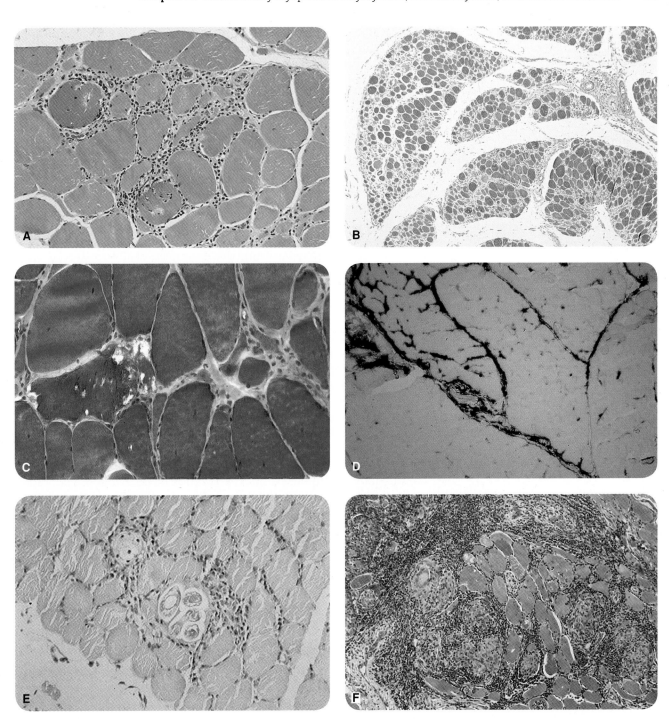

Figure 13.2 Biopsy findings in Myositis. **A:** Muscle biopsies from patients with polymyositis tend to show focal endomysial infiltration by mononuclear cells (hematoxylin and eosin stain). **B:** Muscle biopsies from patients with dermatomyositis show more perivascular and interstitial inflammation with perifascicular myofiber atrophy (modified trichrome stain). **C:** Transverse fresh-frozen section of muscle from a patient with inclusion body myositis displaying purplish granular material lining the multiple vacuoles in several myofibers and the presence of angulated myofibers (modified trichrome stain). **D:** Strong alkaline phosphatase staining of the interstitium is common in the IIM and can help distinguish this condition from other myopathies, even in the absence of inflammation. **E:** Trichinosis parasites in a myofiber surrounded by mononuclear inflammatory cells in a patient originally misdiagnosed with polymyositis (*Courtesy Dr. Lori A. Love*). **F:** Intensely inflammatory granulomatous myositis is characterized by the presence of granulomata and endomysial inflammation in this patient with sarcoidosis (hematoxylin and eosin stain). With permission from Miller W. Frederick. Inflammatory myopathies: Polymyositis, dermatomyositis, and related conditions. In: Koopman WJ, Moreland LW, eds. *Arthritis and Allied Conditions: A Textbook of Rheumatology*. 15th ed. Baltimore: Lippincott Williams & Wilkins; 2005:6–7.

between unaffected cells and fascicles (perimysial); or in the adjacent interstitial tissue, as in the case of CD4+ T cells in DM (Fig. 13.2B). The finding of smaller myocytes at the periphery of the fascicle, called perifascicular atrophy, is also helpful in diagnosing DM. In addition, strong activity of the alkaline phosphatase stain in the interstitium, reflecting regenerating muscle fibers and inflammation, suggests an IIM even if other evidence of inflammation is not prominent (Fig. 13.2D).

Predominance of neutrophils or perineural inflammation usually points to a process other than IIM, whereas predominant plasma cells, eosinophils, or granulomata in an otherwise typical myositis suggest the type of IIM present (i.e., eosinophilic myositis or sarcoidosis; Fig. 13.2F). Irregular red-rimmed inclusions on trichrome stain can identify IBM (Fig. 13.2C). The finding of prominent glycogen (by periodic acid–Schiff stain), fat (by oil red O stain), abnormal mitochondria (the ragged red fiber on hematoxylin and eosin stain), or other inclusions should move one away from the diagnosis of IIM to that of other syndromes. The muscle biopsy can often also be helpful in identifying infectious etiologies, such as trichinosis (Fig. 13.2E).

IMAGING STUDIES

Radiographic studies are useful in screening for and assessing gastrointestinal, cardiac, and pulmonary disease, erosive arthropathy, or calcifications (Table 13.3). There is increasing interest in using MRI, and a related technique called magnetic resonance spectroscopy, to assess muscle disease because these techniques are noninvasive and can sample larger volumes of muscle than EMG and muscle biopsy. Studies suggest that a combination of the T1-weighted image and the STIR (short tau inversion repeat) or other fat-suppressed image should be combined to assess muscle disease in IIM. Multiple cross-sections of the thighs are usually useful views, but the location to be evaluated should be dictated by the location of the most severe the signs and symptoms of the individual. Despite the expense of MRI, it may be a cost-effective adjunct for diagnosing and assessing selected patients by directing the biopsy site. Of note, patients should be instructed to rest for at least an hour prior to the study. Active exercise can cause muscle changes that result in transient elevations in serum CK levels and inflammatory changes seen on MRI.

Treatment

GENERAL CONSIDERATIONS

For the primary care physician, the first step in treatment is to consider early referral to a specialist familiar with muscle diseases (a rheumatologist, or neurologist, with the assistance of a dermatologist, depending on the case). There are many reasons for early referral, including the fact that a delay in diagnosis is associated with increased morbidity and mortality (2); that myositis autoantibody testing as well as specific stains and interpretation of muscle biopsies frequently require expertise from tertiary referral centers; that the IIM are multiorgan diseases that usually necessitate multispecialty evaluation and coordination of care; and that dedicated tertiary referral centers have ongoing research efforts that are invaluable for patients with these very rare diseases.

Therapy should be individualized on the basis of prognostic factors, severity of disease, and risk factors for adverse events associated with therapeutic agents. The past decade has seen a shift from the traditional approach of stepped therapy—in which a structured series of first-line, second-line, and third-line agents are prescribed in chronologic order as disease severity increases—to more individualized, and often more aggressive, forms of therapy.

WHEN TO REFER

- Initial diagnosis of IIM.

- Patient with IIM not responding to maximal doses of prednisone.

- Patient with IIM with suspected interstitial lung disease, cardiac involvement, or severe GI involvement.

- Patient with chronic IIM with new weakness, suspected to have flared.

- Patient with DM with skin involvement only, not responding to standard therapy.

- For patients with IIM with a newly discovered malignancy, refer promptly to an oncologist, as treatment of the malignancy will usually also treat the IIM.

However, assessing disease severity remains a major challenge, especially in chronic cases. It is often difficult to distinguish myositis disease activity (defined as inflammatory changes that may respond to immunosuppressive therapy) from disease damage (defined as irreversible changes that have resulted from prior disease activity), since both manifest primarily as muscle weakness. To this end, the International Myositis Assessment and Clinical Studies Group (IMACS), an international consortium of myositis experts, has developed disease activity and disease damage indices, which incorporate physical examination findings as well as laboratory values in order to better quantify and distinguish active disease from damage, and thus better tailor therapy (10).

REHABILITATION

The goal of all therapy is to optimize the functional levels of patients and, if possible, to return them to normal. In this regard, physical and occupational therapy remain underutilized modalities. Graded rehabilitation that takes into account the stage and severity of the patient's myositis is the best approach. Although bed rest is often necessary during periods of severe disease, passive range of motion exercises and stretching should be initiated early, especially in very debilitated, hospitalized patients to prevent the formation of contractures. As the degree of myositis decreases, patients should increase their activity through stages: active-assisted range of motion, followed by isometric, then isotonic, and finally, aerobic exercise.

THERAPEUTIC APPROACHES FOR MYOSITIS

Corticosteroids remain the primary therapy for the IIM and should be initiated as early as possible in nearly all patients, with the recognition that they tend to require high doses for long periods of time. Important considerations include an adequate initial dose (in most cases at least 1 mg/kg/day) (1), continuation of prednisone at a high dose until or after the serum CK becomes normal (2), which may last several months, and a slow rate of prednisone tapering (3, 11). Tapering prednisone too quickly leads to relapse. The role of pulse corticosteroids as treatment remains unclear. Individuals with poor prognostic factors should be considered for more aggressive therapy using corticosteroids with an added cytotoxic agent from the beginning of their disease.

During this treatment phase, both the primary care physician and the specialist need to aggressively screen for, prevent, and manage common side effects of high doses of prednisone, such as infections, GI ulcers, diabetes, hypertension, hyperlipidemia, water retention, osteopenia/osteoporosis, anxiety, and psychosis, to name a few. Careful consideration should be given to initiation of *Pneumocystis jirovecii* pneumonia prophylaxis, especially in the elderly or those with decreased renal clearance, since trimethoprim sulfamethoxazole (Bactrim) interacts with methotrexate (one of the cytotoxic agents frequently used for IIM), causing toxic levels of methotrexate and bone marrow suppression.

The treatment of IBM remains controversial and most patients with IBM do not respond to therapy at the level seen in patients with myositis in the other clinical groups. Patients with IBM and evidence of active inflammation, however, may benefit from corticosteroid and cytotoxic therapy in terms of slowing the rate of progression of disease. Retrospective reviews of corticosteroid and cytotoxic therapy, a prospective open trial of intravenous gammaglobulin (IVIg), and a randomized trial of combination oral methotrexate plus azathioprine versus high-dose methotrexate with leucovorin rescue, all suggest that the rate of deterioration may be decreased or stabilized in those patients.

Although most patients with DM or PM have at least a partial response to corticosteroids, some do not respond adequately, many more experience disease activity increases during steroid tapering, and most eventually suffer from the toxicities of corticosteroids. Little is known about optimal therapy in corticosteroid-resistant patients. Oral methotrexate, at doses of 7.5 to 25 mg/week, and azathioprine, at 50 to 150 mg/day, are the major therapeutic options for patients who are corticosteroid resistant and patients with initially moderate to high disease activity. A combination of methotrexate and azathioprine leads to improvement in some patients who have had inadequate responses to either agent given alone. Intravenous gammaglobulin, cyclophosphamide, mycophenolate mofetil, FK506, or other combinations of cytotoxic agents may be beneficial in some patients and warrant further evaluation. A double-blind, placebo-controlled trial has shown that IVIg at least transiently increases strength and decreases CK, rash, and muscle inflammation in some patients with DM. The novel biologic anti-inflammatory agent rituximab has been studied in one multicenter, placebo-controlled randomized clinical trial that is nearing completion and shows early promising results in some patients.

Many organ systems may be affected in IIM and cause significant morbidity and mortality. General symptoms of fatigue, fever, and weight loss often respond to corticosteroid or cytotoxic therapy for the underlying myositis. Raynaud's phenomenon may respond to cold avoidance or calcium channel blockers. The rash of DM may be a very troublesome problem for the patient and may persist long after the myositis has resolved. Avoidance of sun and photosensitizers—as well as topical sunscreens and steroids—may be helpful, but often the use of hydroxychloroquine or methotrexate is required. Some authors have used quinacrine successfully, and isotretinoin, despite teratogenic concerns, may be useful in the treatment of IIM rashes. Subcutaneous calcifications, more common in children than adults, can be very troubling. No treatment, other than therapy for the underlying myositis, has been shown to improve calcifications.

Pulmonary fibrosis is a worrisome complication in patients with IIM, can develop rapidly, and in some patients does not improve with any therapy. Nevertheless, pulse corticosteroids, cyclosporine A with careful drug level monitoring, tacrolimus, and cyclophosphamide are often tried in an attempt to treat this cause of great morbidity and mortality. The role of pulmonary transplantation in pulmonary dysfunction associated with systemic autoimmune disease remains unclear, but anecdotal reports suggest successful outcomes in some patients. Symptomatic heart failure should be treated in the standard manner, and if conduction system abnormalities are present, antiarrhythmics and/or pacemaker implantation should be considered. If myocarditis is present, corticosteroids and cytotoxic agents should be used.

Some patients have such severe dysphagia and are at such high risk of aspiration that tube feedings are necessary. Reflux esophagitis is common (as in the clinical case above) and should be treated by the usual approaches of elevating the head of the bed, prescribing antacids, or H2-receptor antagonists. Cricopharyngeal dysfunction can be the cause of significant dysphagia and odynophagia, and may improve with myotomy.

Clinical Course

The IIM are serious and sometimes life-threatening diseases. Survival of patients with myositis has been increasing during the past few decades from 50% prior to the introduction of corticosteroid therapy, to 5-year survival rates of 65% in 1947 to 1968, to approximately 80% more recently (12). Large cohort series with long follow-up have shown that, in general, approximately 20% to 30% of patients with IIM have a monophasic illness (and no longer require any therapy after 2 years of treatment), 20% to 30% have a polyphasic illness characterized by flares punctuated with periods of remission, while the rest have a chronic progressive course and require sustained treatment (13).

The rarity and heterogeneity of myositis has limited the collection of such data, yet a number of studies have attempted to define prognostic factors in the IIM. Adverse prognostic factors include PM as opposed to DM, older age, associated malignancy, cardiopulmonary disease, severe weakness, longer duration of weakness prior to diagnosis, fever, dysphagia, IBM, or the presence of antisynthetase or antisignal recognition particle autoantibodies. Some serologic findings predict a more benign myositis course. These include anti-Mi-2, anti-PM-Scl, and anti-U1RNP autoantibodies (3).

Acknowledgments

We thank Dr. Steven Ytterberg for many useful discussions about myositis. This work was supported by the intramural program of the National Institute of Environmental Health Sciences, NIH.

 Refer to Patient Education

> *ICD9*
> *710.3* **Dermatomyositis** *(acute) (chronic)*
> *729.1* **Myositis**
> *729.1 rheumatic*
> *729.1 rheumatoid*
> *729.1 traumatic (old)*
> **Polymyositis** *(acute) (chronic)*
> *710.4 (hemorrhagic)*
> *with involvement of*
> *710.4 [517.8] lung*
> *710.3 skin*

References

1. Plotz PH, Dalakas M, Leff RL, et al. Current concepts in the idiopathic inflammatory myopathies: polymyositis, dermatomyositis, and related disorders. *Ann Intern Med* 1989;111:143–157.
2. Airio A, Kautiainen H, Hakala M. Prognosis and mortality of polymyositis and dermatomyositis patients. *Clin Rheumatol* 2006;25:234–239.
3. Targoff IN. Dermatomyositis and polymyositis. *Curr Probl Dermatol* 1991;3:131–180.
4. Bohan A, Peter JB. Polymyositis and dermatomyositis (parts 1 and 2). *N Engl J Med* 1975;292:344–347, 403–407.
5. Miller FW. Myositis-specific autoantibodies. Touchstones for understanding the inflammatory myopathies. *JAMA* 1993;270:1846–1849.
6. Fraser DD, Frank JA, Dalakas M, et al. Magnetic resonance imaging in the idiopathic inflammatory myopathies. *J Rheumatol* 1991;18:1693–1700.
7. Hill CL, Zhang Y, Sigurgeirsson B, et al. Frequency of specific cancer types in dermatomyositis and polymyositis: A population-based study. *Lancet* 2001;357:96–100.
8. Greenberg SA. Proposed immunologic models of the inflammatory myopathies and potential therapeutic implications. *Neurology* 2007;69:1966–1967.
9. Vancsa A, Gergely L, Ponyi A, et al. Myositis-specific and myositis-associated antibodies in overlap myositis in comparison to primary dermatopolymyositis: Relevance for clinical classification: retrospective study of 169 patients. *Joint Bone Spine* 2010;77:125–130.
10. Isenberg DA, Allen E, Farewell V, et al., for the International Myositis and Clinical Studies Group (IMACS). International consensus outcome measures for patients with idiopathic inflammatory myopathies. Development and initial validation of myositis activity and damage indices in patients with adult onset disease. *Rheumatology* 2004;43:49–54.
11. Hengstman GJD, Van Den Hoogen FHJ, van Engelen BGM. Treatment of the inflammatory myopathies: Update and practical recommendations. *Expert Opin Pharmacother* 2009;10:1183–1190.
12. Lundberg IE, Forbess CJ. Mortality in idiopathic inflammatory myopathies. *Clin Exp Rheumatol* 2008;26:S109–S114.
13. Bronner IM, Van Der Meulen MFG, de Visser M, et al. Long-term outcome in polymyositis and dermatomyositis. *Ann Rheum Dis* 2006;65:1456–1461.

SECTION 3 Specific Rheumatic Diseases

CHAPTER 14 Vasculitis

Bao Quynh N. Huynh and S. Louis Bridges, Jr

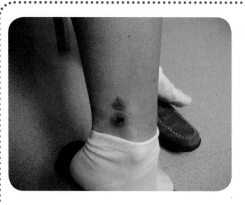

A 39-year-old female with an antinuclear antibody titer of 1:320, speckled pattern is referred to a rheumatologist for painful erythematous lesions on her lower extremities. Despite being on antibiotics for presumed cellulitis, her symptoms progressed, with additional similar lesions developing over the left ankle, left calf, right foot, and right lower leg. Her physical examination was remarkable for multiple 0.3- to 1-cm raised, palpable, tender purpuric lesions over the ankle and posterior aspect of the calves (Fig. 14.1). The remainder of the examination was within normal limits. Laboratory evaluation including complete blood count (CBC), chemistry profile, sedimentation rate, liver function tests, hepatitis serologies, and serum cryoglobulins was normal or negative. A skin biopsy of an active lesion was consistent with leukocytoclastic vasculitis. She was treated with prednisone, but had an incomplete response, so azathioprine was added. Over a course of several months, her lesions resolved completely, leaving only scarring (Fig. 14.1).

Clinical Presentation

Vasculitis is a heterogeneous group of disorders characterized by inflammation of blood vessels. One system of classification of vasculitides is based on the size of the predominant vessels involved (Table 14.1). For example, giant cell arteritis (GCA) involves large-sized blood vessels such as the aorta and its branches, whereas polyarteritis nodosa involves medium-sized vessels containing an internal elastic membrane, muscular media, and adventitia. Small-vessel vasculitis involves capillaries, and postcapillary venules and arterioles. Prior to the 1990s, a formal classification system of vasculitic syndromes did not exist because of a lack of consensus in evidence-based classification of individual patients with vasculitic syndromes (1). This was addressed by the American

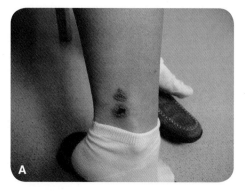
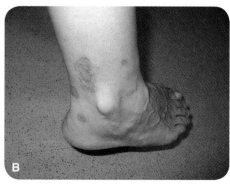

Figure 14.1 Skin lesions at presentation **(A)** and after resolution **(B)**. By permission of Devore AE and Jorizzo JL. Chapter 39: Cutaneous small vessel vasculitis. In: *Vasculitis*, 2nd ed. Ball GV and Bridges SL Jr., eds. New York: Oxford University Press, Inc.; 2008.

Table 14.1 Classification of More Common Forms of Vasculitis, Emphasizing the Predominant Size of Involved Vessels

Large vessel
Giant cell (temporal) arteritis
Takayasu's arteritis

Medium vessel
Polyarteritis nodosa
Hepatitis B virus related
Familial Mediterranean fever
Cutaneous polyarteritis nodosa
Kawasaki's disease

Medium- to small vessel
Wegener's granulomatosis
Churg–Strauss syndrome
Microscopic polyangiitis (polyarteritis)
Vasculitis of connective tissue diseases
Behçet's syndrome (may be large)

Small vessel
Cutaneous leukocytoclastic angiitis
Henoch–Schönlein purpura
Cryoglobulinemic vasculitis

Adapted from Reference (4).

College of Rheumatology (ACR) in 1990, which proposed criteria for the classification of seven different vasculitides (2). These criteria are not meant as diagnostic criteria, as they compared patients with different types of vasculitis, but not patients with other systemic or connective tissue diseases.

The ACR classification criteria do not include microscopic polyangiitis (MPA) or consider antineutrophil cytoplasmic antibodies (ANCA) as diagnostic criteria. In 1994, the Chapel Hill Consensus Conference (CHCC) produced definitions for vasculitis (3) and included MPA in its classification criteria. They also recognized that histological data would not be available for all patients, especially when the clinical condition of the patient might preclude obtaining appropriate biopsies. Furthermore, the sample might not be representative or the salient histological features may not be found because of sampling error. The classification scheme in Table 14.1 embodies features of both ACR and CHCC criteria, and is now widely used for epidemiological studies.

Epidemiology of Vasculitis

The vasculitides affect individuals of all ages, but are predominately seen in the extremes of age groups. Furthermore, the exact etiology is unknown, but it has been demonstrated to be multifactorial with factors such as ethnicity, genes, gender and ultraviolet light, infections, toxins, drugs, smoking, and surgery influencing disease expression (1).

Large-Vessel Vasculitis

GIANT CELL ARTERITIS

There is an increasing incidence with age, with very few cases occurring in those younger than 50 years of age. There is a greater incidence in women, with a female-to-male ratio of around 2:1 (1). Giant cell arteritis is more common in Caucasians than in African-Americans and Hispanics. Interestingly, the incidence of GCA varies with latitude with increasing incidence with higher latitude.

Despite intensive investigation, no specific infectious agent has been identified. As the immune system ages it becomes more vulnerable to infections. Reinfection with the human parainfluenza virus (HPIV) was associated with the onset of GCA. Viruses such as hepatitis B, herpes zoster, Epstein–Barr virus (EBV), herpes simplex virus (HSV 1 and 2), respiratory syncytial virus, and adenovirus have been thought to cause GCA; however, there has been no evidence supporting the association between these organisms and the development of GCA (1).

TAKAYASU'S ARTERITIS

This form of vasculitis occurs worldwide, but it is more common in Asia. The annual incidence in most populations is 1 to 3 per million, with the peak age of the onset of disease in the third decade. The disease is more common in women (1).

Medium-Vessel Vasculitis

The annual incidence of polyarteritis nodosa (PAN) is 2 to 9 per million, with the highest incidence of 16 per million in Kuwait and 14.8 per million in Japan. Where there has been more attention to hepatitis B vaccination, the prevalence of PAN has decreased.

The prevalence of Behçet's syndrome is highest in the regions extending from Eastern Asia to the Mediterranean basin and lowest in Western countries. The highest prevalence is seen in Turkey with 80 to 370 cases per 100,000 people. In Asian countries such as Japan, Korea, China, and Middle Eastern countries such as Iran and Saudi Arabia, the prevalence is between 13.5 and 20 cases per 100,000 people. Behçet's syndrome is more common among females in Asian countries and among males in Middle Eastern countries. It occurs frequently in third and fourth decade of life.

Medium- to Small-Vessel Vasculitis

The incidence of antineutrophil cytoplasm antibody (ANCA)-associated (Wegener's granulomatosis (WG), Churg–Strauss syndrome, and MPA) is approximately 10 to 20 per million per year, with onset peaking between ages 65 and 74 years (5). Wegener's granulomatosis—a disease with necrotizing granulomata of respiratory tract, necrotizing vasculitis, and focal glomerulonephritis—is more common in men and is rarely seen in children (0.3 per million per year). Various studies have demonstrated that WG is not as common as microscopic angiitis in non-European populations, that is, Japanese and Chinese. Familial cases of WG have been reported, albeit rare. HLA DPB1*0401 has been associated with WG. Environmental factors such as seasonality and drugs have been previously thought to contribute to the development of WG. However, studies conducted by Lane et al. did not confirm the seasonal effect on developing this disease. No single drug has been shown to lead to the development of WG; however, certain drugs—including cocaine—can result in ANCA-associated conditions that mimic primary ANCA-associated vasculitis. *Staphylococcus aureus* infections have been associated with WG and a higher risk of relapse (5).

The incidence of MPA is highest in Kuwait, with an incidence of 24 per million. The annual incidence of MPA is also high in the Japanese population, with an incidence of 14.8 per million from 2000 to 2004. Within Europe, MPA is more common in Southern Europe, whereas WG is more common in the northern part of the continent. Churg–Strauss syndrome, the least common of the ANCA-associated vasculitides, has an annual incidence of 1 to 3 per million and is more common in females than males. It has a peak age of onset of 65 to 75 years (5).

Small-Vessel Vasculitis

HENOCH–SCHONLEIN PURPURA

Henoch–Schonlein purpura is more commonly seen in children and less seen in adults with an incidence of 3 to 10 per million (1).

CUTANEOUS SMALL-VESSEL VASCULITIS

Our patient was diagnosed with cutaneous small-vessel vasculitis, also referred to as leukocytoclastic vasculitis (a histologic description) and hypersensitivity vasculitis. This is more common than many other forms of vasculitis. In Norwich from 1990 to 1994, the annual incidence of biopsy-proven cutaneous leukocytoclastic vasculitis was 15.4 per million, with a higher incidence in females. The German study reported that the incidence of CHCC-defined cutaneous leukocytoclastic angiitis was 4 to 9 per million between 1998 and 2002.

Clinical History

At present, there is not a specific set of guidelines to help the clinician in the evaluation of a patient with suspected vasculitis. The current classification criteria are intended mainly for research purposes. While they are helpful for framing the diagnostic approach in the general practice setting, not every patient with a given disease will satisfy these criteria (6). Thus, the practitioner often relies on the clinical history and other modalities, including laboratory data, radiographs, and histopathology in the diagnosis of a vasculitic condition.

The initial assessment includes a thorough history and physical examination of the patient, who may present only with nonspecific constitutional symptoms. This makes the workup of systemic vasculitides quite challenging; however, pattern recognition of signs and symptoms that have been demonstrated in various vasculitic conditions can provide the clinician a good starting point in the diagnostic process (6).

A detailed history of the nature of the condition provides clues that aid in the final diagnosis of the underlying vasculitis. For example, a patient with MPA may present with nonspecific flulike symptoms and arthralgia that can be present months to years before a diagnosis can be made. Microscopic polyangiitis can also present acutely, with the onset of symptoms within days to weeks. Patients with alveolar hemorrhage with pulmonary involvement in ANCA-associated vasculitis may report dyspnea, hemoptysis, and pleuritic chest pain (7). A history of chronic sinusitis, hemoptysis, and hematuria suggests WG, a pulmonary–renal syndrome with medium- to small-vessel involvement. Similarly, a complaint of hearing loss warrants further evaluation for WG as the mucosa of the middle ear or of the nasopharynx may be involved in this condition (8). A report of headaches, jaw claudication, loss of vision, and muscle stiffness may suggest GCA with or without polymyalgia rheumatica.

Age and other risk factors such as smoking history should also be kept in mind in the evaluation process. For example, Kawasaki's disease is more common in children, whereas GCA is seen more frequently in the older population, usually older than 50 years (6).

Physical Examination of the Patient

Certain physical examination findings may also help the clinician arrive at a diagnosis of vasculitis. Furthermore, they provide an idea of the degree of multisystem involvement, such as lungs, kidneys, and type of blood vessels, that is, aorta. The presence of bruits may point toward Takayasu's arteritis, GCA, or Behçet's syndrome. Abdominal pain in the setting of new-onset high blood pressure and peripheral neuropathy raises the possibility of polyarteritis

NOT TO BE MISSED

- Rule out mimickers of vasculitis.
- For visual symptoms and high ESR in patients older than 50 years, have a high clinical suspicion for GCA.
- Recognize life-threatening pulmonary, renal, neurologic, or ocular manifestations.

nodosa. The presence of blood pressure difference or lack of pulse in the arms suggests Takayasu's arteritis.

Churg–Strauss syndrome is another pulmonary–renal syndrome in which a patient with asthma may present with eosinophilia. Certain viral infections have been associated with systemic vasculitides. For example, hepatitis C infection has been demonstrated in cryoglobulinemic vasculitis, especially when associated with Raynaud's phenomenon and palpable purpura. Moreover, hepatitis B infection has been linked to polyarteritis nodosa. Behcet's syndrome is characterized by recurrent oral aphthous and genital ulcers, erythema nodosum, arthritis, and uveitis. Recurrent ocular episodes of uveitis can lead to retinal damage and blindness. The mucosal ulcers in Behcet's syndrome are round, painful lesions with erythematous margins and are covered with a yellow pseudomembrane.

Diagnostic Studies

After performing a complete history and physical examination, the clinician should consider ordering a few basic laboratory tests, such as complete blood cell count with differential, chemistry profile—including transaminases and creatinine, erythrocyte sedimentation rate (ESR), and urinalysis—to gain a better idea of which organ systems may be involved. Anemia of chronic disease and thrombocytosis are commonly seen in vasculitis, whereas thrombocytopenia and leucopenia are suggestive of a disease process other than vasculitis (6). Abnormal aspartate aminotransferase (AST) and alanine aminotransferase (ALT) suggest liver involvement, possibly hepatitis B or C infections that point toward a medium-vessel vasculitis such as polyarteritis nodosa or small-vessel cryoglobulinemic vasculitis, respectively. However, elevated transaminases are not specific to the liver and can be seen in other inflammatory conditions such as myositis. Serum creatinine may give an idea of the examined patient's renal function. The presence of hematuria or proteinuria suggests glomerular involvement and raises the possibility of vasculitic syndromes, that is, WG. Microscopic examination of a urine sample should be performed to look for cellular casts. For example, the presence of red blood cell (RBC) casts or dysmorphic RBCs is highly suggestive of glomerular injury.

An elevated ESR is not specific to vasculitis. Furthermore, a normal ESR does not rule out a diagnosis of vasculitis, as a patient with GCA can have a normal ESR. The presence of cytoplasmic and perinuclear ANCA (c-ANCA and p-ANCA) by indirect immunofluorescence suggests WG and microscopic angiitis, respectively. Antibodies to serine proteinase 3 and myeloperoxidase can be detected with enzyme-linked immunosorbent assays with higher positive predictive value and are highly suggestive of WG and microscopic angiitis, respectively. However, there is overlap as the presence of c-ANCA can be seen in microscopic angiitis and Churg–Strauss syndrome, whereas p-ANCA can be associated with WG (6). Other rheumatologic laboratory tests commonly ordered include serum complement levels. C3 and C4 are usually normal in the systemic vasculitides. Although antinuclear antibodies and rheumatoid factor may be useful in screening for other inflammatory conditions such as systemic lupus erythematosus and rheumatoid arthritis, they are not useful in the evaluation of vasculitis as they are nonspecific and can be associated with both vasculitis and its mimickers, that is, endocarditis.

Used in conjunction with laboratory data, imaging is a useful tool in the evaluation of suspected vasculitis. Cavitary nodules on chest x-ray films might suggest WG. High-resolution chest CT is more sensitive than chest radiography and often used if the chest radiographs are normal while the clinical suspicion for vasculitis is high. Other imaging modalities to be used at the clinician's discretion include brain MRI, head CT, angiography, color duplex ultrasound, and positron emission tomography.

Laboratory tests and imaging modalities are suggestive only of a vasculitic syndrome; they are not diagnostic. Tissue biopsy remains the gold standard of diagnosis (6). The biopsy sites are largely determined by the organs involved.

For example, if the pulmonary or renal systems are involved as in pulmonary–renal syndromes, tissues from lungs or kidneys would be the next logical steps. However, if GCA is suspected, a temporal artery biopsy is indicated. If there is cutaneous involvement as in the patient presented at the beginning of this chapter, then a skin biopsy is necessary. For the patient who presents with neuropathy or myopathy, nerve conduction study or electromyography with muscle biopsy should be performed.

Treatment

Since vasculitis has high morbidity and mortality, it is important to diagnose accurately and early so that appropriate treatments are instituted. Drugs used to treat vasculitis vary from corticosteroids to immunosuppressive agents, such as azathioprine (Imuran) in our described patient, to cytotoxic agents, such as cyclophosphamide (Cytoxan). Newer agents such as rituximab (Rituxan) are available, which was recently demonstrated to be noninferior to cyclophosphamide, as demonstrated in the Rituximab for ANCA-Associated Vasculitis (RAVE) trial (9). The treatment of vasculitis should include patient education. With knowledge of their diseases, patients are more likely to make informed decisions and comply with treatment plans and follow-up as the medications used in the treatment of vasculitis are not harmless. Numerous online resources are available to the patient; a few are provided here (see box to left) as a starting point.

Clinical Course

The differential diagnosis of vasculitis is broad, including many conditions that may mimic true vasculitis. Infections, thromboembolic phenomena, and malignancies cause inflammation and damage to blood vessels, leading to clinical presentation similarly seen in vasculitis (10). The various diseases that cause injury to blood vessels, incite an inflammatory process, and mimic a vasculitic process are provided in Table 14.2.

Furthermore, cutaneous manifestations as seen in our patient presented at the beginning of this chapter can be misdiagnosed initially as infections such as cellulitis. The clinician should bear in mind that imitators of vasculitis exist, order any necessary tests to rule out mimickers of vasculitis, and refer to rheumatology for further evaluation if a diagnosis is still in question.

Infectious organisms such as bacteria, viruses, and fungi often lead to conditions that imitate vasculitis by either causing direct vascular injury or indirectly altering the vascular structure via immune-mediated or toxic mechanisms, resulting in changes similarly seen in vasculitis. For example, *Salmonella* has been implicated in aortitis. Often, central nervous system vasculitis is secondary to bacterial or viral meningitis or due to bacterial endocarditis. Cutaneous infections such as panniculitis and cellulitis can present clinically, very similar to true vasculitis.

Malignancies can create a clinical picture similar to vasculitis via different mechanisms: (a) induction of immune-mediated inflammation, (b) occlusion of blood vessels by either cancer cells or creation of a hypercoagulable state, or (c) invasion of nerves innervating blood vessels, producing a neuropathy mimicking true vasculitis. Other nonmalignant occlusive processes such as atheroemboli and antiphospholipid antibody syndrome should also be considered in the evaluation of suspected vasculitis (10).

Once mimickers of vasculitis have been ruled out and treatments have been instituted for true vasculitis, the clinical course of disease varies from complete remission to relapse to refractoriness to death. Nowadays, the rates of remission in ANCA-associated vasculitis treated with modern therapy are greater than or equal to 90%. Outcome measures in ANCA-associated vasculitis include various assessment tools such as Vasculitis Damage Index and Birmingham Vasculitis Activity Score (BVAS), with the BVAS being the standard.

SECTION 3 Specific Rheumatic Diseases

Table 14.2 Noninflammatory Causes of Vascular Damage

Occlusive processes	Atheroembolic disease
	Thrombotic disorders
	Antiphospholipid antibody syndrome
	Thrombotic thrombocytopenic purpura
	Sickle cell anemia
	Thromboembolism
	Abnormal proteins
	Cryoglobulins
	Cryofibrinogens
	Paraproteins
Neoplasia	Cardiac myxoma
	Other neoplasms
External injury	Exposure to cold
	Radiation exposure
Internal injury	Hypertension, arterial dissection
Infection	Bacterial
	Fungal
	Mycobacterial
	Viral
	Spirochetal/Rickettsial
	Parasitic
Congenital or inherited abnormalities	Pseudoxanthoma elasticum
	Ehlers–Danlos syndrome
	Neurofibromatosis
	Fibromuscular dysplasia
Miscellaneous conditions	Drug effects
	Moyamoya disease
	Nonvascular

Adapted from Reference (10).

During the course of treatment of vasculitis with different immunosuppressive drugs and glucorticoids, drug toxicity remains a concern. Adverse events such as acute allergic reactions, leukopenia, infections, malignancy, diabetes, and osteoporosis have been observed.

Vasculitis is a heterogeneous group of disorders involving blood vessels that can affect multiple organs with dire consequences. However, the prognosis of these conditions, when diagnosed and treated early, is generally positive.

WHEN TO REFER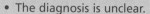

- The diagnosis is unclear.
- Treatment with immuno-suppressive drugs and cytotoxic drugs may be indicated.

ICD9

447.6 **Arteritis**
 446.5 giant cell
 446.0 necrosing or necrotizing
 446.5 temporal
 446.1 Kawasaki
716.9 **Arthropathy•**
 136.1 [711.2] Behçet's•
686.1 **Granulomatosis** *NEC*
 446.4 Wegener's (necrotizing respiratory)
446.0 **Polyarteritis** *(nodosa) (renal)*
Purpura
 287.0 Schönlein (-Henoch) (allergic)
Takayasu (-Onishi) disease or syndrome
 446.7 (pulseless disease)
447.6 **Vasculitis**

References

1. Watts R, Scott DGI. Epidemiology of vasculitis. In: Ball G, Bridges S, Jr, eds. *Vasculitis*. 2nd ed. New York: Oxford University Press, Inc; 2008:7–22.
2. Fries JF, Hunder GG, Bloch DA, et al. The American College of Rheumatology 1990 criteria for the classification of vasculitis. Summary. *Arthritis Rheum* 1990;33(8):1135–1136.
3. Jennette JC, Falk RJ, Andrassy K, et al. Nomenclature of systemic vasculitides. Proposal of an international consensus conference. *Arthritis Rheum* 1994;37(2):187–192.
4. Ball G, Bridges S, Jr. Classification of Vasculitis. In: Ball G, Bridges S, Jr, eds. *Vasculitis*. 2nd ed. New York: Oxford University Press, Inc; 2008:3–6.
5. Ntatsaki E, Watts RA, Scott DG. Epidemiology of ANCA-associated vasculitis. *Rheum Dis Clin North Am* 2010;36(3):447–461.
6. Fessler B. Approach to the diagnosis of vasculitis in adult patients. In: Ball G, Bridges S, Jr, eds. *Vasculitis*. 2nd ed. New York: Oxford University Press, Inc; 2008:277–285.
7. Chung SA, Seo P. Microscopic polyangiitis. *Rheum Dis Clin North Am* 2010;36(3):545–558.
8. Holle JU, Laudien M, Gross WL. Clinical manifestations and treatment of Wegener's granulomatosis. *Rheum Dis Clin North Am* 2010;36(3):507–526.
9. Stone JH, Merkel PA, Spiera R, et al. Rituximab versus cyclophosphamide for ANCA-associated vasculitis. *N Engl J Med* 2010;363(3):221–232.
10. Chung S, Sack K. Imitators of vasculitis. In: Ball G, Bridges SL, Jr, eds. *Vasculitis*. 2nd ed. New York: Oxford University Press, Inc; 2008:599–621.

CHAPTER 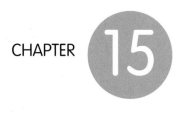 Giant Cell Arteritis and Polymyalgia Rheumatica

Angelo Gaffo

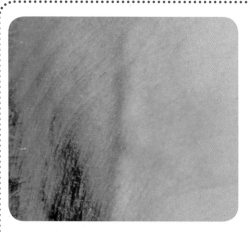

A 76-year-old white woman presents to her primary care physician with a 3-month history of progressive fatigue, malaise, poor appetite, and a 10-lb weight loss. She also reports bilateral shoulder and hand pain. No visual complaints are reported, and on examination, she is noticed to have mild bilateral metacarpophalangeal swelling and pain with palpation. Laboratory findings include a normochromic, normocytic anemia (hematocrit of 28%) and increased inflammatory markers with an erythrocyte sedimentation rate (ESR) of 60 mm/hour. No erosions are noted on hand radiographs, and a tentative diagnosis of seronegative rheumatoid arthritis is made. While the patient waits for a rheumatology referral she is placed on a 10-mg dose of oral prednisone.

Two weeks later when she is seen by a rheumatologist, the fatigue, malaise, poor appetite, and arthritis are mildly improved, but still present. No visual complaints are reported, but the patient has developed persistent jaw discomfort and weakness while chewing as well as headaches, with scalp tenderness noted while laying on a pillow or wearing glasses. On physical examination there is a palpable temporal artery (Fig. 15.1) and significant scalp tenderness. Additional findings include continued shoulder and pelvic girdle pain on palpation. Laboratory findings are largely unchanged, with an ESR at 56 mm/hour.

A temporal artery biopsy is scheduled in the next days and is shown in Figure 15.2.

Clinical Presentation

Polymyalgia rheumatica (PMR) and giant cell arteritis (GCA) are two clinical conditions that share multiple pathophysiologic and clinical characteristics. Both almost exclusively affect individuals older than 50 years, are characterized by musculoskeletal pain and stiffness, and are usually accompanied by prominent constitutional symptoms such as malaise, weight loss, and elevated inflammatory markers. In addition, both the diseases have a good response to different dosages of glucocorticoid therapy. Whereas PMR limits its involvement to the musculoskeletal system, GCA is a pan-arteritis that affects the aorta and its main branches with a special, but not exclusive, predilection for the extracranial branches of the carotid artery. As a consequence, early recognition of GCA is essential to avoid its more feared ischemic consequences, including irreversible vision loss. Polymyalgia rheumatica can evolve into GCA, with this clinical continuum leading many authors to consider PMR a forme fruste of GCA in which overt vasculitis has not developed.

Both PMR and GCA appear to be more common in whites of northern European descent than

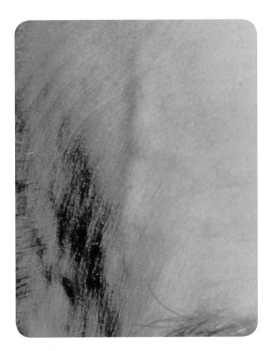

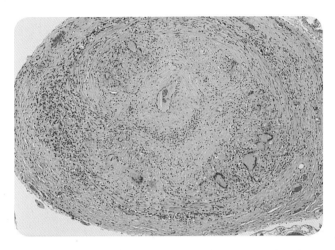

Figure 15.1 A prominent, tender temporal artery. Reproduced with permission from Gold DH, Weingeist TA. *Color Atlas of the Eye in Systemic Disease.* Baltimore: Lippincott Williams & Wilkins; 2001.

Figure 15.2 Temporal artery biopsy in giant cell arteritis reveals a chronically inflamed artery with marked narrowing of the lumen. Hematoxylin and eosin stain; original magnification × 310. With permission from Tasman W, Jaeger E. *The Wills Eye Hospital Atlas of Clinical Ophthalmology.* 2nd ed. Philadelphia: Lippincott Williams & Wilkins; 2001.

in other racial groups. The incidence rate of GCA in whites of northern European descent has been estimated at around 20 to 30/100,000. Reports from other groups including southern Europeans, African Americans, Asians, and Arabs describe a much lower incidence rate at 1 to 11/100,000. Polymyalgia rheumatica is approximately three times more common than GCA, which in turn has been reported as the most common form of vasculitis in the older than 50 years age group and the incidence increases with age until the ninth decade of life. These conditions are exceedingly rare in individuals younger than 50 years. Women have an increased frequency of both PMR and GCA when compared to men (1.7:1 for PMR and 3.5:1 for GCA).

The central histologic feature of GCA is the presence of an inflammatory infiltrate with predominance of CD4+ T cells and macrophages that can extend across the whole elastic artery vessel wall, but usually concentrates around the internal elastic lamina (Fig. 15.2) (1). Destruction of the internal elastic lamina is a pathognomonic feature of GCA. Giant cells can be present, but are an inconsistent feature of the disease, reported in about 50% of biopsy-proven cases. Large numbers of giant cells in the biopsy specimen have been associated with a higher risk of ischemic complications. Although fibrinoid necrosis could be seen in rare cases, its presence is so unusual that it should raise suspicion for alternative diagnoses. No characteristic histopathologic features have been reported for PMR, and the main role of biopsy is workup of suspected accompanying GCA.

Polymyalgia rheumatica and giant cell arteritis, very likely being part of a common pathophysiologic syndrome, share many clinical characteristics. Polymyalgia rheumatica itself is considered a clinical manifestation of GCA. Nevertheless, a majority of patients with PMR never develop other manifestations of GCA and PMR is still widely considered a stand-alone condition. Giant cell arteritis is mostly recognized by its cranial arteritis and musculoskeletal

Table 15.1 Clinical Features of Giant Cell Arteritis Syndromes[a]

Cranial arteritis	• Headache and scalp tenderness • Jaw claudication • Ophthalmic ischemia: vision loss, blurred vision, visual hallucinations, diplopia • Trismus, facial pain, tongue claudication or infarction, carotidynia, dysphagia • Posterior circulation transient ischemic attacks or strokes: confusion, cortical blindness, ataxia
Polymyalgia rheumatica	• Pain and stiffness around the shoulders, neck, and/or hips • Fatigue • Peripheral arthritis
Wasting and cachexia	• Fever or night sweats • Malaise or anorexia • Weight loss • Depression
Aortitis and peripheral artery occlusion	• Limb claudication • Bruits or decreased pulses • Raynaud's phenomenon • Dry cough • Chest pain or dyspnea • Sudden death

[a]Including polymyalgia rheumatica.

manifestations. However, other manifestations of the disease can easily go unnoticed, including those secondary to aortitis (limb claudication, aneurysms, Raynaud's phenomenon) and wasting with cachexia (fever, night sweats, weight loss, anorexia; Table 15.1) (2). It is very important to note that these clinical subsets are not mutually exclusive, and the clinical presentation can have considerable overlap.

Examination

CRANIAL ARTERITIS

Cranial arteritis is a result of the inflammatory involvement of the extracranial branches of the carotid artery. Headache is the most common manifestation. The specific characteristics of this headache are variable, without a specific type (could be dull, sharp, or throbbing), location (bilateral or unilateral, temporal, occipital, or diffuse), or intensity (from mild to severe). It is usually the persistence of this complaint that brings it to the attention of the clinician. Another feature that should raise a flag is the increased sensitivity of the scalp to tactile stimuli: suddenly the patient has discomfort with routine activities such as wearing glasses, combing their hair, or laying their head on a pillow. The correlation of this on physical examination is temporal tenderness on palpation, with the additional finding of a pulsating, enlarged, or nodular temporal artery in a few cases. Jaw claudication is one of the most specific symptoms of the disease. It is believed to be caused by demand ischemia in the masseter muscles. Nevertheless, the onset of pain can sometimes happen swiftly after the initiation of mastication. Trismus, facial pain, tongue claudication or infarction, scalp necrosis, and carotidynia are additional manifestations of ischemia in this circulatory bed.

The most feared complication of GCA is the vision loss caused by ischemic compromise of the optic nerve and the choroid induced by posterior ciliary artery occlusion (a branch of the ophthalmic, which is itself a branch of the internal carotid artery). In half of the patients the onset of vision loss is sudden and, in almost all cases, painless. An important proportion of patients can have premonitory symptoms, including blurred vision, transient monocular visual loss (*amaurosis fugax*), visual hallucinations, and diplopia. Visual loss caused by GCA is very often irreversible, and its premonitory symptoms can be considered a true medical emergency. On fundoscopic examination, disk edema followed by disk pallor is prominent.

Central nervous system ischemia in the form of transient ischemic attacks or strokes can occur as a consequence of GCA and, preferentially, affect the posterior circulation. These are believed to be secondary to thromboembolic disease, narrowing or occlusion of the carotid or vertebrobasilar arteries.

POLYMYALGIA RHEUMATICA

The main clinical characteristic of PMR is pain and stiffness around the muscles of the shoulder and pelvic girdle. Usually the onset is sudden and the shoulder girdle is affected first. Nighttime pain is common, but in the mornings, the symptoms could be so pronounced that the patient has marked difficulty caring for themselves and can end up confined to bed. There is evidence that the proximal painful manifestations of PMR in the shoulder and pelvic girdle are consequence of inflammation of multiple periarticular shoulder and hip bursas. Peripheral joint swelling that can progress to involve the whole hand is commonly described. True peripheral arthritis heralds more resistant disease. Disuse muscle atrophy can develop in long-standing untreated patients.

WASTING AND CACHEXIA

A prominent systemic inflammatory response leading to a presentation with fever, malaise, and weight loss resembling a fever of unknown origin can occur. It is important to emphasize that GCA accounts for about 20% of cases of fever of unknown origin in individuals older than 65 years. Fever is usually low grade, but spikes of up to 39°C or 40°C are not uncommon. Paradoxically, a presentation with these features accompanied with concomitant high levels of inflammatory markers seems to be protective against the development of cranial arteritis, but it is unclear if this is because of an earlier diagnosis with concurrent earlier exposure to glucocorticoid therapy or the predominance of inflammatory factors that may protect against arterial occlusion.

AORTITIS AND PERIPHERAL ARTERIAL OCCLUSION

This is by far the most under-recognized manifestation of GCA, but it affects approximately 10% of patients. Many more may be affected subclinically. Peripheral arterial occlusions affect vascular beds in a manner similar to Takayasu's arteritis, with a preference for the subclavian, axillary, and brachial arteries. Giant cell arteritis rarely involves other vessels such as the femoral, coronary, or mesenteric arteries. Presentation includes limb claudication, Raynaud's phenomenon, decreased pulses, and bruits over the involved vessels. An additional symptom that can be attributed to peripheral arterial involvement, in this case of the respiratory tract, is a persistent dry cough. Patients with peripheral arterial compromise are usually not affected by concomitant cranial arteritis.

Aortitis tends to preferentially affect the thoracic aorta, leading to aneurysm formation, dissection, and aortic incompetence. Common clinical presentations include dyspnea and chest pain (caused by aortic insufficiency, leading to demand coronary ischemia), along with the finding on routine chest radiographs of an enlarged aortic shadow. Sudden death can also occur, usually as a consequence of aortic dissection.

SECTION 3 Specific Rheumatic Diseases

Studies

In both PMR and GCA, the clinical assessment provides most of the elements necessary for the diagnosis, with some support provided by laboratory data, histopathology from a temporal artery biopsy, and very uncommonly radiologic studies.

Giant cell arteritis should be suspected in any patient older than 50 years with symptoms of PMR or tissue ischemia in the head, neck, or upper thorax. A high erythrocyte sedimentation rate (ESR) or C-reactive protein (CRP) titer are supportive of the diagnosis, but it is very important to note that around 25% of biopsy-proven cases do not have abnormal values of either at presentation. Elevated levels of interleukin 6 are promising markers of disease activity, as they are part of the pathophysiologic pathway of the disease. However, their use has not been standardized yet. Other common laboratory findings include microcytic anemia, thrombocytosis, leukocytosis, abnormalities in biochemical liver test (alkaline phosphatase and transaminases), and low levels of albumin.

The role of imaging in the diagnosis of GCA is still largely undetermined. Patients who present with cranial arteritis could be considered for a Doppler ultrasound examination of the temporal arteries, where a hypoechoic rim around the vessel lumen (known as the "hypoechoic halo") could be a useful finding in the prediction of vessel inflammation and in finding an adequate site for biopsy. However, the procedure is highly operator dependent, and subsequent studies have not proved its usefulness for diagnostic purposes. Doppler ultrasound techniques could be useful for the assessment of stenosis in other vascular beds, such as the vertebral or subclavian arteries. In patients who present with limb claudication or signs of aortic compromise (aortic insufficiency or aneurysmal dilatation), an angiogram or a less invasive magnetic resonance imaging angiography (MRA) could be considered. A smooth, uniform tapering in the affected peripheral vessel lumen is the characteristic finding in GCA. Magnetic resonance imaging angiography has the additional benefit of allowing the assessment of the vessel wall for thickening and edema that can precede occlusion. Positron emission tomography with F^{18}-fluorodeoxyglucose can demonstrate increased uptake in affected vessels and is a promising, but still not widely adopted, technique for assessment of disease activity.

The mainstay of the diagnosis of GCA is the histopathologic examination of the temporal artery. It is important to note that some patients do not have any temporal artery involvement, mainly the subset of patients who present as aortitis or peripheral arterial occlusion, and may not benefit from the procedure. However, the biopsy of the temporal artery remains as a time-honored confirmatory test in a great majority of cases and should be pursued whenever possible. Many misconceptions exist about the timing and technical aspects of the procedure (Table 15.2) (3, 4). The inflammatory compromise induced by GCA is often patchy and could be missed even in properly performed biopsies. The way to minimize this possibility is by obtaining a generous segment of the artery for study. At the very least 1 cm is required, but segments of 3 cm or more are preferred. Bilateral samples, although not usually feasible, have been shown to improve the diagnostic yield by 20% to 40%. Multiple cuts of the artery specimen should be performed and studied. Temporal artery biopsies are useful even 4 weeks into high-dose glucocorticoid therapy. The finding most commonly affected by this therapy is the disappearance of the inflammatory infiltrates from the vessel wall, but fragmentation of the elastic lamina, endothelial proliferation, and even the empty "nests" where giant cells were located (in cases that present with giant cells) can still be useful and supportive of the diagnosis. As a consequence, lack of prompt access to a physician who could perform the procedure should not be a deterrent for starting appropriate high-dose therapy in reasonably high suspicion cases. Even in properly performed and processed temporal artery biopsies, the result can be negative in up to 15%

Table 15.2 Important Considerations Regarding Temporal Artery Biopsies for Giant Cell Arteritis

- The length of the artery segment obtained should be at least 1 cm, but lengths of 3–4 cm are preferred
- Bilateral temporal artery biopsies increase the diagnostic yield by 20%–40%
- Process and cut the entire arterial segment, as the disease has a patchy distribution
- Do not strip the arterial sample off its periarterial connective tissue. Several times the diagnosis can be found in periarterial vessels rather than the temporal artery biopsied
- Despite being the preferred diagnostic test, false negatives in temporal artery biopsies are common (about 15% of cases)
- Temporal artery biopsies should be performed as soon as possible. However, they can be useful even after 4 weeks of glucocorticoid therapy

cases of confirmed GCA. Physicians encountering this difficult scenario should consider promptly enrolling the help of a rheumatologist, assessing the compromise of other vascular beds through imaging, and guiding treatment decisions on the basis of clinical symptoms and the overall level of suspicion for GCA.

Polymyalgia rheumatica has no specific diagnostic markers and the approach is essentially clinical. Similar to GCA, the inflammatory markers are usually elevated, but there is no threshold that can differentiate the two conditions. The use of ultrasound or magnetic resonance imaging to identify the periarticular bursitis of the shoulder and hips that are characteristic of the condition has been advocated. However, these procedures have failed to demonstrate a clear differentiation with other conditions that can resemble PMR.

DIFFERENTIAL DIAGNOSES

The American College of Rheumatology developed classification criteria for GCA in 1990 (Table 15.3) (5). As most classification criteria, these were created in order to help to include patients in studies in a uniform fashion and should not be applied to the diagnosis of individual patients. These criteria perform reasonably well in differentiating GCA from other vasculitides, but their usefulness is diminished when trying to differentiate it from conditions other than vasculitides. These criteria focus heavily on the cranial arteritis presentation pattern, and other presentation patterns could be missed when these are utilized.

CLINICAL POINTS

- Polymyalgia rheumatica is a clinical diagnosis, and therefore, there is no confirmatory test.
- Cranial arteritis is the better recognized form of GCA. However, other clinical presentations include wasting syndromes, PMR, aortitis, and peripheral arterial occlusions. These are often missed, and clinicians should maintain a high index of suspicion.
- Temporal artery biopsy is the gold standard for the diagnosis in most cases of GCA. It should be pursued whenever possible, even after the patient has been exposed to glucocorticoids.
- When there is suspicion of visual symptoms related to GCA, high-dose glucocorticoid therapy should be initiated as soon as possible. This should not be delayed while waiting for a temporal artery biopsy.
- Patients on high-dose glucocorticoid therapy for GCA should be closely monitored and treated for expected complications of therapy, most notably bone mass loss, hyperglycemia, and hypertension.

Table 15.3 Traditional Format of the 1990 American College of Rheumatology Criteria for the Classification of Giant Cell Arteritis[a]

- Age at disease onset equal to or older than 50 years
- New onset of or new type of headache
- Temporal artery tenderness to palpation or decreased pulsation (unrelated to atherosclerosis)
- Erythrocyte sedimentation rate greater than 50 mm/h
- Biopsy of the temporal artery showing vasculitis consistent with giant cell arteritis

Adapted from reference 5.
[a]The presence of three or more criteria yields a sensitivity of 93.5% and a specificity of 91.2%.

Table 15.4 Differential Diagnosis of Polymyalgia Rheumatica and Giant Cell Arteritis

POLYMYALGIA RHEUMATICA	GIANT CELL ARTERITIS
Seronegative rheumatoid arthritis	Vasculitides including Wegener's granulomatosis, microscopic polyangiitis, polyarteritis nodosa
Cervical and hip osteoarthritis	Atherosclerosis
Fibromyalgia	Temporal–mandibular joint disease and odontogenic problems
Inflammatory muscle disease, including inclusion body myositis and polymyositis	Trigeminal neuralgia
Amyloidosis	Amyloidosis
Malignancy	Malignancy, including multiple myeloma, Waldënstrom's macroglobulinemia, and myelodysplastic syndromes
Infections including chronic viral conditions or endocarditis	Infections including otitis media, sinusitis, pharyngitis, endocarditis, and osteomyelitis
Hypothyroidism	Subacute thyroiditis
Depression	Nonarteritic anterior ischemic optic neuropathy
Parkinson's disease	Chronic kidney disease with uremia or calciphylaxis
Late-onset systemic lupus erythematosus	
Drug reactions, e.g., myositis from statins, Parkinsonian symptoms from neuroleptics	
Lumbar spinal stenosis	
Crystal arthropathies, including polyarticular gout and calcium pyrophosphate deposition disease	

The differential diagnosis of both GCA and PMR is extensive and should be weighed carefully before committing patients to long-term glucocorticoid therapy (Table 15.4). Of all the signs and symptoms discussed for GCA, only jaw claudication and abnormal temporal arteries on palpation helped to reliably distinguish GCA from other items in the differential diagnosis.

The main consideration in the differential diagnosis of PMR is usually seronegative rheumatoid arthritis. Both the diseases can be very difficult to differentiate, given that PMR can sometimes cause peripheral joint swelling. Response to glucocorticoid therapy is not a reliable way of differentiating between the two conditions. The predominance of discomfort affecting the shoulder and pelvic girdle is the better way to differentiate the two in favor of PMR, although these elements of the history could often be difficult to obtain from certain patients. Fibromyalgia and related myofascial pain disorders tend to occur in younger individuals, but could be extremely difficult to differentiate from PMR when the inflammatory markers are not elevated. The preferential location of the discomfort in the shoulders and hip girdle, along with a rapid response to a low dose of glucocorticoids, could be clues in differentiating PMR from fibromyalgia. Polymyalgia rheumatica lacks the muscle enzyme elevations of the inflammatory myopathies, and if the patient's symptoms allow a proper muscle strength examination, the results should be very close to normal.

A condition that could closely resemble both PMR and GCA is amyloidosis. Patients could present with proximal pain, fatigue, weakness, very high inflammatory markers, and hardened temporal arteries. A temporal artery biopsy is very often the test that provides the diagnosis, showing the characteristic Congo red stain in the affected vessel wall. Other vasculitides such as Wegener's granulomatosis, microscopic polyangiitis, and polyarteritis nodosa could mimic GCA in their presentation. It is very important to note that all of these vasculitides can also affect the temporal artery and present with inflammatory infiltrates, leading inexperienced pathologists to diagnose GCA when this is the main condition suspected. Absence of fibrinoid necrosis and fragmentation of the elastic lamina are findings expected from biopsies in patients with GCA. Atherosclerosis and giant cell arteritis could be differentiated by their angiographic patterns in case of a vascular obstruction. Smooth tapering of the blood vessel lumen is expected in GCA, as opposed to sudden blocks in branching points in atherosclerosis.

Treatment

To date, glucocorticoid therapy is the only approach that has been proved to be effective in both PMR and GCA. The initial dose of glucocorticoids in GCA without current or recent findings suggestive of vision loss is of 40 to 60 mg/day of prednisone or its glucocorticoid equivalent. In cases of impending vision loss, high doses of intravenous glucocorticoids (1,000 mg of intravenous methylprednisolone for 3 days followed by 60 mg a day of prednisone) is a common approach although clear evidence of its benefit over prednisone 40 to 60 mg/day is lacking. Even this aggressive approach very rarely salvages vision when more than 24 hours have elapsed since the vision loss. For this reason, it is important to emphasize the emergent nature of this aggressive treatment when premonitory signs of vision loss are present. If a temporal artery biopsy cannot be obtained within a few hours, glucocorticoid therapy should be started and followed by a biopsy as soon as possible. Apart from vision loss, symptoms of GCA usually respond dramatically within 48 hours, but it may take up to 5 days in some cases.

The treatment of PMR should be initiated at a dose of 10 to 20 mg of prednisone or its glucocorticoid equivalent per day. As with GCA, the response is usually so dramatic that some use it as a confirmatory diagnostic element. In both PMR and GCA, tapering of glucocorticoids should be slow, starting somewhere between 2 and 4 weeks after the initiation of treatment, and only after the reversible manifestations of the disease have responded and inflammatory marker titers have normalized. Recommendations for glucocorticoid tapering can be found in Table 15.5 (3). The role of inflammatory markers in the tapering of glucocorticoids is supportive, and treatment decisions are primarily based on the presence or absence of clinical manifestations. Patients who are asymptomatic but see their ESR or CRP titers increase should have their glucocorticoid taper slowed down, but may not need to have their glucocorticoid dosage increased again. On the other hand, patients with normal ESR or CRP but with clinical manifestations of relapse need to have their glucocorticoid dose increased again. Patients typically stay on glucocorticoids an average of 2 years, and most of that period should be at low doses. Caregivers should monitor and aggressively treat complications of glucocorticoid therapy, including but not limited to glucocorticoid-induced osteoporosis, diabetes, hyperlipidemia, depression, and peptic ulcer disease. Large doses of intravenous glucocorticoids as a standard induction therapy in patients with GCA could lead to a more rapid response and decrease the future need for oral glucocorticoids to treat the

SECTION 3 Specific Rheumatic Diseases

PATIENT ASSESSMENT

- Polymyalgia rheumatica and giant cell arteritis are seen in people older than 50 years.

- Elevated sedimentation rates and/or C-reactive protein levels are found in a large majority but not all cases.

- Other abnormal, but less specific, laboratory findings are microcytic anemia, thrombocytosis, leukocytosis, elevated alkaline phosphatase and transaminase, and hypoalbuminemia.

- Temporal artery biopsy specimens must be of sufficient length, at least 1 cm and preferably 3 cm, to avoid sampling error.

Table 15.5 **Recommendations for Glucocorticoid Tapering in Polymyalgia Rheumatica and Giant Cell Arteritis**

	GIANT CELL ARTERITIS	POLYMYALGIA RHEUMATICA
Initial dose in milligrams of prednisone[a]	1 mg/kg/d	10–20 mg/d
When to start tapering	After at least 2 weeks of treatment, and only when symptoms have resolved and inflammatory markers have normalized	
Tapering recommendations[b]	• Reduce daily dosage by 5–10 mg every 2–4 weeks until reaching 20 mg/d; *then* • Reduce daily dosage by 2.5–5 mg every 2–4 weeks until reaching 10 mg/d; *then* • Reduce daily dosage by 1–2.5 mg every 1–2 months until discontinuation	• Reduce daily dosage by 2.5–5 mg every 2–4 weeks until reaching 10 mg/d; *then* • Reduce daily dosage by 1–2.5 mg every 1–2 months until discontinuation

Adapted from reference 3.

[a]Does not apply to optic ischemia, where high doses of intravenous glucocorticoids are preferred.

[b]Proceed and continue tapering only if the patient remains asymptomatic. Disease relapses are common for both giant cell arteritis and polymyalgia rheumatica during this phase.

NOT TO BE MISSED

- Elderly patients with marked functional decline and difficulty caring for themselves may have PMR or GCA as the underlying diagnosis.

- Jaw claudication is a relatively specific symptom of the disease and should be asked about during the evaluation of patients suspected of having GCA.

- Vision loss is the most feared complication of GCA. Symptoms suggestive of ophthalmic compromise should always be explored; these mainly include blurry vision, transient visual loss, visual hallucinations, and diplopia.

- A thorough peripheral vascular examination (pulses and blood pressure) should always be performed in patients suspected of having PMR or GCA as this may reveal findings indicative of aortitis or peripheral arterial occlusions.

- The presence of normal inflammatory markers (ESR and/or CRP), while unlikely, does not exclude the diagnosis of PMR or GCA.

condition. Failure to respond to glucocorticoid therapy should prompt a reassessment of the diagnosis.

Acetylsalicylic acid (aspirin), at a dose between 81 and 325 mg/day, is an important adjuvant therapy in patients with GCA who do not have contraindications to it. Studies support its role in preventing visual loss and ischemic complications, but its mechanism of action is unclear as thrombosis does not play a big role in vascular occlusions caused by GCA. Trials of glucocorticoid-sparing agents have been unsuccessful. Azathioprine, antimalarials, cyclophosphamide, dapsone, and statins all had disappointing results in keeping the disease in remission and in their glucocorticoid-sparing effect. Despite initial enthusiasm with methotrexate, its efficacy in maintaining remission and as a glucocorticoid-sparing agent could not be confirmed in a large randomized controlled trial (6). A similar disappointing result was obtained with the tumor necrosis factor receptor antibody infliximab, which showed no effect as a glucocorticoid-sparing agent (7). In conclusion, the current approach remains to keep the lowest dose of glucocorticoids for the shortest period of time, in order to avoid side effects.

Clinical Course and Conclusions

The prognosis for the great majority of patient with PMR is good, as the disease is usually treatment responsive and most patients discontinue glucocorticoids after 1 to 2 years. A subset of patients could develop a seronegative inflammatory polyarthritis requiring a treatment approach similar to rheumatoid arthritis, but this arthritis is not aggressive or erosive.

The most ominous manifestations of GCA are the development of vision loss or other cranial ischemic manifestations, principally strokes. If this is avoided, patients respond well to high-dose glucocorticoid therapy. The main long-term morbidity is secondary to a prolonged exposure to glucocorticoids. A majority of patients have at least one relapse of disease, usually in the form of PMR. No clear picture about life expectancy in GCA has been obtained, with contradicting studies supporting both a premature mortality and a normal life expectancy.

WHEN TO REFER

- All patients suspected of having GCA should be referred to a rheumatologist.

- If the initial symptoms of GCA are suggestive of impending vision loss, patients should be started immediately on high doses of glucocorticoids while urgently requesting a consultation from a rheumatologist and a surgical specialist capable of performing a temporal artery biopsy. These are usually ophthalmologists, ENT surgeons, or general surgeons. Specifications about the biopsy specimen management should be provided.

- Patient suspected of having GCA with vision symptoms should see an ophthalmologist as soon as possible for a fundoscopic examination and to rule out other reversible causes of vision loss.

- Patients with PMR who have symptom recurrence after an appropriate glucocorticoid course and taper should be referred to a rheumatologist.

ICD9

447.6 **Arteritis**
   446.5 giant cell
725 **Polymyalgia**
   725 rheumatica

References

1. Ashton-Key M, Gallagher PJ. Surgical pathology of cranial arteritis and polymyalgia rheumatica. *Baillieres Clin Rheumatol* 1991;5(3):387–404.
2. Weyand CM, Goronzy JJ. Giant-cell arteritis and polymyalgia rheumatica. *Ann Intern Med* 2003;139(6): 505–515.
3. Nesher G, Nesher R. Polymyalgia rheumatica and giant cell arteritis. In: Ball V, Bridges SL, eds. *Vasculitis*. New York: Oxford University Press; 2008:xviii, 629, 16 pp. of plates.
4. Seo P, Tone JH. Large-vessel vasculitis. *Arthritis Rheum* 2004;51(1):128–139.
5. Hunder GG, Bloch DA, Michel BA, et al. The American College of Rheumatology 1990 criteria for the classification of giant cell arteritis. *Arthritis Rheum* 1990;33(8):1122–1128.
6. Hoffman GS, Cid MC, Rendt-Zagar KE, et al. A multicenter, randomized, double-blind, placebo-controlled trial of adjuvant methotrexate treatment for giant cell arteritis. *Arthritis Rheum* 2002;46(5):1309–1318.
7. Hoffman GS, Cid MC, Hellmann DB, et al. Infliximab for maintenance of glucocorticosteroid-induced remission of giant cell arteritis: A randomized trial. *Ann Intern Med* 2007;146(9):621–630.

SECTION 3 Specific Rheumatic Diseases

16 Overlap Syndromes and Unclassified or Undifferentiated Connective Tissue Disease

Iris Navarro-Millán and Graciela S. Alarcón

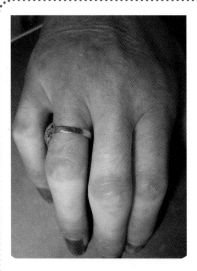

A 48-year-old Hispanic woman with symmetric polyarthritis, anemia, myalgias, and proximal muscle weakness. Over time she developed sclerodactyly and skin thickening over arms, hands, and face. She was found to be antinuclear antibody (ANA), anti-double stranded DNA (anti-dsDNA), anti-Smith, anti-Sjogren's syndrome A (SSA), Sjogren's syndrome B (SSB), and anticardiolipin IgG and IgM antibodies positive, without a history of thrombosis or miscarriages. Rheumatoid factor (RF) and anti-CCP antibodies were negative; however, radiographs of the hands and feet showed large erosions on both hands and feet. Her CK was elevated and a muscle biopsy was consistent with an inflammatory myopathy. Because of progressive dyspnea, a high-resolution computed tomography was performed, which demonstrated interstitial lung disease (ILD).

Introduction

Despite significant gains in the understanding of the immunopathogenesis of the different connective tissue diseases (CTDs), their etiology remains elusive. The diagnosis of the different CTDs is thus a matter of clinical judgment as patients present with constellations of symptoms, physical findings, and laboratory features that permit their recognition (1). Oftentimes, however, patients present with manifestations of more than one different CTD or with manifestations that defeat classification. The term "overlap" is used in this chapter for the first group of patients, whereas the terms "unclassified" or "undifferentiated" are used for the second group; the term mixed (M) CTD is reserved for patients with a defined overlap syndrome (*vide infra*). As our understanding of the etiopathogenesis of the CTDs improves, more precise labels will certainly be used.

The term atypical (A) CTD has arisen from the consensus reached by nonphysicians working with patients with silicone breast implants; the "legal" definition of ACTD is such that almost any individual presenting with some (subjective, for the most part) neuropsychologic or musculoskeletal manifestation may be diagnosed with this "entity."

Table 16.1 Terminology or Nomenclature

ACR	American College of Rheumatology
CTD	Connective tissue disease
Defined CTD	Clear-cut diagnosis of systemic lupus erythematosus, rheumatoid arthritis, polydermatomyositis, or scleroderma
Overlap syndrome	Presence of two defined CTDs (see Table 16.2)
Undifferentiated CTD	Patients with clinical features of CTDs who do not meet criteria for a defined CTD
Mixed CTD	A particular form of overlap syndrome (see Table 16.2)
Atypical CTD	Term used in the silicone breast implant litigation (not sanctioned by the ACR)

The rheumatologic community has not validated the existence of such disorder; thus, ACTD is not discussed.

The terminology or nomenclature used in this chapter is summarized in Table 16.1.

CLINICAL POINTS

- While there are patients with an autoimmune rheumatic disease who may develop manifestations of another, there are some patients who fully develop two or more diseases simultaneously or sequentially.

- These patients may be classified as having an overlap syndrome.

- Common overlap syndromes include rhupus, sclerodermatomyositis or scleromyositis, and MCTD.

- Mixed connective tissue disease is a term coined nearly 40 years ago to refer to patients with features of more than one disease (arthritis, scleroderma, lupus, myositis) with high anti-U1RNP antibodies; with time, however, these patients usually evolve into a more defined CTD.

- There is no consensus on how to diagnose unclassified or undifferentiated CTD; such a label may represent the prodrome of lupus; however, some of these patients may remain undifferentiated or incomplete or evolve into a fibromyalgia-like syndrome with ANA positivity.

The Overlap Syndromes

The following overlap syndromes have been described in the literature: rhupus or the overlap between rheumatoid arthritis (RA) and systemic lupus erythematosus (SLE); sclerodermatomyositis (or scleromyositis) or the overlap between scleroderma and myositis; and MCTD or the overlap between poly/dermatomyositis, scleroderma, SLE, and RA in the presence of anti-U1RNP antibodies and HLA-DR4. Other "overlaps" are considered subsets of defined CTDs rather than overlaps; such is the case for patients with SLE or RA who also have myositis or vasculitis, as well as for patients with SLE who have clinical and laboratory features of the antiphospholipid antibody syndrome (APS). Other patients with a defined CTD present overlapping manifestations with non-CTD disorders; such is the case of patients with luposclerosis as the overlapping clinical syndrome of SLE, and multiple sclerosis has been called. Finally, patients with primary APS may also present with manifestation of multiple sclerosis. Table 16.2 summarizes these different conditions by categories.

The first three overlap syndromes are now described in some detail.

RHUPUS

Arthralgias and arthritis are rather common in patients with SLE; however, in some patients with SLE, the most prominent clinical manifestation is a symmetric polyarthritis. These patients may or may not have a positive RF. That was the case of our patient whose clinical presentation was a symmetric inflammatory arthritis with radiographic evidence of erosions that resemble RA, yet her serologies were more suggestive of SLE. Patients with RA may present some extra-articular features and a positive ANA test that may suggest the diagnosis of SLE. The term rhupus, however, is reserved for those patients who clearly meet criteria for both SLE and RA, and who present characteristic clinical features of both the disorders. These patients usually have a seropositive, erosive, symmetric polyarthritis, which antedates the onset of unequivocal clinical features of SLE. They also present autoantibodies characteristic of both the disorders; these include IgM-RF, ANA, anti-dsDNA, and in about half the patients, antibodies to Ro. Most recently highly specific antibodies for RA

PATIENT ASSESSMENT

- Our patient had symmetric polyarthritis in a rheumatoid-like distribution with serologies that were more consistent with SLE rather than with RA.

- Hands and feet radiographs demonstrated an erosive arthritis highly suggestive of RA.

- There was biopsy-proven polymyositis.

- Sclerodactyly and ILD suggested the diagnosis of systemic sclerosis (SSc).

- These findings represent the overlap of four rheumatic diseases: RA, SLE, SSc, and polymyositis; however, she lacked anti-U1RNP antibodies, the hallmark of MCTD.

Table 16.2 Overlap Connective Tissue Diseases and Related Syndromes

Recognized overlap CTDs

SLE/RA: Rhupus
Myositis/scleroderma: Sclerodermatomyositis or scleromyositis
Myositis/scleroderma/RA/SLE: MCTD

Subsets within defined CTDs

SLE/myositis
RA/myositis
SLE/APS
RA/vasculitis
SLE/vasculitis

Overlap CTD and a nonrheumatic disorder

SLE/multiple sclerosis

Overlap CTD-like and a nonrheumatic disorder

APS/multiple sclerosis

CTD, connective tissue disease; SLE, systemic lupus erythematosus; RA, rheumatoid arthritis; APS, antiphospholipid antibody syndrome.

such as anticyclic citrullinated peptide antibodies have also been described in patients with rhupus (2). Some of the extra-articular features these patients present may be related to the presence of rheumatoid nodules rather than to SLE; this distinction may have therapeutic implications.

In patients with rhupus, RA usually presents first and is not until an average of 15 to 18 years that symptoms and serologies for SLE may ensue (3). Patients with rhupus should be distinguished from those patients with SLE who develop deforming nonerosive arthropathy which resembles that occurring in patients with recurrent rheumatic fever (Jaccoud's arthropathy). These patients initially present with correctable subluxation of the metacarpophalangeal joints with ulnar deviation, as well as swan-neck and boutonniere fingers and Z-thumb deformities. These abnormalities appear to be the result of ligamentous laxity and compression of hand musculature rather than result from the presence of pannus. The magnitude of the above-described features was the basis for the development of an index to aid in the diagnosis of Jaccoud's arthropathy. Van Vugt et al. have developed an algorithm to classify the deforming hand arthropathy of patients with lupus; a revision of this algorithm is presented in Figure 16.1.

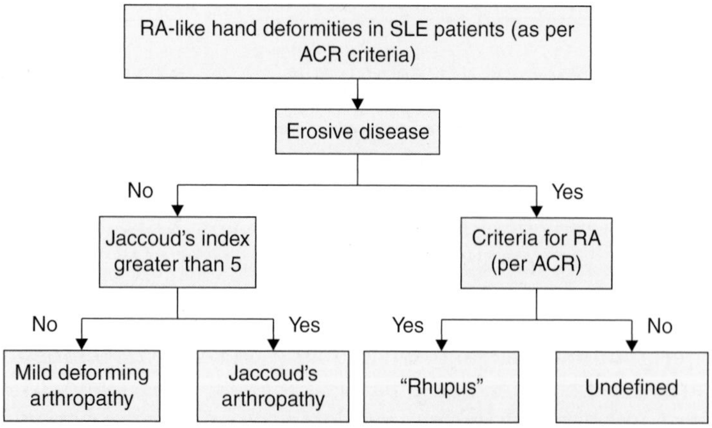

The frequency of rhupus at the population level is unknown. Since most of these cases have been recognized at tertiary care centers, this probably reflects the degree of awareness about this condition, rather than its true frequency. The lack of clinical criteria creates confusion in the characterization of this syndrome (4). It is also unclear whether the coexistence of SLE and RA is the result of the random association of these disorders or the result of genetic predisposition for both, as postulated by Brand et al.

Figure 16.1 Flow diagram for the diagnosis of the deforming arthropathies of SLE. RA, rheumatoid arthritis; SLE, systemic lupus erythematosus; ACR, American College of Rheumatology. Modified from Van Vugt et al. (1).

From the practical point of view, patients with rhupus should be treated according to their clinical manifestations (and their severity), utilizing compounds proved to be effective in both RA and SLE. Thus, antimalarial drugs may be needed to prevent SLE flares, but methotrexate or leflunomide may be needed to prevent joint damage. Antitumor necrosis factor α (TNF-α) therapy has been associated with the development and exacerbation of SLE as well as exacerbation of the SLE component of this overlap syndrome (5, 6). This therapy should, therefore, be used very carefully in patients where the "arthritis" is refractory to disease-modifying antirheumatic drugs (DMARDs), yet there are features that suggest the presence of a more systemic CTD (see RA Chapter 9).

SCLERODERMATOMYOSITIS OR SCLEROMYOSITIS

These are patients with manifestations of scleroderma and poly/dermatomyositis that exhibit variable cutaneous, muscular, and organ system manifestations; although this overlap syndrome was originally described in adults, pediatric cases have also been reported. Common manifestations characteristic of SSc are also frequently found in sclerodermatomyositis or scleromyositis, including Raynaud's phenomenon, myalgias or arthralgias, dysphagia, and in about 30% of the patients, ILD. Features of dermatomyositis such as periorbital edema and erythema, Gottron's papules, and erythematous and poikilodermatous lesions on the trunk and arms or the "shawl sign" may occur over the course of the disease (7). While there are authors who stress the importance of the presence of "mechanic's hands" (hyperkeratotic chronic eczema of the hands) (8), others suggest that this might be present in all types of myopathies and thus this finding is not specific for sclerodermatomyosistis or scleromyositis. Our own experience with this rare disorder, however, is quite different; the patients (children and adults) we have followed have had severe and generalized skin involvement with the consequent occurrence of flexion contractures. Pulmonary, gastrointestinal, and renal involvement, as the one described in scleroderma, is characteristically mild, but severe megacolon and restrictive lung function have been described.

Patients with sclerodermatomyositis usually exhibit high ANA titers in a homogeneous pattern, which correspond to the presence of the PM-Scl antigen (a nucleolar antigenic complex of 11 to 16 polypeptides); anti-U1RNP antibodies are characteristically absent. PM-Scl antibodies are not, however, specific for scleromyosistis, but in different case series, they have been the most frequently found antibodies; in fact, they have been described in up to 83% of patients with this disease, but only in 10% to 17% with other CTDs (9). From the immunogenetic point of view, patients with sclerodermatomyositis are either HLA-DR3 homozygous or HLA-DR3/DR4 heterozygous. They are thus quite different from patients with MCTD.

The frequency of this disorder is largely unknown; as with rhupus, most publications on sclerodermatomyositis come from tertiary care facilities and include small case series and case reports; thus, population-based figures are unavailable.

The treatment of these patients should be aimed at controlling the inflammatory process in muscles and other tissues involved. While SSc associated with myositis is usually a very severe form of the disease, scleromyositis has, in general, a protracted and rather benign course. The difference lies on its visceral involvement and not infrequently by the visual signs of dermatomyositis (7). Muscle inflammation is usually mild and steroid responsive. Aggressive treatment such as the one used in SSc and dermatomyositis could be more harmful than the disease itself, and is rarely required (7). This is an important reason for recognizing patients with this overlap syndrome. The prognosis of patients with this overlap syndrome depends on the degree of organ system involvement they have, but overall, the prognosis is more favorable than SSc or dermatomyositis by themselves (9).

SECTION 3 Specific Rheumatic Diseases

MIXED CONNECTIVE TISSUE DISEASE

The first description of MCTD dates back to 1972 when Sharp described 25 patients with overlapping clinical manifestations of RA, SLE, myositis, and scleroderma occurring predominantly in adult women; similar cases have been described in children and older adults (1). These patients also exhibited extremely high titers of antibodies to extractable nuclear antigen (ENA), later identified as antibodies to U1RNP and HLA-DR4 positivity. Since then, to date, this syndrome has been at the center of discussion, with some rheumatologists favoring its recognition and others not. There are those who argue that patients with MCTD, including the ones originally described by Sharp, tend to evolve into one of the more defined CTDs, such as SLE, myositis, or scleroderma, and should not be considered to have a defined syndrome. There are others, however, who propose that patients with anti-U1RNP antibodies, but no clear-cut manifestations of MCTD, represent early or undefined MCTD and that as time goes on they evolve into the full-blown MCTD syndrome. So the presence of antibodies to U1RNP, although characteristic of MCTD, does not, in the absence of other clinical features, suffice to make this diagnosis. The fact that some patients evolve into a more defined CTD has been postulated to have genetic basis. Patients who start as MCTD and are HLA-DR3 or HLA-DR5 evolve into SLE or scleroderma, whereas those who are HLA-DR4 remain as MCTD.

Table 16.3 shows the distinct clinical features of MCTD: Raynaud's phenomenon, sclerodactyly, sausage digits, lymphoadenopathy, malar rash, myositis, pulmonary involvement, esophageal dysmotility, symmetric polyarthritis (in an RA-like distribution), and serositis. Organ system involvement, particularly gastrointestinal and pulmonary, occurs with variable frequency, but renal and central nervous system involvements are conspicuously absent. Raynaud's phenomenon severe enough to produce severe digital ischemia and necrosis, sausage digits, swollen hands, polyarthritis, and rash are the more common presenting manifestations of MCTD. Criteria for the diagnosis of MCTD have been proposed by Sharp and subsequently by other investigators; they include, in addition to the clinical manifestations described, the presence of antibodies to ENA (anti-U1RNP) at very high titers (in the millions) in the absence of anti-Smith antibodies. A pathogenic role for anti-U1RNP antibodies has not been determined to date; it is quite possible (and in fact has been proposed) that these antibodies modify the clinical expression of a CTD.

Treatment in patients with MCTD is directed toward the clinical manifestations present, and to the prevention of structural damage in affected organs, using standard pharmacologic compounds commonly used in the more defined CTDs, such as corticosteroids, methotrexate, and other immunosuppressive drugs. The prognosis in patients with MCTD is variable; patients who evolve into a defined CTD adopt the clinical course and outcome of the new entity, whereas those who remain as an overlap may develop prominent digital

Table 16.3 Clinical and Laboratory Features of Mixed Connective Tissue Disease	
MAJOR	**MINOR**
Swollen fingers and/or hands	Arthritis
Raynaud's phenomenon	Alopecia
Esophageal dysmotility	Myositis
Sclerodactyly	Trigeminal neuropathy
Myositis	Cytopenias
Serositis	
Pulmonary involvement	
Anti-U1RNP antibodies	
Negative anti-Sm antibodies	

ischemic or necrotic events, as well as pulmonary hypertension or significant gastroesophageal reflux.

THE UNCLASSIFIED OR UNDIFFERENTIATED CONNECTIVE TISSUE DISEASES

There is no consensus on how exactly to diagnose these patients. Some authors consider these patients to be the preamble of MCTD, others of lupus (prelupus, latent lupus, incomplete lupus); others, including our group, may consider these patients as having an ANA-positive, fibromyalgia-like syndrome (see Fibromyalgia chapter). Others prefer to call these patients unclassified or undifferentiated CTDs only to indicate the fact that these patients tend to evolve into a defined CTD. Indeed a large effort by rheumatologists at different U.S. academic centers took place between 1982 and 1995; they constituted the largest cohort of "unclassified" patients with disease manifestations of up to 12 months in duration and followed these patients over time. The aim was to identify among these patients the predictors of a given outcome. Three subgroups of patients were recognized within this cohort of unclassified patients: (a) those with isolated Raynaud's phenomenon, (b) those with unexplained polyarthritis (patients quite not meeting criteria for the diagnosis of RA), and (c) those with truly undefined manifestations (as provided in Table 16.4). It can be argued that not all patients entering the undefined category would have been included as such to date; indeed some of these patients probably could have been considered as having an ANA-positive, fibromyalgia-like syndrome as described by our group several years ago. This multicentric group also constituted a second cohort of patients with well-defined CTDs that served as a comparison for the unclassified patients.

Patients in this study were followed longitudinally in an effort to determine the patients' final diagnosis. Yearly visits were done during the first 5 years; an additional visit was conducted at 10 years. The protocol required only an update interval history, a physical examination, and a core of laboratory tests. Any other laboratory test or more sophisticated ancillary procedure required the presence of clinical manifestations that could justify ordering or performing them. The results of this study are worth discussing. First, the overwhelming majority of patients entering the study as defined CTDs kept the same diagnosis at a later time point; this contrasts with less than 50% for those with undifferentiated disease that kept the same diagnosis. Among those with unclassified diseases, there were some differences depending on the subgroup within this cohort at enrollment. Of those who started as unexplained polyarthritis,

NOT TO BE MISSED

- Not all patients with symptoms of more than one rheumatic disease represent an overlap.
- Symptoms such as Raynaud's phenomenon, arthritis, sclerodactyly, and alveolitis may be present in patients with different rheumatic diseases and are still more commonly explained by one entity (one disease) than several occurring simultaneously.

Table 16.4 Clinical Features of Patients with Unclassified or Undifferentiated Connective Tissue Disease

Arthralgias/arthritis

Myalgias

Rashes

Sicca

Pericarditis/pleuritis

Pulmonary involvement

Peripheral neuropathy

Elevated acute-phase reactant(s)

Positive serologic test for syphilis

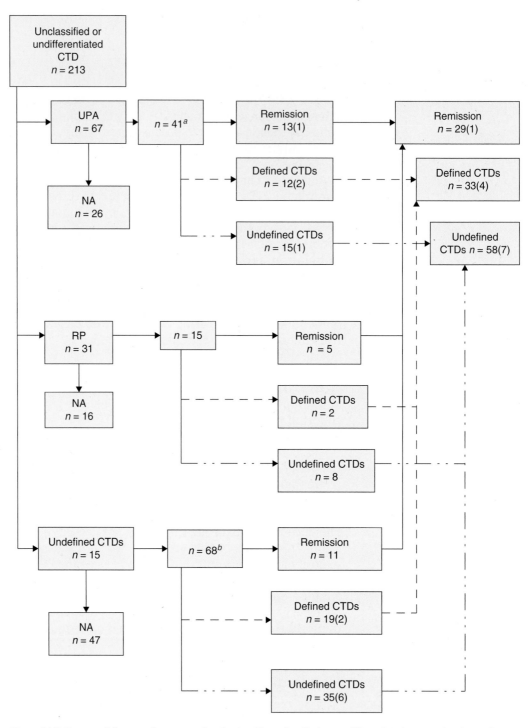

Figure 16.2 Ten-year follow-up diagnoses of patients with unclassified or undifferentiated connective tissue disease (CTD); UPA, unexplained polyarthritis; NA, nonavailable; RP, Raynaud's phenomenon. [a]One patient developed psoriatic arthritis; [b]one patient each developed psoriatic arthritis, sarcoidosis, and myasthenia gravis. Modified from Alarcón (1).

about one third remained undifferentiated, one third went into remission, and the other third evolved into a defined CTD. In contrast, of those patients who entered the cohort as isolated Raynaud's phenomenon or as undefined manifestations of a CTD, about one half remained as undifferentiated; patients with Raynaud's phenomenon were more likely to go into remission, whereas those with undefined manifestations were more likely to evolve into a defined CTD. Figure 16.2 summarizes the initial and final diagnoses of patients from this undifferentiated CTD cohort.

WHEN TO REFER

- Inflammatory arthritis.

- Skin changes characterized by thickening, sclerodactyly, and Raynaud's phenomenon.

- Positive serologies for CTD in the setting of appropriate clinical manifestations.

- Referral allows the rheumatologist to define the diagnosis (as much as possible) and recommend proper management; this is of paramount importance if the possible deleterious impact of the CTD is to be lessened.

The examination of socioeconomic–demographic and clinical parameters for predictors of a given outcome among patients from the entire undifferentiated cohort rendered some interesting data. Young patients of African-American ethnicity with alopecia, serositis, discoid lupus, positive ANAs, and anti-Smith antibodies were more likely to evolve into SLE; those with small hand joints involvement were more likely to evolve into RA. Of course it can be argued that in both these cases patients could have been diagnosed as having SLE and RA, respectively, but following the strict guidelines established a priori for this study they could not, since they did not meet criteria for either disorder.

Recently, few studies have shown that low levels of vitamin D in patients with UCTD may play a role in the subsequent progression into a well-defined CTD. Supplementation of these patients with vitamin D as well as measurement of vitamin D levels might be considered (10).

In summary, more than a precise diagnosis, the generalist should follow patients with manifestations suggestive, but not diagnostic, of a CTD with a very open mind and be ready to diagnose and treat a CTD if clear-cut manifestations of such evolve. Patients should be treated according to their clinical manifestations, trying to minimize the impact of the disorder as well as that of the therapies utilized.

Refer to Patient Education

ICD9

710.9 **Connective tissue, diffuse**

References

1. Alarcon G. Unclassified or undifferentiated connective tissue disease. In: Koopman WJ, Boulware DW, Heudebert GR, eds. *Clinical Primer of Rheumatology.* Lippincott Williams and Wilkins. 2003:213–219.
2. Amezcua-Guerra LM, Springall R, Marquez-Velasco R, et al. Presence of antibodies against cyclic citrullinated peptides in patients with "rhupus": A cross-sectional study. *Arthritis Res Ther* 2006;8(5):R144.
3. Rodriguez-Reyna TS, Alarcon-Segovia D. Overlap syndromes in the context of shared autoimmunity. *Autoimmunity* 2005;38(3):219–223.
4. Pipili C, Sfritzeri A, Cholongitas E. Deforming arthropathy in SLE: Review in the literature apropos of one case. *Rheumatol Int* 2009;29(10):1219–1221.
5. Levine D, Switlyk SA, Gottlieb A. Cutaneous lupus erythematosus and anti-TNF-alpha therapy: A case report with review of the literature. *J Drugs Dermatol* 2010;9(10):1283–1287.
6. Soforo E, Baumgarter M, Francis L, et al. Induction of systemic lupus erythematosus with tumor necrosis factor blockers. *J Rheumatol* 2010;37(1):204–205.
7. Jablonska S, Blaszyk M. Scleromyositis (scleroderma/polimyositis overlap) is an entity. *J Eur Acad Dermatol Venereol* 2004;18(3):265–266.
8. Torok L, Dakó K, Cserin G, et al. PM-SCL autoantibody positive scleroderma with polymyositis (mechanic's hand: clinical aid in the diagnosis). *J Eur Acad Dermatol Venereol* 2004;18(3):356–359.
9. Jablonska S, Blaszczyk M. Scleromyositis: A scleroderma/polymyositis overlap syndrome. *Clin Rheumatol* 1998;17(6):465–467.
10. Zold E, Szodoray P, Kappelmayer J, et al. Impaired regulatory T-cell homeostasis due to vitamin D deficiency in undifferentiated connective tissue disease. *Scand J Rheumatol* 2010;39:490–497.

CHAPTER 17 Fibromyalgia

Graciela S. Alarcón

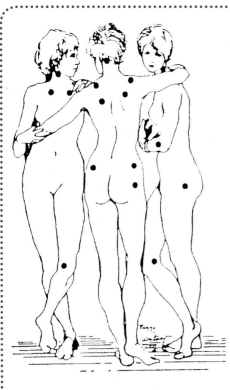

A 40-year-old obese, sedentary, Caucasian woman presents to a rheumatologist with a 6-month history of generalized myalgias, arthralgias, swelling of small hand joints, and morning stiffness of unspecified duration. Her primary care physician had run some tests and referred her for possible rheumatoid arthritis (RA). (IgM rheumatoid factor was positive at 24 units.) Other symptoms elicited by the rheumatologist included fatigue, unrefreshed sleep, intermittent abdominal pain, and increased urinary frequency. Morning stiffness lasted about 30 minutes. Physical examination revealed an obese white woman in no distress. There were multiple tender areas over the upper and lower back, and around the shoulder and pelvic girdles. The hands were puffy (fat), but no synovitis was detected in any of the joints. A complete blood count and a urinalysis were normal. Radiographs of the affected areas were not obtained.

Introduction

Fibromyalgia (FM) is a condition affecting preferentially middle-aged white women; men, children of either gender, and older adults can be affected, however (1). Fibromyalgia has been recognized primarily in the middle and upper socioeconomic strata. Whether this reflects only access to health care or true differences in the incidence and prevalence of the disorder among disadvantaged populations has not been determined.

The true incidence and prevalence of FM is unknown. Population-based studies are difficult to interpret; issues such as the criteria used to diagnose FM, whether primary and secondary cases are included, and the demographic characteristics of the population that is being surveyed need to be considered. Studies from North America and Europe, imperfect as they may be, reveal overall prevalence rates between 1% and 5%, but figures as high as 13% have been reported. These population-based studies confirm the gender distribution (predominantly female) of the FM syndrome. In the clinical setting, the frequency of FM depends, to a certain extent, on the degree of awareness about this condition. Figures between 2% and 4% have been reported in the primary care setting. In rheumatology clinics, the frequency of FM fluctuates between 3% and 20%. These figures probably reflect the rheumatologists' interest in FM and the level of awareness about this condition among community physicians and the public at large (1).

Like many other rheumatic disorders, the etiopathogenesis of FM is probably multifactorial (1). Susceptible individuals may develop FM as a result of the interaction of peripheral and central factors. Familial aggregation of FM does not itself prove genetic susceptibility; in fact, it can be argued that familial aggregation reflects only learned behavior among the offspring of adult patients with FM. However, the familial pattern of FM (affecting primarily the female gender) suggests an autosomal-dominant transmission (1). Animal data indeed suggest that genetic factors may influence pain sensitivity and pain modulation; human data are just emerging (1).

In some patients, FM evolves in an insidious manner. It is impossible to determine precisely when symptoms really started. Other patients, however, can time the onset of their symptoms to a traumatic event (physical or emotional) or to a well-defined infectious process. In fact, these postinfectious cases were called in the past "reactive FM" (comparing them to other postinfectious rheumatic disorders (reactive arthritis)) (1), but this term is no longer used. With regard to trauma, the nature of the trauma does not really matter (severity of injury or even if the event was predominantly physical, but perceived as emotional by the patient) (1). Numerous infectious processes have been described as capable of precipitating FM. They include infections with the human immunodeficiency virus, hepatitis C virus, Coxsackie virus, and Parvovirus B19 (1). Infections with *Borrelia burgdorferi* (Lyme disease) have also been recognized as capable of precipitating FM. It should be noted that, unfortunately, many cases of post-Lyme FM are erroneously diagnosed as chronic Lyme disease and patients are subjected to costly, unnecessary, and lengthy treatments (see Chapters 27 to 30).

Clinical Presentation

Fibromyalgia is a chronic musculoskeletal disorder characterized by generalized pain and tenderness at specific anatomic sites, called *tender points* (1).

Fibromyalgia can occur in isolation or in the setting of other musculoskeletal or rheumatic disorder (primary vs. secondary FM) (1). In fact, in some patients with rheumatoid arthritis (RA) or systemic lupus erythematosus (SLE), the overwhelming clinical manifestations are those of FM, and not the ones we typically attribute to either RA or SLE. These FM symptoms are, by and large, unresponsive to therapies commonly used for the treatment of the underlying condition.

MUSCULOSKELETAL MANIFESTATIONS

Patients with FM often present to their physicians complaining of diffuse arthralgias and myalgias as well as of joint swelling, particularly in the small joints of the hands and feet (1). Some patients also complain of morning stiffness, lasting from minutes to hours; others exhibit joint hypermobility. It should be noted, however, that joint swelling is not present in these patients.

OTHER CLINICAL MANIFESTATIONS

Patients with FM may experience numerous other clinical manifestations. In fact, these other manifestations may be the ones that bring these patients to seek medical help. Symptoms referred to all organ systems have been described. In some cases, these other manifestations, rather than pain, may be the predominant ones.

Fatigue
Patients with FM often complain of some degree of fatigue; rarely, however, is fatigue so intense as to be the factor determining incapacitation, unlike the situation of patients with chronic fatigue syndrome (CFS) (1). In turn, patients

SECTION 3 Specific Rheumatic Diseases

with CFS may experience arthralgias and myalgias, and may exhibit some tender points. Rarely, the patients may meet criteria for both the disorders. Like pain, fatigue is a subjective manifestation, which can only be quantified by self-report.

Sleep Disturbances

Patients with FM, regardless of the intensity of their pain, usually complain of poor sleep; they may have difficulty falling asleep or may wake up throughout the night. As a result, they awake in the morning unrefreshed and tired. Some investigators have postulated that the musculoskeletal pain in FM results from sleep deprivation. Sleep studies conducted in patients with FM have indeed shown abnormal recordings during deep sleep. This pattern, called "non–rapid eye movement anomaly," is characterized by a relative fast frequency (alpha waves) superimposed in a slower delta frequency (1). Similar findings have been obtained in normal individuals subjected to sleep deprivation; these abnormalities are neither specific nor sensitive for FM. Another abnormality, sleep apnea, described in some patients with FM, primarily overweight men, can be considered a marker for this disorder. However, only a careful assessment of sleep (including the spouse or bed partner) may uncover the presence and severity of sleep apnea.

Other Manifestations

Table 17.1 provides other clinical manifestations described in patients with FM. These patients may be under the care of different physicians for their various symptoms and may be subjected to extensive, expensive, and even invasive tests and procedures in order to rule out more serious or different disorders. Imaging and nuclear medicine studies, endoscopies, and exploratory surgeries are, unfortunately, not uncommonly performed. Table 17.1 provides procedures and tests commonly obtained in patients with FM.

Rheumatologists see patients with possible FM in consultation in different situations. One scenario is that of patients with FM who have failed numerous treatments and who come seeking a cure for their ailment. A second scenario is that of patients who want to legitimize their diagnosis for legal purposes (e.g., workman's compensation or disability determination) (1). Still others are patients with different musculoskeletal disorders, who had been diagnosed as having FM but whose diagnoses have been overlooked. Examples include spinal stenosis, peripheral neuropathies, systemic vasculitis, myositis, and polymyalgia rheumatica, among others. A fourth scenario is that of patients who have been diagnosed as having "refractory RA" and have received multiple medications, but have significant joint complaints (pain primarily). If patients are obese, the differentiation between puffy or fatty hands and true arthritis may not be readily evident to the nonrheumatologist. Lastly, other patients have been diagnosed as having SLE or referred for evaluation of possible SLE. They present FM-like manifestations and a positive test for antinuclear antibodies (ANA). They may also have subjective, but not objective, clinical manifestations that render the diagnosis of SLE plausible, until the history is examined more critically (1). For example, patients may present after having had oral or nasal ulcers, photosensitivity, and photosensitive rashes. Similarly, they may complain of Raynaud's phenomenon–like manifestations, alopecia, chest pain (which worsens in inspiration), and of course, arthralgias and myalgias. A positive ANA in this setting reinforces the diagnosis of SLE and, unfortunately, may prompt the initiation of potentially toxic pharmacologic compounds. Although it is never possible to be sure whether such patients may eventually develop SLE, it is preferable to wait until objective evidence of SLE becomes evident and to not alarm these patients unduly.

Table 17.1 Symptoms, Diagnostic Tests or Procedures, and Diagnoses in Patients with Fibromyalgia Seeking Health Care

SPECIALIST	REASONS FOR CONSULTATION	POTENTIAL TESTS/ PROCEDURES	POSSIBLE DIAGNOSES[a]
Internist	Malaise, fatigue, weakness	Various	Various
Cardiologist	Palpitations, chest pain, syncope, hypotension	ECG, exercise test, echocardiogram, conventional and MR angiograms, cardiac catheterization, tilt-table evaluation	Mitral valve prolapse, atypical angina, dysautonomia
Pulmonologist	Dyspnea, snoring	Pulmonary function tests, arterial blood gases, polysomnogram	Asthma, sleep apnea
Gastroenterologist	Dysphagia, dyspepsia, abdominal pain, bloating, constipation, diarrhea	Upper and lower GI tract endoscopies, radiographs and/or biopsies, abdominal CT and/or ultrasound, abdominal angiogram	Noncardiac chest pain, irritable bowel syndrome, gastroesophageal reflux
Endocrinologist	Weakness, faintness	Fasting blood sugars, serum hormone levels	Hypoglycemia
Rheumatologist	Myalgias, arthralgias, Raynaud's phenomenon, weakness, neck and/or back pain, fatigue	Serologic tests, electrophysiologic studies	"Latent," "variant," or "prelupus"; costochondritis; polymyalgia rheumatica; "undifferentiated" CTD
Dermatologist	Pruritus, hives, skin rashes, "photosensitivity"	Skin biopsies	Dermatitis
Allergist	"Allergies"	Skin tests, suppression tests	Allergies Multiple chemical sensitivities
Neurologist	Dizziness, dysesthesias, vertigo, headache, syncope, seizures	CT scans and/or MRIs, MR angiograms, electrophysiologic studies, lumbar puncture, biopsies	Migraine, restless leg syndrome, dysautonomia, anxiety
Gynecologist	Polyuria, dysuria, dyspareunia, "vaginitis," pelvic pain	Cystoscopies, colposcopies	UTI, cystitis, vaginitis, endometriosis
Otorhinolaryngologist	Tinnitus, cough, headache, hoarseness, snoring, vertigo, dizziness	Audiograms, CT scans or MRIs, polysomnogram	Rhinitis, sinusitis, Menièrie, sleep apnea
Orthopedist	Neck and/or back pain	Radiographs, MRIs, and/or CT scans	"Arthritis"
Neurosurgeon	Headache, neck and/or back pain, dysesthesias	CT scans and/or MRIs, electrophysiologic studies	Spinal stenosis, radiculopathy
Ophthalmologist	Dry eyes, blurred vision, double vision	Schirmer test, fluorescein test	Sicca syndrome
Psychiatrist	Anxiety, depression, insomnia, decreased memory, sexual and/or physical abuse	MMPI, neurocognitive evaluation, other psychologic tests	Anxiety, depression, abuse (sexual and/or physical)
Dentist	Dry mouth	Salivary gland biopsy	Sicca syndrome

Modified from Alarcón GS. Fibromyalgia: Dispelling diagnostic and treatment myths. *Wmn Health Pri Care (Orth Ed)* 1999;2:11–22.

CT, computerized tomography; CTD, connective tissue disease; ECG, electrocardiograms; GI, gastrointestinal; MMPI, Minnesota Multiphasic Personality Inventory; MR, magnetic resonance; MRI, MR imaging; UTI, urinary tract infection.

[a]Some of these diagnoses represent true associations. Others, unfortunately, are given to patients in an effort to explain their symptoms, but lack organic basis.

SECTION 3 Specific Rheumatic Diseases

NOT TO BE MISSED

- Sleep apnea
- Systemic lupus erythematosus
- Rheumatoid arthritis
- Polymyalgia rheumatica
- Peripheral neuropathy
- Spinal stenosis
- Depression

Examination

A careful history (multitude of somatic complaints, fatigue, poor sleep, and impaired cognition) and a complete physical examination (not limited to tender points) should point to the correct diagnosis. The examination typically does not identify any organic musculoskeletal cause of pain and typically only tenderness in typical tender points and hyperalgesia at times.

Studies

At this time, the inclusion of either imaging brain studies (particularly SPECT) or the study of serum and CSF levels of neuropeptides in all patients with FM is not recommended (Fig. 17.2). As useful as these studies have been and continue to be in clarifying the nature of this mysterious condition, their diagnostic properties (sensitivity, specificity, and negative, positive, and overall predictive value) have not been determined, and their risk and cost make them currently unjustifiable. Other ancillary studies including laboratory tests should be ordered only as clinically indicated or to exclude other conditions that present with clinical features similar to FM, such as sleep studies to exclude sleep apnea or thyroid function tests to exclude hypothyroidism.

Although the condition had been recognized for decades under other names (*nonarticular rheumatism*, *psychogenic rheumatism*, and *fibrositis*), it was not until 1990 that the ACR defined criteria for the classification of these patients and FM was "officially" borne. Generalists, however, never felt quite comfortable with the examination of tender points (Fig. 17.1); the ACR has recently published revised diagnostic criteria that encompass a measure of symptom severity, reflecting the nonarticular manifestations of FM (2). According to the new diag-

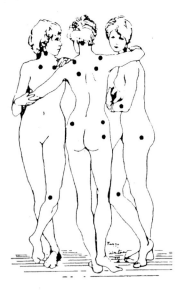

Figure 17.1 Tender point locations for the 1990 American College of Rheumatology classification criteria for fibromyalgia. Adapted from Wolfe F, Smythe HA, Yunus MB, et al. The American College of Rheumatology 1990 criteria for the classification of fibromyalgia: Report of the multicenter criteria committee. *Arthritis Rheum* 1990;33:160–172, by permission.

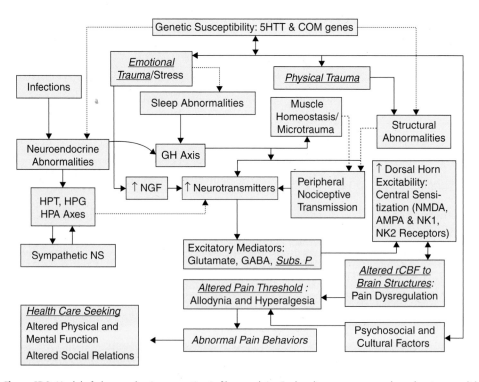

Figure 17.2 Model of abnormal pain perception in fibromyalgia. *Broken lines* are proposed mechanisms; *solid lines,* defined mechanisms. *HPT,* hypothalamic–pituitary–thyroid axis; *HPG,* hypothalamic–pituitary–gonadal axis; *HPA,* hypothalamic–pituitary–adrenal axis; *GH,* growth hormone axis; *NGF,* nerve growth factor; *NS,* nervous system; *NO,* nitric oxide; *rCBF,* regional cerebral blood flow. Modified from Weigent DA, Bradley LA, Blalock JE, et al. Fibromyalgia; Dispelling diagnostic and treatment myths. *Am J Med Sci* 1998;315:405–412.

Table 17.2 Criteria and Ascertainment of Fibromyalgia

Criteria

A patient satisfies diagnostic criteria for fibromyalgia if the following three conditions are met:

1. Widespread Pain Index (WPI) ≥7 and Symptom Severity (SS) scale score ≥5 or WPI 3–6 and SS scale score ≥9
2. Symptoms have been present at a similar level for at least 3 months
3. The patient does not have a disorder that would otherwise explain the pain

Ascertainment

1. If WPI: note the number of areas in which the patient has had pain over the last week. In how many areas has the patient had pain? Score will be between 0 and 19

Shoulder girdle, left	Hip (buttock, trochanter), left	Jaw, left	Upper back
Shoulder girdle, right	Hip (buttock, trochanter), right	Jaw, right	Lower back
Upper arm, left	Upper leg, left	Chest	Neck
Upper arm, right	Upper leg, right	Abdomen	
Lower arm, left	Lower leg, left		
Lower arm, right	Lower leg, right		

2. SS scale score:
   Fatigue
   Waking unrefreshed
   Cognitive symptoms

For the each of the three symptoms above, indicate the level of severity over the past week using the following scale:
   0—no problem
   1—slight or mild problems, generally mild or intermittent
   2—moderate, considerable problems, often present and/or at a moderate level
   3—severe: pervasive, continuous, life-disturbing problems

Considering somatic symptoms in general, indicate whether the patient has:
   0—no symptoms
   1—few symptoms
   2—a moderate number of symptoms
   3—a great deal of symptoms

The SS scale score is the sum of the severity of the three symptoms (fatigue, waking unrefreshed, cognitive symptoms) plus the extent (severity) of somatic symptoms in general. The final score is between 0 and 12

With permission from reference 2.

nostic criteria, FM is present if the following conditions are met: (a) Widespread Pain Index (WPI) ≥7 and symptom severity (SS) scale ≥5 or WPI between 3 and 6 and SS ≥9; (b) symptoms have been present for at least 3 months; and (c) the patient does not have other disorder to explain his or her symptoms. Widespread Pain Index is defined by points given to different body regions (range: 0 to 19) and SS comprises four domains: fatigue, unrefreshed sleep, cognitive impairment, and somatic complaints—each one measured in a scale from 0 to 3 for a total of 12 possible points (Table 17.2). These criteria correctly classified between 89% and 95% of patients with FM. Either the 1990 or 2010 criterion can be used in the clinical and research settings.

Treatment

Given that we are just beginning to understand this disorder, it should not come as a surprise that we have limited effective therapies to manage these patients. Primary care physicians have the tremendous responsibility of steering patients away from unproved (and often risky) treatments. Patients with FM need to first believe that we, their health care providers, acknowledge that their pain is real and causes suffering (1). Second, realistic goals should be established from the outset. Third, it should be emphasized that pharmacologic compounds constitute only one element of the overall treatment plan. Other elements include a balance between exercise and rest; a diet aimed at achieving or maintaining an ideal body weight; avoidance of alcohol, caffeine, nicotine, and recreational drugs; and modification of abnormal sleep behaviors or habits (3).

Patients with FM are so often overweight and deconditioned that they have to start an exercise program very gradually. Aquatic exercises rather than land exercises are better tolerated; unfortunately, year-round aquatic programs exist only in urban areas and are not accessible to all patients. If these facilities exist, however, patients should be strongly advised to enter aquatic exercise programs under proper supervision. Low-impact aerobics is an alternative for patients lacking aquatic facilities. Recently, favorable results in terms of the Fibromyalgia Impact Questionnaire and the SF-36 have been reported with classic Young-style Tai Chi in a small 12-week single-blinded study; although a larger and longer confirmatory study is needed, these data are certainly relevant (4).

Unfortunately, many patients with FM present to rheumatologists with a (sometimes very large) sac or box, which includes current and past medications (in addition to a binder with medical records and a stack of radiographs and imaging studies). Once patients have reached this level of polypharmacy, it is extremely difficult to simplify their therapeutic regimen. Moreover, the rationale for the use of some compounds is virtually lacking. That is the case, for example, for nonsteroidal anti-inflammatory drugs (NSAIDs) usually detailed to generalists and specialists alike as the panacea for "arthritis" and prescribed quite often to patients with FM (5). Other than their possible central effect (purely analgesic), there is no reason to use them. Narcotic analgesics (of different strength and quality) are, unfortunately, also commonly used, even in children and young adults. It is my experience that once patients with FM start this type of analgesic, they rarely are able to discontinue it. Muscle relaxants are also commonly used for a prolonged time. Nonsteroidal anti-inflammatory drugs, narcotic analgesics, and muscle relaxants, if used, need to be prescribed judiciously and for limited time periods (e.g., during exacerbation of background pain or after trauma in patients with joint hypermobility). This should be discussed with the patient from the outset (1). Patients need to understand that FM per se does not produce physical deformities and that despite pain, a relatively normal life—including work, family, and recreational activities—is possible. Living with pain can, however, exert a toll on patients and families with studies suggesting that FM is a risk factor for self-inflicted death (6, 7).

Pharmacologic compounds found to be beneficial in patients with FM include the tricyclic antidepressants (TCAs) as well as the selective serotonin reuptake inhibitors (SSRIs), independent of whether patients are depressed (1). Among the TCAs, amitriptyline is the most commonly used (1). The starting dose varies between 10 and 25 mg/day and can be escalated to 50 to 75 mg/day. In terms of the SSRIs, the most commonly used is fluoxetine; the most frequent dose is 20 mg/day, but higher doses have been used. Other SSRIs including citalopram, sertraline hydrochloride, and have also been used. Double reuptake inhibitors such as milnacipran venlafaxine and duloxetine have also been shown to be of benefit in patients with FM (8). Finally, a meta-analysis of the effectiveness of antidepressants in FM for the outcome of pain has shown them to be beneficial (9). The newest "kid on the block" is pregabalin (10). In the landmark 2005 study of Crofford et al., 529 patients with FM were randomized to either 150, 300, 450 mg or placebo, with the 450 mg group demonstrating improvement in terms of pain, fatigue, and sleep. A number of other pregabalin studies have now been performed with one of them being of longer duration

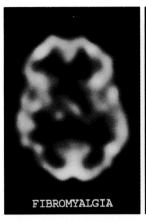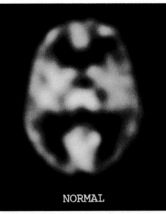

FIBROMYALGIA   NORMAL

Figure 17.3 Single-photon-emission computerized tomography of the brain in a normal individual and one with fibromyalgia. There is decreased regional cerebral flow to the thalamus and caudate nuclei in the patient with fibromyalgia. Modified from Alarcón GS. Fibromyalgia: Dispelling diagnostic and treatment myths. *Wmn Health Pri Care (Orth Ed)* 1999;2:11–22.

WHEN TO REFER

- When the diagnosis is in doubt and a more serious rheumatic disorder is being considered.

- When the patient would like to have a second opinion to confirm diagnosis.

(11); overall, these studies support the original report of Crofford et al. Anxiolytics and other psychopharmaceutical drugs should be restricted to patients with clear-cut indications for their use (concomitant psychopathology).

The role of liniments and other topical preparations (substance P antagonists, such as capsaicin) in the treatment of FM is probably limited to those circumstances in which there is definite added local pathology to a region or area of the musculoskeletal system (e.g., a shoulder, elbow, trochanteric or anserine bursa). In the past, rheumatologists frequently injected several tender points with corticosteroids and anesthetics every so often. Some patients indeed reported these injections to be beneficial. This effect probably relates to the use of steroids and their systemic absorption, rather than to their local effect. The rationality for performing periodic soft-tissue injections in all patients with FM is nonexistent, other than perhaps "needling" these patients in much the same way as is done with acupuncture, now a recognized alternative treatment for FM (1). The role of soft-tissue massages, hypnotherapy, relaxation, and spinal manipulations for the treatment of FM is undetermined for now.

Claims have appeared on the Internet of the successful treatment of FM with decompressive surgery of the craniocervical junction (1). This surgery is based on the reported possible association of FM with Chiari malformation (protrusion of the tonsils below the level of the foramen magnum). Although we recognize that patients with cervical spinal stenosis may exhibit some FM-like manifestations, searching for this association should be done only if clinical manifestations are indicative of canal stenosis and compressive myelopathy, but not otherwise (1). Unfortunately, the Internet has favored the dissemination of unfiltered information capable of directly reaching many more patients than with methods used in the past. (Millions of Web sites are found.) PCPs should be properly informed so that patients receive adequate counseling and unnecessary and risky surgical procedures are avoided.

Clinical Course

Although patients with FM do not develop obvious physical deformities or impairments, this disorder can affect several domains of their lives (pain, iatrogenesis, employment, and financial and family stability) (1, 6, 7). Patients who remain employed, physically active, and trim; take few medications; and have adequate coping skills and a supportive family tend to do better than those who are physically inactive, unemployed, overweight, and already taking many medications.

Conclusions

Although we do not completely understand all the mechanisms involved in the musculoskeletal pain patients with FM have, we have made significant strides toward understanding them. Drawing from our studies and those of other investigators, we have put together a testable pain model. The contributions of peripheral and central factors to the pathogenesis of pain in FM are shown in Figure 17.3, which is an iteration of the model our group has published before (1). This model should be modified as new evidence emerges from research conducted worldwide. Figure 17.4 summarizes the main points discussed in this chapter.

SECTION 3 Specific Rheumatic Diseases

*Fibromyalgia is not a psychiatric disorder. The misconception that fibromyalgia may be an affective disorder arose from the fact that patients seen in tertiary care centers (patients included in most clinical trials and studies) often have a concomitant psychiatric illness. However, they are not typical of all persons with fibromyalgia.

*Criteria for the classification of fibromyalgia (2000) patients include widespread and persistent musculoskeletal pain and the presence of soft tissue tender points in at least 11 of 18 anatomic sites called "tender points" (See Figure 20.1). However, these criteria were developed for research and not so much for clinical practice. In fact, a new set of criteria have been proposed (2010) which do not include these tender points but, in addition to widespread pain, include a symptom severity scale (See Table 20.1).

*The following findings help support the diagnosis of fibromyalgia (and some of them are considered in the symptom severity scale of the 2010 preliminary diagnostic criteria, as noted in Table 20.1): fatigue, difficulty sleeping, arthralgias, headache, chest, abdominal, pelvic and/or perineal pain, cognitive impairment, weakness, and dysesthesias.

*Why patients with fibromyalgia experience chronic pain remains unknown, although evidence points out to aberrations in CNS processing of stimuli. Abnormalities of the endocrine system, sleep disturbances, altered cerebral blood flow to the thalamus and caudate nucleus, bilateral activation of the somatosensory cortices on painful stimulation, increase resting brain activity within multiple brain networks and altered neuropeptide serum and CSF levels are seen in these patients (See Fig. 17.3 for a model of fibromyalgia etiopathogenesis).

*Although the etiology of fibromyalgia remains unknown, several triggers have been identified: bacterial (i.e., *Borrelia Burgdorferi*) or viral (i.e., Parvovirus) infections, physical and/or emotional trauma, and sleep deprivation. However, in some patients the onset of fibromyalgia is insidious, and no triggers can be identified. A genetic predisposition is supported by studies in twins and siblings.

*Managing patients with fibromyalgia is challenging. A combination of pharmacological and non-pharmacological options is recommended. Non-pharmacological options include cognitive-behavioral therapy, exercise (combined with periods of rest). Newer pharmacological options including the double reuptake inhibitors and pregabalin have been shown to be beneficial. Antidepressants, in general, have shown to be beneficial as well.

*NSAIDs and glucocorticoids are not indicated for the treatment of patients with fibromyalgia except under specific circumstances (localized area of pain of clear inflammatory nature). However, NSAIDs can be used sporadically for their analgesic effects. Narcotic analgesics and other psychotropic drugs should be avoided if at all possible.

Figure 17.4 Important practical issues in fibromyalgia. Modified from Alarcón GS. *Wmn Health Pri Care (Orth Ed)* 1999;2:11–22.

ICD9

729.1 **Fibromyalgia**

References

1. Alarcon G. Fibromyalgia. In: Koopman WJ, Boulware DW, Heudebert GR, eds. Lippincott Williams and Wilkins; 2003:226–235.
2. Wolfe F, Clauw DJ, Fitzcharles MA, et al. The American College of Rheumatology preliminary diagnostic criteria for fibromyalgia and measurement of symptom severity. *Arthritis Care Res* 2010;62:600–610.
3. Bernardy K, Füber N, Köllner V, et al. Efficacy of cognitive-behavioral therapies in fibromyalgia syndrome— a systematic review and meta-analysis of randomized controlled trials. *J Rheumatol* 2010;37:1991–2005.
4. Wang C, Schmid CH, Rones R, et al. A randomized trial of tai chi for fibromyalgia. *N Engl J Med* 2010;363(8):743–754.
5. Bennett RM, Jones J, Turk DC, et al. An internet survey of 2,596 people with fibromyalgia. *BMC Musculoskelet Disord* 2007;8:27.
6. Wolfe F, Hassett AL, Walitt B, et al. Mortality in fibromyalgia: An 8,186 patient study over 35 years. *Arthritis Care Res* 2011;63:94–101.
7. Dreyer L, Kendall S, Danneskiold-Samsøe B, et al. Mortality in a cohort of Danish patients with fibromyalgia: Increased frequency of suicide. *Arthritis Rheum* 2010;62:3101–3108.
8. Goldenberg DL, Clauw DJ, Palmer RH, et al. Durability of therapeutic response to milnacipran treatment for fibromyalgia. Results of a randomized, double-blind, monotherapy 6-month extension study. *Pain Med* 2010;11:180–194.
9. Häuser W, Bernardy K, Uçeyler N, et al. Treatment of fibromyalgia syndrome with antidepressants: A meta-analysis. *JAMA* 2009;301:198–209.
10. Crofford LJ, Rowbotham MC, Mease PJ, et al. Pregabalin for the treatment of fibromyalgia syndrome: Results of a randomized, double-blind, placebo-controlled trial. *Arthritis Rheum* 2005;52:1264–1273.
11. Crofford LJ, Mease PJ, Simpson SL, et al. Fibromyalgia relapse evaluation and efficacy for durability of meaningful relief (FREEDOM): A 6-month, double-blind, placebo-controlled trial with pregabalin. *Pain* 2008;136:419–431.

18 Pregnancy and Rheumatic Diseases

Michael Lockshin

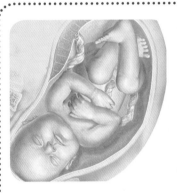

A 39-year-old woman with long-standing rheumatoid arthritis, which she believes is now quiescent, consults you because she is planning a pregnancy. She has not been under regular medical care, but instead has taken ibuprofen or naproxen on an as-needed basis for joint pain. A prior pregnancy 3 years earlier was successfully delivered at term. She comes now at the insistence of her colleague. She asks for your advice regarding risks to her and her potential child, particularly those imparted by treatment. You point out that anti-inflammatory medications interfere with cilial motion that transports the ovum through the Fallopian tube and, thus, modestly inhibits fertility.

Your evaluation shows moderately active synovitis in her wrists (with signs of early carpal tunnel syndrome), elbows, and knees. Her laboratory studies show strong positive rheumatoid factor, anticyclic citrullinated peptide, and anti-Sjogren's syndrome A (SSA), also known as anti-Ro. Anti-Sjogren's syndrome B (SSB) antibodies, also known as anti-La, anticardiolipin, anti-β_2-glycoprotein I, and lupus anticoagulant tests are negative. Lateral cervical spine x-ray in flexion and extension shows 11-mm displacement of the odontoid process from the anterior arch of the atlas in flexion.

Clinical Presentation

That the patient has not been in medical contact despite ongoing disease is a matter of concern. Her choice may reflect misunderstanding about her illness, conflicts with her physicians, social or financial issues, denial, or other issues. Whatever the reason, her earlier choice to avoid medical care raises flags for management of a future pregnancy.

EXAMINATION

Immediate things to assess include careful joint examination, focusing especially on joint instability, because of potential worsening as pregnancy-associated relaxin loosens ligaments in late pregnancy. Cervical spine subluxation and C1 to C2 instability are especially important because of potential cord injury. It may be necessary to provide the patient with a rigid collar during late pregnancy and during delivery, when intubation is a possibility. Ligament loosening at the hip and knee may cause gait problems as pregnancy progresses. Carpal tunnel symptoms typically worsen in late pregnancy.

STUDIES AND TREATMENT

Infants of mothers with anti-SSA and anti-SSB antibodies are at risk for neonatal lupus (rash, about 20%; congenital heart block, about 3%) (1). Pregnancies characterized by these autoantibodies require special monitoring of fetal cardiac status (by fetal echocardiogram looking for ventricular contraction strength, pericarditis, and atrial–ventricular conduction delay) between weeks 15 and 26 (2).

However, effective treatment for in utero heart block is not available (3); early delivery may be required. Neonatal lupus rash, if it occurs, will appear after delivery. Hydroxychloroquine may be protective (4).

Patients with any rheumatic illness may have antiphospholipid antibodies. Low-titer antiphospholipid antibodies do not appear to impart risk and need not be treated; lupus anticoagulant and possibly high-titer IgG anticardiolipin may lead to early, severe preeclampsia, premature delivery, and fetal growth restriction or death (5). For this patient, the negative tests and the prior successful pregnancy are reassuring that she is not at risk. Evidence is unclear whether pregnant patients *with lupus anticoagulant* who have *not* had a prior thrombosis or fetal loss should be prophylactically treated with heparin (prophylactic doses, usually 1 mg/kg enoxaparin per day or its equivalent). Evidence is weak that it is necessary to treat patients who have anticardiolipin antibody without lupus anticoagulant, but not prior thrombosis or fetal loss. Patients with prior fetal losses and high-titer anticardiolipin or lupus anticoagulant but no prior thromboses should receive prophylactic dose treatment; those with prior thromboses should receive therapeutic dose treatment (1 mg/kg enoxaparin every 12 hours or its equivalent).

CLINICAL COURSE

Your patient achieves pregnancy through ovarian stimulation, ovum retrieval, in vitro fertilization, and embryo implantation. This process involves daily injections of follicle-stimulating hormone followed by human chorionic gonadotropin, laparoscopic removal of mature ova, fertilization in vitro, examination of the growing embryo for chromosomal abnormalities, and implantation into the uterine cavity. During this procedure, the patient is at risk for ovarian hyperstimulation syndrome, in which multiple ova mature simultaneously. In mild cases, this results in abdominal pain; in severe cases, fluid retention, cytokine storm, and renal failure. Other than hyperstimulation syndrome, the risks of assisted reproductive techniques are not unduly high for patients with rheumatic disease, even those with antiphospholipid antibodies (6).

During her pregnancy, because she has anti-SSA antibodies, her fetus should be monitored, by fetal echocardiography, between weeks 15 and 26 for signs of the carditis associated with neonatal lupus. If such occurs, treatment of the fetus with dexamethasone or betamethasone or intravenous immunoglobulin may be attempted, but success rates are low (3); delivery may be indicated to prevent progression. Although not relevant for this patient, pregnancies of women with antiphospholipid antibodies must also be monitored for fetal growth rate, placental size and health, and amniotic fluid volume. Women at highest risk are those with lupus anticoagulant, very high titer anticardiolipin antibody, or systemic lupus erythematosus. Patients with low-titer antibody who lack lupus anticoagulant are likely not at risk, nor are those with isolated other autoantibodies, such as antibody to β_2-glycoprotein I or antiphosphatidylserine. Patients with high-titer antiphospholipid antibodies who have had prior pregnancy loss should be prophylactically treated with heparin, prophylactic doses, for example, 1 mg/kg enoxaparin plus 81 mg aspirin daily, from conception to delivery; patients with prior thrombosis should receive therapeutic doses, for example, 1 mg/kg enoxaparin every 12 hours. The need to treat patients with high-titer anticardiolipin or lupus anticoagulant with no prior pregnancy losses is not established; because some physicians may advise treatment and others not, negotiation with the patient, her obstetrician, and other concerned family members is necessary. Sometimes acceding to treatment requests of older or infertile women who may not meet treatment criteria, but who have limited opportunity for future pregnancies, is required.

Patients with high-titer antiphospholipid antibodies are additionally at risk for early, severe preeclampsia. In rheumatoid arthritis and other rheumatic diseases, differential diagnosis is not difficult, but proteinuria, thrombocytopenia, and hypertension closely resemble systemic lupus erythematosus flare (7). Distinguishing features between lupus and preeclampsia are as follows: urinary erythrocyte casts occur in lupus nephritis, but not preeclampsia; normocomplementemia is unusual in lupus nephritis, but hypocomplementemia may occur in both. Lupus rash, arthritis, fever, and lymphadenopathy do not occur in preeclampsia. However, painful palmar erythema ("vasculitis") occurs in both.

For patients with destructive arthritis, delivery merits special care. Cervical spine disease and temporomandibular disease may complicate intubation or other handling on the delivery table. Shoulder and elbow disease may complicate emergency placement of intravenous lines; hand and wrist disease may interfere with tight gripping of handles during the "push" stage of vaginal delivery. Normal vaginal delivery requires full hip flexion and abduction, and full knee flexion. In the heat of delivery, obstetric staff may overestimate mobility and dislocate or fracture joints with limited range of motion. The risk is especially high for patients with hip replacements.

A normal labor may take 18 or more hours, during which the patient may not be able to take her normal medications. Especially for maintenance corticosteroids, the rheumatologist should remind the obstetric staff to give these medications intravenously.

CONCLUSIONS

Postpartum issues include relatively slow recovery because of the mother's chronic illness. (The contemporary "in-and-out in 1 day" practice for delivery should be avoided.) Medications should be resumed quickly, with attention to those medications acceptable for breast-feeding if the mother chooses to do this. (Several sources of information about acceptable medications are available; 8, 9.) Mothers with upper extremity arthritis may be unable to cradle a baby for nursing. Mothers with any chronic illness may be unable to breast-feed or care for their infants in the way they wish, potentially leading to depression or family conflict or both.

Because familiarity with the many potential complications of rheumatic disease pregnancy is not widespread, referral to an expert in the field for consultation at least once is advisable. Some patients, for instance those with no serologic warning signs or anatomic risks, may be considered low risk and need no further evaluation. Those with antiphospholipid antibodies, anti-SSA/Ro and anti-SSB/La antibodies, with prior fetal loss or complicated pregnancies, anatomic disabilities, renal or cardiopulmonary disease, thrombocytopenia, and requiring potentially toxic medications should all receive specialized care.

References

1. Brucato A, Cimaz R, Caporali R, et al. Pregnancy outcomes in patients with autoimmune diseases and anti-Ro/SSA antibodies. *Clin Rev Allergy Immunol* 2011;40(1):27–41.
2. Buyon JP, Clancy RM, Friedman DM. Cardiac manifestations of neonatal lupus erythematosus: Guidelines to management, integrating clues from the bench and bedside. *Nat Clin Pract Rheumatol* 2009;5(3):139–148. [Review]
3. Friedman DM, Llanos C, Izmirly PM, et al. Evaluation of fetuses in a study of intravenous immunoglobulin as preventive therapy for congenital heart block: Results of a multicenter, prospective, open-label clinical trial. *Arthritis Rheum* 2010;62(4):1138–1146.
4. Izmirly PM, Kim MY, Llanos C, et al. Evaluation of the risk of anti-SSA/Ro-SSB/La antibody-associated cardiac manifestations of neonatal lupus in fetuses of mothers with systemic lupus erythematosus exposed to hydroxychloroquine. *Ann Rheum Dis* 2010;69(10):1827–1830, epub May 6, 2010.
5. Salmon J, Girardi G, Lockshin MD. The antiphospholipid syndrome—a disorder initiated by inflammation: Implications for therapy of pregnant patients. *Nat Clin Pract Rheumatol* 2007;3(3):140–147.

SECTION 3 Specific Rheumatic Diseases

6. Guballa N, Sammaritano L, Schwartzman S, et al. Ovulation induction and in vitro fertilization in lupus and antiphospholipid antibody syndrome. *Arthritis Rheum* 2000;43:550–556.
7. Ruiz-Irastorza G, Khamashta M, Gordon C, et al. Measuring systemic lupus erythematosus activity during pregnancy: Validation of the scale Lupus Activity Index in Pregnancy (LAI-P). *Arthritis Care Res* 2004;51:78–82.
8. Ostensen M, Lockshin M, Doria A, et al. Update on safety during pregnancy of biological agents and some immunosuppressive anti-rheumatic drugs. In: Cutolo M, Matucci-Cerinic M, Lockshin MD, Ostensen M, co-eds. *Pregnancy in the Rheumatic Diseases. Rheumatology* 2008;47(Suppl 3):28–31.
9. Østensen M, Khamashta M, Lockshin M, et al. Antirheumatic drug therapy and reproduction. *Arthritis Res Ther* 2006;8:209.

Osteoarthritis and Metabolic Bone and Joint Disease

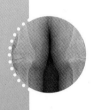

Chapter 19 **Osteoarthritis**

Mary S. Walton, Carlos J. Lozada, and Seth M. Berney

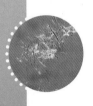

Chapter 20 **Gout and Crystal-Induced Arthropathies**

Angelo Gaffo

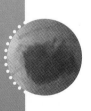

Chapter 21 **Osteopenic Bone Diseases and Osteonecrosis**

Kenneth G. Saag, Gregory A. Clines, and Sarah L. Morgan

Chapter 22 **Arthropathies Associated with Systemic Diseases**

Leann Maska and Amy C. Cannella

(19) Osteoarthritis

Mary S. Walton, Carlos J. Lozada, and Seth M. Berney

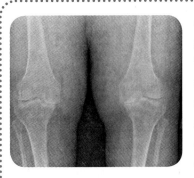

A 60-year-old male former professional football player with a history of multiple knee injuries complains of bilateral knee pain for 10 years. The patient also complains of bilateral wrist pain and 15 to 20 minutes of morning stiffness. He denies joint swelling, Raynaud's phenomena, sicca symptoms, fever, or chills.

On physical examination, he is a non–ill-appearing male with a nontender nodule on the right index distal interphalangeal (DIP) joint and bony enlargement of right long and left ring proximal interphalangeal (PIP) and DIP joints. He also has tenderness on palpation at the base of bilateral thumbs' carpometacarpal (CMC) joints and enlargement of his bilateral knees with pain and crepitus on passive range of motion. His wrists, metacarpophalangeal (MCP) joints, elbows, hips, and ankles are normal (Fig. 19.1).

Introduction

Osteoarthritis (OA), also referred to as degenerative joint disease (DJD), is the most common form of joint disease in humans. Because of physician visits, medications, surgical intervention, and time missed from work, OA appears to cost as much as 30 times more than rheumatoid arthritis (RA) (1).

Osteoarthritis was once thought to be the result of aging. However, we now believe that it develops as a consequence of multiple factors, including biochemical and biomechanical abnormalities, as well as genetic predispositions manifesting clinically as OA.

EPIDEMIOLOGY

Osteoarthritis can be defined radiographically or clinically (radiographs plus clinical symptoms or signs). Utilizing radiographic criteria, 30% of individuals between the ages of 45 and 65 are affected, and more than 80% are affected by their eighth decade of life.

The prevalence of OA increases in both men and women as they age, but gender differences exist. Osteoarthritis affects men more commonly among patients younger than 45 years and women more commonly among patients older than 55 years. Additionally, DIP OA is ten times more likely in women than in men. Mothers and sisters of women with DIP OA are two to three times more likely to be affected by it (2).

Obesity in women has been linked to OA of the knees and hip (3) and is probably also a risk factor for knee OA in men Obesity is also a risk factor for hand OA in both genders. The mechanisms for this have not been clearly elucidated and may include increase in body mass, altered biomechanics of gait, genetic predisposition, and/or altered metabolism. We also cannot adequately explain the association between obesity and OA of non–weight-bearing joints such as the sternoclavicular and DIP joints.

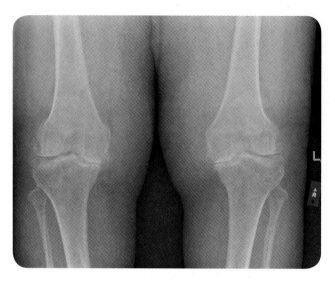

Figure 19.1 Standing (weight-bearing) view of the knees indicates significant bilateral medial joint space narrowing, moderate bilateral lateral compartment joint space narrowing, and medial and lateral joint osteophyte formation.

PATHOGENESIS

Initially thought of as a disease only of articular cartilage, OA involves the entire joint, including the subchondral bone. Because the role of inflammation in OA with increased expression of cytokines and metalloproteinases in synovium and cartilage is becoming more recognized, the term *degenerative joint disease* is no longer appropriate when referring to OA. Furthermore, the contention that OA is "noninflammatory" is incorrect, while "mildly inflammatory" would be a more accurate description.

The etiopathogenesis of OA has been divided into three stages (5). During stage 1, increased production of proteolytic enzymes such as metalloproteinases (e.g., collagenase and stromelysin) destroys the cartilage matrix. During stage 2, the cartilage surface erodes and fibrillates, releasing proteoglycans and collagen fragments into the synovial fluid. Finally, in stage 3, these cartilage breakdown products induce a chronic inflammatory response in the synovium, characterized by macrophage production of interleukin 1 (IL-1), tumor necrosis factor (TNF-α), and metalloproteinases. These substances probably increase the cartilage ulcerations and may stimulate chondrocytes to produce more metalloproteinases, resulting in cartilage loss and bony eburnation and ultimately subchondral bone osteophyte formation.

Clinical Presentation

The initial goal of the health care professional when seeing a patient with joint pain is to differentiate OA from more inflammatory arthritides, such as RA.

In contrast to OA, RA primarily affects the wrists, MCP joints, and PIP joints (PIP), and spares the DIP joints and thoracic and lumbosacral spine. Rheumatoid arthritis is also typically associated with inflammatory morning stiffness (more than 1 hour) and radiographic findings of bone loss (periarticular osteopenia; marginal erosions of bone) rather than bone formation.

Symptomatic hip OA is usually insidious in onset and may cause diminished internal rotation, a limp, and groin or buttock pain. However, not uncommonly, patients may experience low back pain or medial knee pain, representing pain referred from the hip. Pain in the lateral aspect of the thigh, around the greater trochanter that is usually reproducible on palpation, usually represents greater trochanteric bursitis, not OA.

Osteoarthritis of the lumbar spine can cause spinal stenosis. These symptoms may include pseudoclaudication with intermittent or constant pain in the legs worsened by exertion (particularly when the patient stands straight up or hyperextends the back, such as descending stairs) and relieved by flexing the back, sitting, or walking upstairs.

Erosive OA, a disorder occurring primarily in women, causes inflammation of the DIP or PIP joints, resulting in a central joint erosion (described as "seagulls" on radiograph).

Multiple causes of secondary OA exist, including joint trauma (fractures or surgeries), prior inflammatory arthropathy, Paget disease, hemophilia, multiple endocrinopathies, neuropathic or Charcot joints, and congenital or hypermobility disorders.

The disease progression is characteristically slow, over years or decades. Eventually, these events alter the joint architecture, and additional bone grows as it remodels to stabilize the joint.

CLINICAL POINTS

- What Differentiates OA From RA
- Asymmetric joint involvement
- Bony joint enlargement (not joint swelling)
- New bone formation (osteophytes)
- Morning stiffness <45 to 60 minutes
- Involvement of DIP joints, PIP joints, and/or spine; sparing MCP joints

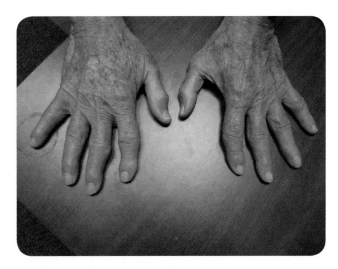

Figure 19.2 Bony joint enlargement of the right thumb interphalangeal joint, bilateral index and long finger proximal interphalangeal (PIP) joints, and multiple distal interphalangeal (DIP) joints with angulations at the right ring finger DIP, long finger PIP and DIP, index finger PIP and DIP, and the left index finger PIP and DIP joints.

Examination

The physical examination findings are limited to the affected joints. On inspection, there may be bony enlargement and malalignment (such as angulation of the PIP, DIP, or knee joints) depending on disease severity. Heberden's and/or Bouchard's nodes (compressed fibrogelatinous cysts) overlying the DIP and PIP joints, respectively, may develop and inflame (Fig. 19.2).

A noninflammatory joint effusion (defined as a WBC count of 200 to 2,000 WBC/mm^3) may occur, usually without significant joint erythema or warmth. Patients have pain on active or passive range of motion of the affected joints. Crepitus (a grating or grinding sensation that occurs as the joint is moving) is characteristic of larger joints, such as the knees. Limitation of joint motion may be present in more advanced cases, as well as periarticular muscle atrophy secondary to disuse.

Diagnostic Studies

Osteoarthritis typically does not cause any conventional laboratory abnormalities other than a noninflammatory synovial fluid analysis (a leukocyte cell count of 200 to 2,000/mm^3, with a mononuclear predominance). In contrast, the laboratory findings in RA correlate with systemic inflammation and commonly include elevated acute-phase reactants (erythrocyte sedimentation rate and C-reactive protein) and the "anemia of chronic disease." Eighty percent of patients eventually have a positive serum rheumatoid factor. Inflammatory joint fluid (WBC >2,000 cells/mm^3 with a polymorphonuclear cell predominance) further differentiates the two diseases.

Radiographic findings most indicative of OA are bony growths at the joint margins known as osteophytes (colloquially known as "bone spurs"). Other findings include asymmetric joint space narrowing, subchondral sclerosis, and subchondral cyst formation. The severity of the radiographic findings often fails to correlate with symptoms until the joint space is obliterated. When radiographing knees and hips, weight-bearing (or upright) views result in a more realistic image of the joint.

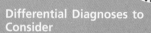

Treatment

The management of OA includes preventive and therapeutic (nonpharmacologic and pharmacologic) *components*.

PREVENTIVE THERAPY

Although many of the presently established risk factors, such as increasing age and genetics, cannot be altered, the single most important modifiable factor emerging from epidemiologic trials is obesity.

Weight loss should be a goal in patients who are obese because even modest weight loss has been accompanied by, at times, a dramatic improvement in back and lower extremity symptoms.

SYMPTOMATIC THERAPY OF OA

The most effective symptomatic therapy combines several simultaneous approaches and may be more effective if a multidisciplinary approach is used (e.g., the rheumatologist, physiatrist, orthopedist, physical therapist, occupational therapist, psychologist, psychiatrist, nurse/nurse coordinator, dietitian, and social worker).

Physical Measures

A variety of physical modalities are valuable for improving the symptoms of OA, and include exercise, supportive devices, alterations in activities of daily living, and thermal modalities (Table 19.1).

Table 19.1 Physical Measures in the Management of Osteoarthritis

Exercise
    Passive range of motion
    Rest periods
    Active: range of motion, isometric, isotonic, isokinetic

Support and orthotic devices
    Canes
    Crutches
    Collars
    Shoe insoles
    Medial taping of the patella
    Knee braces

Modified activities of daily living
    Proper positioning and support when sitting, sleeping, or driving a car
    Adjusting ways of performing such activities as getting dressed, etc.
    Adjusting furnishings around the house or at work (e.g., raising the level of a chair or toilet seat)

Thermal modalities
    Superficial heat (e.g., hot packs and paraffin baths)
    Deep heat (e.g., ultrasound)
    Cold applications (e.g., cold packs and vapocoolant sprays)

Miscellaneous
    Pulsed electromagnetic fields
    Transcutaneous neural stimulation
    Acupuncture
    Chiropractic
    Spa, massage, and yoga therapy

From Lozada CJ, Altman RD. In: Koopman WJ, ed. *Arthritis and Allied Conditions: A Textbook of Rheumatology.* 14th ed. Philadelphia: Lippincott Williams & Wilkins, 2001:2246–2263, with permission.

Exercise may reduce pain and improve function in patients with OA. Although physical and occupational therapy guidance are required in some patients, in most instances, the exercises can be performed by the patient at home after minimal instruction.

Improved strength of the para-articular structure adds stability and support to the joint and appears to reduce symptoms. Strengthening of the quadriceps muscles in a patient with knee OA can improve function and decrease pain for up to 8 months (6). Moreover, a supervised program of fitness walking and education improves the patient's functional status. Health care providers should actively dispel the myth that any exercise worsens arthritis and thus should encourage patients with OA to gradually increase their activity. However, increasing pain may be a warning sign that they have exceeded their exercise tolerance.

Exercises that maximize muscle strengthening while minimizing stress on the affected joints are preferable. Swimming is particularly effective because it causes minimal joint impact and strengthens multiple muscle groups. Unfortunately, certain exercises may actually worsen symptoms (e.g., chondromalacia patella may be worsened by bicycle riding; lumbar facet OA may be worsened by hyper-extension of the spine, as in swimming). Additionally, we no longer recommend bed rest for patients with acute or chronic low back pain.

Supportive devices are also helpful because they partially unload the weight from joints, and may decrease pain and improve balance and mobility. These devices include canes, crutches, walkers, corsets, collars, and orthotic devices for shoes. Canes, when properly used, can increase the base of support, decrease loading, and reduce demands on the lower limb and its joints. The total length of a properly measured cane should equal the distance between the upper border of the greater trochanter of the femur and the bottom of the heel of the shoe. This should result in elbow flexion of about 20 degrees and be held in the hand contralateral to and moved together with the affected limb.

Proper footwear and orthotic shoes can be of great value. A short leg that accentuates lumbar scoliosis may be helped through a unilateral heel or a sole lift. An orthotic device, or shoe insert, may help the patient with subluxed metatarsophalangeal joints. A patient's walking ability and pain in the medial compartment of the knee may improve with a lateral heel-wedged insole. Athletic shoes with good medial and lateral support, as well as good medial arch support, and calcaneal cushion can be of benefit.

Knee braces may be of use in some patients with tibiofemoral disease, especially those with lateral instability and a tendency for the knee to "give out."

Joint supports and orthotic devices allow the patient to participate in more activities, improve compliance, and retain functional independence. These devices should be frequently monitored to ensure proper use, such as the proper sizing and orientation of the cervical collar. Cane and crutch tips should be changed when worn in order to avoid slipping on smooth or wet surfaces.

Patients may need to alter some of their *activities of daily living* because simple adjustments may decrease their symptoms. For example, patients with back pain should avoid sitting on soft couches or recliners, or lying in bed with a pillow under the knees. Instead they should sit in straight-back chairs with good structural support (cushions allowed). Raising the level of a chair or toilet seat can be helpful, because the hip and knees are subjected to the highest pressures during the initial phase of rising from the seated position. However, lift chairs are very rarely helpful or necessary. The patient should also use a firm mattress, perhaps with a bed board, and avoid slouching, even when driving. The car seat should be placed forward so that the knees are flexed during driving.

Thermal modalities can help decrease a patient's pain. The use of heat, cold, or alternating heat and cold is based on the patient's preference. Traditionally, the more acute the process, the more likely cold applications will be of benefit. Heat can be subdivided into superficial and deep, with no proven advantage of one over the other. The therapeutic value of applying heat includes decreasing

SECTION 4 Osteoarthritis and Metabolic Bone

joint stiffness, alleviating pain, relieving muscle spasm, and preventing contractures. The temperatures used range from 40° to 45°C (104° to 113°F) for 3 to 30 minutes. Hot packs, paraffin baths, hydrotherapy, and radiant heat provide superficial heat. Deep heat can be provided by using ultrasound, usually for larger joints, such as hips. However, heat should be used with caution in patients who are anesthetized, somnolent, or obtunded and is contraindicated over tissues with inadequate vascular supply, bleeding, or cancer as well as areas close to the testicles or near developing fetuses. Cold is typically used in the form of cold packs or vapocoolant sprays to relieve muscle spasm, decrease swelling in acute trauma, and relieve pain from inflammation.

Several *miscellaneous* physical modalities that are also utilized include massage, yoga therapy, acupressure, acupuncture, magnets, pulsed electromagnetic fields, transcutaneous neural stimulation, and spa therapy (balneotherapy). **But, many of these programs are of unproven value.**

Psychosocial Measures
Pain and disability are not solely related to physical impairment, but appear associated with the patient's psychosocial conditions. Older age, lower educational level, lower income, and unmarried status have been linked to disability in patients with musculoskeletal complaints (7). Furthermore, patient depression may worsen their perception of pain and thus the effectiveness of the therapy.

Reassurance, counseling, and education by the health care provider are important to mitigate the negative effects of adverse psychosocial factors. Patients must participate in their care, which may lead to better patient compliance and outcomes. Periodic telephone support has been found to be beneficial and to promote self-care among patients with OA (8).

Medication-Based Symptomatic Therapy
Medications used to treat symptoms in OA can be divided into categories of topical agents, systemic oral agents, adjuvant therapies (e.g., antispasmodic and psychoactive drugs), intra-articular agents, and structure- or disease-modifying drugs (no agents yet proved to belong in this latter category; Table 19.2). The

---

Table 19.2 Pharmacologic Therapy for Patients with Osteoarthritis[a]

Oral acetaminophen

COX-2–specific inhibitor

Nonselective NSAID plus misoprostol or a proton pump inhibitor[b]

Nonacetylated salicylate

Other pure analgesics

Tramadol

Opioids

Intra-articular

Glucocorticoids

Hyaluronan

Topical capsaicin

Methylsalicylate

COX-2, cyclooxygenase-2; NSAID, nonsteroidal anti-inflammatory drug.

[a]The choice of agent(s) should be individualized for each patient.

[b]Misoprostol and proton pump inhibitors are recommended in patients who are at increased risk for upper gastrointestinal adverse events.

From reference 11.

treatment regimen should be individualized for each patient and these medications are often used in combinations.

Patients frequently inquire about the benefits of diets, vitamins, minerals, and supplements. However, no conclusive evidence exists that any of these improve the symptoms or the underlying disease. Therefore ingestion of special foods, vitamins, zinc, copper, and home remedies beyond the recommended daily requirements should be discouraged.

Topical Agents

Topical agents can be useful adjuncts in the treatment of OA. Capsaicin, derived from capsicum, the common pepper plant, is available without prescription. It interferes with substance P–mediated pain transmission by reversibly depleting stores of substance P in unmyelinated C-fiber afferent neurons. Until the nerve endings are depleted of substance P, capsaicin (applied two to four times daily) may cause a burning sensation where it is applied. If not used continuously, the nerve endings renew their supply of and sensitivity to substance P. Warn patients to avoid inadvertently getting capsaicin in the eyes, because their eyes will burn tremendously.

A variety of other topical analgesics exist of questionable benefit. These include menthol- and salicylate-based over-the-counter topical preparations, as well as topical nonsteroidal anti-inflammatory drugs (NSAIDs).

Systemic Oral Agents

Non–anti-inflammatory *analgesics* include drugs such as acetaminophen. Despite many years of research, the mechanisms of action of acetaminophen are still not adequately understood. In animals, the actions appear to act at the spinal cord and cerebral levels and interfere with at least cyclooxygenase-3. Nevertheless, acetaminophen may be as effective as ibuprofen for the treatment of knee OA pain (9). Furthermore, acetaminophen is safer than NSAIDs because it does not appear to cause gastropathy or nephropathy at conventional doses, but hepatotoxicity can occur when ingested at high doses.

Tramadol is also an effective analgesic by mildly suppressing the μ-opioid receptor and inhibiting the uptake of norepinephrine and serotonin. It can cause nausea and central nervous system side effects that can be reduced by starting with 50 mg twice daily for 3 days and slowly escalating the dose to the maximum recommended dose of 50 mg QID or until the desired pain relief is achieved.

The OA pain is generally responsive to narcotic analgesics. Mildly potent and minimally addictive narcotic analgesics, such as codeine, have been effective in patients with OA, especially in combination with nonnarcotic analgesics (e.g., acetaminophen and/or NSAIDs). Because of the addictive potential of the stronger opiates and opioids, the risks of oxycodone and hydrocodone should be compared with the benefits of the pain relief achieved. *Anti-inflammatory drugs*, of which NSAIDs are the most commonly prescribed, are used for treating both pain and mild inflammation in OA. With most traditional NSAIDs, analgesia can be achieved at smaller doses than are needed for anti-inflammatory effects. However, for most NSAIDs, the greater the dose, the greater the anti-inflammatory effect (also the greater risk of an adverse reaction). Most rheumatologists recognize that at therapeutic doses, all NSAIDs appear equally effective at providing analgesia.

The major potential adverse effects of nonselective NSAIDs are gastropathy (peptic ulcer disease and gastritis) and renal dysfunction (interstitial nephritis and prostaglandin-inhibition–related renal insufficiency). These adverse effects are more prevalent in the elderly.

Effective strategies have been developed to mitigate the gastrointestinal (GI) toxicity of the NSAIDs: use of lower doses, nonacetylated salicylate, concomitant use of misoprostol (200 μg BID to QID), or a proton pump inhibitor, use of a specific cyclooxygenase (COX)-2 inhibitor, topical analgesics, intra-articular therapy with a depocorticosteroid or hyaluronate, avoiding concomitant use of multiple NSAIDs, glucocorticoids, or systemic anticoagulants. However, antacids and H$_2$ blockers have not been as effective (10). We frequently instruct our patients to take acetaminophen 1 g BID or TID with their NSAID. Anecdotally, this results in improved pain relief compared with either agent individually.

Glucosamine sulfate and chondroitin sulfate have been both tested individually and in combination. Despite their popular use, the available data are inconclusive regarding their benefit on pain or disease.

S-adenosylmethionine (SAM-e) and *methylsulfonylmethane* (MSM) have also been used without conclusive evidence of their efficacy.

Adjuvant Agents

Any analgesic program can be supplemented with *tricyclic antidepressants* or *selective serotonin reuptake inhibitors*. Not only they may accentuate the effect of the other analgesics, they may exert part of their benefit in those patients having sleep disturbances because of nocturnal myoclonus and fibromyalgia-like complaints.

Antispasmodics are useful in reducing muscle pain and spasm in OA. Pain associated with muscle spasm may be reduced with an injection of lidocaine, with or without a depocorticosteroid.

Intra-Articular Therapy

Oral corticosteroids are not indicated for the treatment of OA. However, *intra-articular corticosteroids* may relieve the patient's pain. They have not been consistently helpful in facet joints for treatment of chronic low back pain, but have been useful in many patients as epidural injections for symptomatic spinal stenosis. Despite the clinical impression that they may be of value, no consistent clinical predictors of response to intra-articular depocorticosteroids have been found to aid in patient selection for this therapy.

In general, depocorticosteroid injections should be limited to four injections to any single joint per year (typically no more frequently than at 3-month intervals). However, if patients require multiple injections, they probably require orthopedic surgical intervention.

Complications of intra-articular depocorticosteroids, such as septic arthritis, are rare if proper aseptic technique is employed. Depocorticosteroids are crystalline and can induce a transient synovitis or "postinjection inflammatory reaction." This reaction occurs within several hours of the injection, in contrast to a joint infection, which most often happens 24 to 72 hours after the procedure. The application of cold compresses often reduces the pain until the inflammation resolves. The suspicion of infection should prompt immediate aspiration with subsequent Gram stain and cultures. Furthermore, frequent intra-articular corticosteroids may damage cartilage and bone, and may even contribute to the development of avascular necrosis.

Synthetic and naturally occurring *hyaluronic acid derivatives* are administered intra-articularly. These *viscosupplements* are prepared in a variety of molecular weights (range <100,000 to >1,000,000 Svedberg units) and may reduce pain and improve mobility for prolonged periods of time. The mechanism(s) of action is unknown. However, some evidence exists, suggesting an anti-inflammatory effect (particularly the high-molecular-weight preparation), a short-term lubricant effect, an analgesic effect by directly buffering synovial nerve endings, and a stimulating effect on synovial lining cells into producing normal hyaluronic acid, perhaps through binding to the synovial cell CD44H receptors.

The viscosupplements include Synvisc (HYLAN GF 20) administered as three weekly injections, Hyalgan (hyaluronate sodium) administered as three to five weekly injections, and Orthovisc (hyaluronan) administered as three weekly injections.

SECTION 4 Osteoarthritis and Metabolic Bone

WHEN TO REFER

- If uncertain about the diagnosis
- If pain unresponsive to acetaminophen or NSAIDs
- If the patient has an inflammatory arthropathy
- If the clinician suspects that the patient needs joint replacement

Surgical Intervention

The primary reason for elective orthopedic surgery is intractable pain. The secondary reason for surgery is restoration of compromised joint function. Interventions include removal of loose bodies, stabilization of joints, redistribution of joint forces (e.g., osteotomy), relief of neural impingement (e.g., spinal stenosis and herniated disc), and joint replacement (e.g., total knee replacement).

Osteotomies may serve as alternatives to arthroplasty in younger, overweight patients and in unicompartmental disease of the knee. This may delay progression of disease (hence the need for total joint replacement).

Arthroscopic intervention should be limited to patients in whom an additional diagnosis is suspected, such as cartilaginous or ligamentous damage.

Clinical Course

With adequate pain relief, patients should have an uncomplicated clinical course. There is no good epidemiologic data that OA shortens life expectancy as RA and systemic lupus erythematasus (SLE) have clearly been demonstrated to do. While overall survival is not affected by this condition, the disease tends to have a slow, progressive course often culminating in the need for invasive orthopedic procedures to achieve pain control. As such, aggressive management of modifiable risk factors, such as weight control and supervised exercise programs, are of paramount importance to lengthen the time for an orthopedic procedure.

ICD9

715.9 **Osteoathritis** – *(see also* Osteoarthrosis*)* •
Use the following fifth-digit
subclassification with categories 715:
0 site unspecified
1 shoulder region
2 upper arm
3 forearm
4 hand
5 pelvic region and thigh
6 lower leg
7 ankle and foot
8 other specified sites except spine
9 multiple sites
715.9 **Osteoarthrosis** *(degenerative) (hypertrophic)* •
715.0 [0,4,9] generalized
  715.3 localized •
  715.1 idiopathic •
  715.1 primary •
  715.2 secondary •
715.89 multiple sites, (not generalized)
715.09 polyarticular
721.90 spine (see also Spondylosis)
524.6 temporomandibular joint

References

1. Kramer JS, Yelin EH, Epstein WV. Social and economic impacts of four musculoskeletal conditions: A study using national community-based data. *J Rheumatol* 1983;26:901–907.
2. Lawrence JS. Generalized osteoarthrosis in a population sample. *Am J Epidemiol* 1969;90:381–389.
3. Felson DT. The epidemiology of knee osteoarthritis: Results from the Framingham osteoarthritis study. *Semin Arthritis Rheum* 1990;20:42–50.
4. Pelletier JP, Martel-Pelletier J, Howell DS. Etiopathogenesis of osteoarthritis. In: Koopman WJ, ed. *Arthritis and Allied Conditions: A Textbook of Rheumatology.* 13th ed. Baltimore: Williams & Wilkins, 1997:1969–1984.

5. Fisher NM, Pendergast DR, Gresham GE, et al. Muscle rehabilitation: Its effects on muscular and functional performance of patients with knee osteoarthritis. *Arch Phys Med* 1991;72:367–374.

6. Cunningham LS, Kelsy JL. Epidemiology of musculoskeletal impairments and associated disability. *Am J Pub Health* 1984;74:574–579.

7. Rene J, Weinberger M, Mazzuca SA, et al. Reduction of joint pain in patients with knee osteoarthritis who have received monthly telephone calls from lay personnel and whose medical treatment regimens have remained stable. *Arthritis Rheum* 1992;35:511–515.

8. Bradley JD, Brandt KD, Katz BP, et al. Comparison of an antiinflammatory dose of ibuprofen, an analgesic dose of ibuprofen, and acetaminophen in the treatment of patients with osteoarthritis of the knee. *N Engl J Med* 1991;325:87–91.

9. Yeomans ND, Tulassay Z, Juhasz L, et al. A comparison of omeprazole with ranitidine for ulcers associated with nonsteroidal antiinflammatory drugs. Acid Suppression Trial: Ranitidine versus Omeprazole for NSAID-associated Ulcer Treatment (ASTRONAUT) Study Group. *N Engl J Med* 1998;338:719–726.

10. Altman RD, Hochberg MC, Moskowitz RW, Schnitzer TJ. Recommendations for the medical management of osteoarthritis of the hip and knee: 2000 update. *Arthritis Rheum* 43:1905–1915.

11. Lozada CJ, Altman RD, In Koopman WJ, ed. Arthritis and Allied Conditions: A textbook of Rheumatology. 14th ed. Philadelphia: Lippincott Williams & Wilkins, 2001:2246–2263.

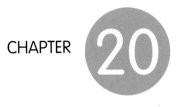 Gout and Crystal-Induced Arthropathies

Angelo Gaffo

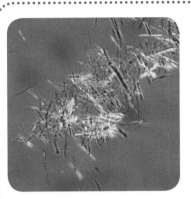

A 65-year-old patient with poorly controlled diabetes, hypertension, heart failure, and a prior diagnosis of gout is hospitalized because of an exacerbation of heart failure with worsening edema and progressive dyspnea. On hospital stay day number 2, symptoms leading to admission were significantly improved. However in the prior 12 hours, he has developed a red, warm, swollen, and extremely tender right ankle.

An arthrocentesis of the affected joint yields cloudy fluid that is positive for the presence of negatively birefringent needle-shaped crystals (Fig. 20.1). A joint glucocorticoid injection was delayed and only analgesic treatment along with low-dose oral colchicine was provided. At 48 hours the synovial fluid culture was reported positive for growth of Klebsiella spp. The patient improved with antibiotic therapy, repeated joint aspirations, low-dose colchicine, and analgesics.

Clinical Presentation

Gout is the clinical manifestation from the tissue deposition of monosodium urate (MSU) crystals. The disease has become more prevalent in Western populations, specifically in certain patient groups such as transplant recipients. It is one of the few medical conditions for which physicians have a nearly complete understanding of the causative and necessary factor for its development, in this case a serum urate concentration above the saturation threshold, or hyperuricemia. This understanding of the etiology and therapeutic target of the disease has not translated into adequate management for the majority of patients with gout because of a combination of factors, including incomplete knowledge of the basic therapeutic principles of the disease and the growing complexity of patients with gout, driven by multiple comorbidities or polypharmacy. Until recently, a scarcity of therapeutic options for gout added to these challenges, but that panorama has started to change.

EPIDEMIOLOGY

Gout is the most common inflammatory arthritis in the United States: according to the most recent estimate by the National Arthritis Data Workgroup, using 1996 data from the National Health Interview Survey (NHIS) and National Health and Nutrition Examination Survey (NHANES), 3.0 million adults older than 18 years had gout in the previous year and 6.1 million adults older than 20 years had gout at some point of their lives. The frequency rates have clearly been increasing in the last decades, with a current estimated prevalence at 940 per 100,000 adults older than 18 years (1).

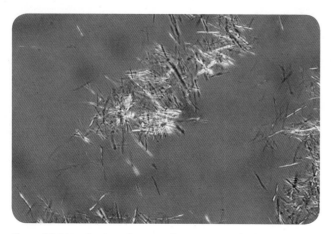

Figure 20.1 Needle-shaped monosodium urate crystals showing characteristic negative birefringence. (Axis of the polarizer points at four O'clock and crystals are predominantly yellow at that direction; perpendicular crystals are predominantly blue.) Courtesy of H. Ralph Schumacher, Jr., M.D., and Janet Dinnella, University of Pennsylvania (http://www.med.upenn.edu/synovium. Accessed June 6, 2011).

CLINICAL POINTS

- Early in the disease course, gout is characterized by acute attacks of arthritis (flares) and asymptomatic intervals. If the disease goes untreated, it morphs into a chronic deforming arthritis with tophi.

- Common precipitants of gout flares include acute illnesses, alcohol intake, starvation, excessive intake of purines, and use of certain medications (allopurinol, diuretics, cyclosporine).

- Gout flares initially involve the lower extremity joints and peak in intensity within 24 hours.

- When starting urate-lowering therapy for gout, it should always be accompanied by prophylactic therapy for gout flares (nonsteroidal anti-inflammatory drugs (NSAIDs), glucocorticoids, or low-dose colchicine).

- Calcium pyrophosphate deposition disease can present as acute arthritis (*pseudogout*), an inflammatory subacute polyarthritis (*pseudorheumatoid arthritis*), degenerative joint disease (*pseudo-osteoarthritis*), spinal disease, and a destructive arthritis resembling a neuropathic arthritis.

Worldwide, data about measures of disease frequency and time trends are heterogeneous. It is unclear if these variations are because of true differences in frequencies or heterogeneous gout definitions and methods of data collection. The prevalence of gout in the United Kingdom in 1993 seemed to have tripled when compared with that in the 1970s. Other gout high-prevalence populations are the Malayo-Polynesians and New Zealand Maoris (close to 10%). On the other hand, relatively low disease frequencies have been reported in China.

HYPERURICEMIA

Uric acid, found in serum as urate, is the end product of purine metabolism in humans. The accumulation of urate beyond its solubility point of 6.8 mg/dL defines hyperuricemia, a necessary but not sufficient factor for the development of gout. Gout is the clinical manifestation of the deposition of MSU crystals in tissues.

The importance of hyperuricemia as a causative factor for gout has been corroborated in prospective studies. As part of the Normative Aging Study, a cohort of 2,046 men was followed for 15 years (2). The risk for gout followed a gradient depending on the initial urate level: with an initial level of more than 9 mg/dL, the annual incidence rate was 4.9%. When the initial level was between 7.0 and 8.9 mg/dL, the annual incidence rate was 0.5%, and finally, it was 0.1% with urate levels less than 7.0 mg/dL. The importance of hyperuricemia in predicting gout attacks is limited not only to the initial diagnosis, but also to the management, as it has been demonstrated that low serum urate levels predict freedom from recurrence of gout flares.

Uric acid is synthesized in the liver from purine compounds provided by diet and the endogenous pathway of purine synthesis de novo. It is then released into the circulation almost exclusively in its soluble-form MSU, which is readily available for filtration in the proximal tubules of the kidney. Two mechanisms exist through which an individual could develop hyperuricemia: overproduction (excretion of more than 600 mg/day in the urine while on a purine-free diet, accounting for 10% to 15% of cases) and underexcretion (excretion of less than 400 mg/day, accounting for 85% to 90% of cases). In both cases the problem could be primary (secondary to enzymatic inherited disorders of urate production or defects in renal excretion) or secondary to excessive purine turnover (diet, malignancies), medications, or toxins. For an expanded overview of causes of hyperuricemia, see Table 20.1.

After a nearly complete filtration in the glomerulus, urate undergoes an extensive reabsorption in the proximal tubule largely mediated by a specific organic anion transporter. After the first round of reabsorption, a second cycle of secretion and further reabsorption occurs in the distal portions of the proximal tubules. These final steps determine the net urate excretion, typically 8% to 12% of the initially filtered load.

Once hyperuricemia ensues, the probability of developing gout depends on the concentration of urate in the tissue or joint and other predisposing factors such as a low pH, low temperature, previous trauma to the joint, and lack of mobility (e.g., during sleep, when there is an increased water reabsorption, and concentration of urate). Recent advances in understanding how MSU crystals cause the characteristic gout inflammatory response have been made. Along with other crystals, such as calcium pyrophosphate, silica, and asbestos, MSU is internalized into phagocytes and sensed by the innate immune system as a

Table 20.1 Causes of Hyperuricemia

INCREASED URIC ACID PRODUCTION	IMPAIRED URIC ACID EXCRETION
Primary	
Idiopathic	Idiopathic or genetically determined renal hyperuricemia
Enzyme deficiencies leading to accelerated purine nucleotide synthesis: hypoxanthine-guanine phosphoribosyltransferase (cause of Lesch–Nyhan syndrome), phosphoribosylpyrophosphate synthetase (PRPP) overactivity	
Secondary	
Excessive purine diet intake	Reduced renal functional mass because of chronic kidney disease
Increased purine nucleotide turnover: myeloproliferative and lymphoproliferative diseases, psoriasis	Inhibition of tubular urate secretion (organic acidosis): lactic acidosis, keto-acidosis, ethanol, preeclampsia
Accelerated adenosine triphosphate (ATP) degradation: ethanol intake, tissue hypoxia, glycogen storage diseases	Inhibition of tubular urate secretion (drugs): salicylates, thiazides, cyclosporine, etc.
	Enhanced tubular urate reabsorption: dehydration, diuretic use, insulin resistance
	Unknown mechanism: chronic lead exposure, hypertension, hyperparathyroidism, sarcoidosis, berylliosis

danger signal indicative of tissue damage and recognized by a series of sophisticated cytosolic receptors (3).

The effect of diet as a risk factor for hyperuricemia and gout has been clarified by epidemiologic evidence. Cross-sectional analyses reveal that total beer, liquor, meat, and seafood consumption were associated with higher serum uric acid levels. However, the magnitude of the increase in serum urate in most individuals per unit of intake is relatively small. Wine, total protein, and dairy intake have not been found to be associated with higher serum urate levels. The effect of alcohol intake in inducing flares in patients with established gout is significant.

Fructose intake has gathered much attention as a factor associated with higher levels of serum urate, renal disease, and the development of hypertension. Fructose may induce hyperuricemia through depletion of adenosine triphosphate and its rapid conversion into adenosine monophosphate, which will be later catabolized into uric acid. Epidemiologic studies have established an association between fructose intake and hyperuricemia and gout.

There are several medications and toxins that influence the renal handling of uric acid. Aspirin has a dual effect on serum uric acid levels, with high levels of intake (more than 3 g/day) being uricosuric and lower levels of intake (75 to 2,000 mg/day) promoting uric acid retention. Diuretics (both loop and thiazides) are well known to be associated with higher serum urate levels, possibly through volume contraction and concurrent stimulation of urate reabsorption at the level of the urate absorption receptor in the proximal tubules. Cyclosporine and tacrolimus are widely used drugs for posttransplant immunosuppression and are strongly associated with the development of hyperuricemia and gout;

•••••••••••••••••••••••••••
PATIENT ASSESSMENT

- When approaching patients in which a crystal arthritis is in the differential, a joint aspiration with microscopic examination under polarized light should be performed whenever possible.

- Serum urate levels should not be utilized for the evaluation or assessment of suspected gout flares.

- As septic arthritis is usually in the differential of crystal arthritides, gram stain and culture of fluid aspirates should usually be performed, even in cases in which crystals are readily identified.

- The diagnosis of calcium pyrophosphate deposition disease can be supported by the finding of fine cartilage calcification (chondrocalcinosis) in radiographs of the affected joints.

other chemicals associated with hyperuricemia and gout include lead, pyrazinamide, ethambutol, and niacin.

Examination

Gout is a chronic disease that, if untreated, typically progresses over four phases: (a) asymptomatic hyperuricemia, (b) gout flares, (c) intercritical periods, and (d) chronic, usually tophaceous gout. This progression is illustrated in Figure 20.2. Typically, gout flares present as warmth, swelling, erythema, and pain of abrupt onset in the involved joint, with symptoms peaking over 8 to 12 hours. Patients usually describe the pain as excruciating, and even the slightest physical contact with the affected area (like that produced by a bedsheet) can induce marked suffering. Nighttime onset of symptoms is frequent. Fever, chills, and malaise are commonly part of the presentation in patients with polyarticular flares. In the elderly, atypical presentations that include delirium are frequent. Commonly, the involved joints are in the feet (with the first metatarsophalangeal being eventually involved in more than 90% of cases), ankles, knees, elbows, wrists, and fingers. The predilection for the lower extremities is because of lower temperatures in these joints that favor the precipitation of MSU crystals. Extra-articular sites are also involved, including the bursas (mainly the olecranon and prepatellar bursas) and tendons. The first attack is usually monoarticular, and locates at the first metatarsophalangeal joint in 50% of the cases. Precipitants of gout flares include acute illness (trauma, sepsis, surgery), alcohol intake, starvation, excessive intake of certain food groups (mainly purines), and medications. Drugs such as allopurinol, thiazides, and cyclosporine—which affect serum urate levels or cause body fluid shifts—have been associated with gout flares. Untreated attacks frequently resolve over 3 to 10 days, sometimes with exfoliation of the overlying skin.

The clinical course of gout is characterized by an amelioration or complete disappearance of symptoms during the intercritical period. However, if the disease progresses into chronic gout, the length of these intercritical periods shortens and chronic joint pain persists even during these intercritical periods (Fig. 20.2). It is not infrequent to recover MSU crystals from aspirates of a previously affected joint during the intercritical period.

Chronic gout is characterized by the unremitting nature of the symptoms, destructive arthritis, and the identifiable deposition of solid uric acid in tissues

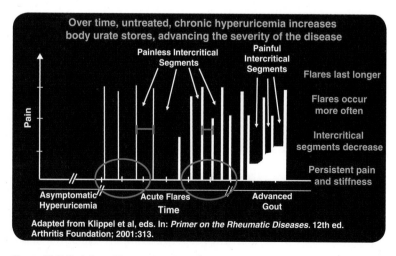

Figure 20.2 Evolution of hyperuricemia and gout.

(tophi). At this stage the involved joints remain persistently uncomfortable, stiff, and swollen. The condition may mimic other inflammatory arthritides, such as rheumatoid arthritis. Superimposed acute flares, which are usually polyarticular and additive, still occur. Tophi appear as a function of the degree and duration of untreated hyperuricemia, usually over extensor surfaces (forearms and the Achilles tendon) and pressure points, typically in the fingers, wrists, knees, and olecranon bursas.

Studies

The diagnosis of gout is strongly supported by the combination of a classical clinical presentation (monoarthritis and tophi) along with evidence of hyperuricemia and clinical response to colchicine, NSAIDs, or glucocorticoids. However, it is very important to emphasize that each one of these diagnostic considerations are imperfect and that the diagnosis can only be reliably established by the identification of negatively birefringent needle-shaped MSU crystals from an affected joint or tissue.

The most common way of identifying MSU crystals in patients suspected of having a gout flare is through synovial fluid aspiration from an affected joint. The fluid obtained from joints affected by gout is usually turbid with a yellow tinge, but in extreme cases, it is thick and chalky, with a white coloration. The cell counts are usually in the inflammatory range from 3,000/mm^3 up to greater than 50,000/mm^3, more than 90% of these cells being polymorphonuclear. Often, needle-shaped MSU crystals can be identified under standard light microscopy. However, the optimal way to visualize MSU is through polarized light microscopy, in which needle-shaped MSU crystals will appear with a bright-yellow or blue coloration (depending on if the axis of the polarizer is parallel or perpendicular to the crystal) against a purple background (Fig. 20.1). Many times the MSU crystals are found inside a leukocyte that is attempting phagocytosis. Despite being the standard way of determining the presence of a gout flare, synovial fluid analysis with crystal identification has some drawbacks. For example, patients with gout and hyperuricemia that are not having a gout flare could have MSU crystals in their joint synovial fluid (usually in the context of a noninflammatory cell count). Also, the aspiration of small joints could be technically challenging and the procedure could be difficult to perform for untrained practitioners. Another potential issue is that synovial fluid has to be promptly analyzed as cells counts decline and crystals degenerate when sample processing is delayed. Finally, the identification of MSU crystals in partially treated patients or those in which the gout flare is resolving can be challenging and requires lots of patience on part of the examiner. Bursal fluid, tophi aspirates, and tissue samples can also be analyzed with the purpose of identifying MSU crystals.

Measurement of serum urate is an unreliable predictor of gout flares and should not be used with diagnostic purposes as up to 40% of cases of acute gout occur in the setting of normouricemia. On the other hand, hyperuricemia is frequent in the general population and could be present in the setting of an acute arthritis secondary to rheumatoid disease, psoriasis, infection, and so on. Other ancillary investigations such as the measurement of urine urate excretion and plain radiographs have a limited role in diagnostic and management decisions.

The American College of Rheumatology (formerly American Rheumatism Association) proposed preliminary criteria for the diagnosis of acute gouty arthritis in 1977 (Table 20.2; 4). Despite their widely adopted use and citation, those were never validated, and important limitations in their performance have been recognized. More recently, the European League Against Rheumatism has proposed recommendations for the diagnosis of gout that translate

Table 20.2 Rules for the Classification and Diagnosis of Gout

	ARA PRELIMINARY CLASSIFICATION CRITERIA FOR ACUTE GOUTY ARTHRITIS (1977)	EULAR EVIDENCE-BASED RECOMMENDATIONS FOR GOUT DIAGNOSIS (2006)	DIAGNOSIS OF GOUT IN PATIENTS WITH ACUTE MONOARTHRITIS (2010)
Context	Acute arthritis (flares)	Any gout	Community-based undiagnosed monoarthritis
Rule or recommendations	1. Monosodium urate crystals in the joint fluid; *or* 2. Tophus proven to contain urate crystals; *or* 3. Six of the following: • More than one attack of acute arthritis • Maximal inflammation developed within 1 day • Attack of monoarticular arthritis • Joint redness • First MTP joint painful or swollen • Unilateral attack involving first MTP joint • Suspected tophus • Hyperuricemia • Asymmetric swelling within a joint (radiographs) • Subcortical cysts without erosions (radiographs) • Negative cultures during acute episode	1. Rapid (6–12 hours) development of severe pain, swelling, erythema is highly suggestive, but not specific for gout 2. For typical presentations, clinical diagnosis is reasonably accurate 3. MSU crystals in synovial fluid of tophus confirms gout 4. Routine search for MSU crystals in diagnosed joints is recommended 5. Identification of MSU crystals from asymptomatic joints allows diagnosis in intercritical periods 6. Gram stain and culture should be done in joints suspected to have gout 7. Serum urate do not confirm or exclude gout 8. Renal urate excretion should be considered in certain patients 9. Radiographs seldom are not useful in acute gout 10. Risk factors and comorbidities should be assessed	1. Male sex (2 points) 2. Previous patient reported—attack (2 points) 3. Onset within 1 day (0.5 points) 4. Joint redness (1 point) 5. First MTP involvement (2.5 points) 6. Hypertension or ≥1 cardiovascular diseases[a] (1.5 points) 7. Serum urate >5.88 mg/dL (3.5 points) • Less than 4 points: gout prevalence 2.8% • More than 4 to <8 points: gout prevalence 27% • More than 8 points: gout prevalence 80.4%
Performance	Sensitivity 88% Specificity 80%	Not provided	Area under the curve 0.87

ARA, American Rheumatism Association (currently American College of Rheumatology); EULAR, European League Against Rheumatism; MSU, monosodium urate; MTP, metatarsophalangeal.

[a]Angina pectoris, myocardial infarction, heart failure, cerebrovascular accident, transient ischemic attack, or peripheral vascular disease.

Table adapted from references 4–6.

into a diagnostic rule (5). In addition, a Dutch primary care group developed a diagnostic rule for identification of gout in patients with monoarthritis without the need of an arthrocentesis that could be of great usefulness to clinicians in communities without access to prompt synovial fluid analysis (Table 20.2; 6).

DIFFERENTIAL DIAGNOSIS

Gout flares can be mimicked by other inflammatory and infectious conditions, mainly septic arthritis (Table 20.3). The clinical differentiation between these conditions can be difficult in the immune-suppressed, elderly, or subjects with multiple comorbidities. In these settings, both conditions can be polyarticular and associated with prominent systemic manifestations such as fever, chills,

NOT TO BE MISSED

- Tophi are MSU tissue deposits that usually locate subcutaneously over extensor surfaces (arms and Achilles tendons), and pressure points in the hands, wrists, knees, and olecranon bursas.

- In patients who are elderly, chronically ill, and hospitalized, gout flares frequently are polyarticular and can be accompanied by prominent systemic symptoms, including fever and chills.

- Medication noncompliance is a very frequent cause of gout that is resistant to urate-lowering therapy.

Table 20.3 Differential Diagnosis of Gout

GOUT FLARES	CHRONIC GOUT
Septic arthritis	Rheumatoid arthritis
Pseudogout and other crystal arthritides	Osteoarthritis
Trauma	Calcium pyrophosphate deposition disease (pseudorheumatoid arthritis)
Rheumatoid arthritis	Psoriatic arthritis
Acute seronegative arthritis	Polymyalgia rheumatica
Neuropathic arthritis	

and confusion. It is important to notice that both entities can coexist in the same patient, as joint aspirates containing gout or pseudogout crystals have also been reported positive for bacterial cultures. Septic arthritis can also present in patients with established gout, mimicking a new flare of the disease. For this reason, gram stain and cultures are recommended as part of the routine laboratory work-up of synovial fluid aspirated from a patient in whom gout is suspected.

Other conditions that can mimic gout flares include trauma, pseudogout and other crystal arthritides, or flares of other inflammatory arthritides, such as seronegative spondyloarthropathies and rheumatoid arthritis. Chronic gout could be difficult to differentiate from other inflammatory arthritides, most notably rheumatoid arthritis. Tophi could be mistaken as rheumatoid nodules in that same context. In elderly patients with extreme disability caused by chronic polyarticular gout, the clinical picture could be confused with polymyalgia rheumatica, seronegative arthritis, or depression.

Treatment

The management goals in gout differ depending on the setting. In acute gout the treatment is aimed at resolving the flares of prominent pain and inflammation. In the intercritical periods the goals are to maintain uric acid at subsaturation levels, preventing the occurrence of new flares and the development of chronic tophaceous gout. A list of the agents available for management of gout is presented in Table 20.4.

MANAGEMENT OF GOUT FLARES

Success in promptly and completely aborting gout flares depends on how early the pharmacologic management is initiated and continuing it for an appropriate amount of time. As a general rule, long-term urate-lowering therapy should not be initiated until joint inflammation has completely resolved. Patients should be informed about resolution of a flare not being a cure for the disease.

Multiple oral and parenteral nonselective NSAIDs have proved to be effective therapies for gout flares. High dosages are used in the first 3 to 4 days, followed by a lower maintenance dose for a total of 7 to 10 days. These lower doses can also be used to prevent recurrence of attacks, although there is no controlled evidence to support this approach. Caution should be exercised because of the well-known gastric, renal, cardiac, hematologic, and hepatic toxicities of NSAIDs. Close monitoring or complete avoidance of NSAIDs is recommended in elderly patients, users of warfarin, and those with cardiac, renal, or hepatic dysfunction.

Table 20.4 Therapeutic Agents for Management of Gout

MANAGEMENT OF ACUTE GOUT FLARES
- Nonsteroidal anti-inflammatory drugs
- Oral colchicine
- Oral or intravenous glucocorticoids
- Cosyntropin (ACTH)

PROPHYLAXIS DURING INITIATION OF URATE-LOWERING THERAPY
- Nonsteroidal anti-inflammatory drugs
- Oral colchicine
- Oral glucocorticoids

URATE-LOWERING THERAPY
- Xanthine oxidase inhibitors: allopurinol, febuxostat
- Uricosurics: probenecid, sulfinpyrazone
- Uricases: pegloticase

IN DEVELOPMENT
- Interleukin 1β inhibitors for gout flares and urate-lowering prophylaxis: rilonacept, canakinumab
- Selective uricosurics: RDEA 594 (URAT-1)

Among the selective COX-2 inhibitors, etoricoxib and lumiracoxib have been found to be efficacious and well tolerated for management of gout flare episodes. Neither agent is available in the United States, but it suggests that agents in this category, such as celecoxib, could be useful for the treatment of gout flares. Scheduled maintenance doses of NSAIDs can be used as prophylactic therapy during initiation of urate-lowering therapy.

Colchicine interferes with microtubule assembly and through this mechanism with phagocytosis and chemotaxis. It is most effective in controlling gout flares when taken within the first 24 hours after symptom onset. The commonly advocated dosage of 0.6 mg orally every hour until "symptom resolution or diarrhea" (to a maximum of 6.0 mg in 12 hours) is very often limited by prominent gastrointestinal side effects, with nausea, vomiting, and diarrhea leading to dehydration and an incomplete resolution of the flare. This approach to management of gout flares has been progressively falling out of favor.

The issue of colchicine dosing for gout flares has been clarified by a randomized controlled trial which established that a "low-dose" approach of colchicine (1.2 mg by mouth followed by 0.6 mg 1 hour later) achieved comparable serum concentrations of the drug and efficacy in the resolution of gout flare symptoms when contrasted with the "high-dose" approach described above. This "low-dose" approach had a significantly lower rate of gastrointestinal and total adverse events (7). Intravenous colchicine has been linked to multiple fatalities and its use is strongly discouraged.

Colchicine is commonly used as a prophylactic agent to prevent flares. The dosages used in this setting are between 0.6 to 1.2 mg/day orally, but dose reductions must be performed if the drug needs to be used in the setting of kidney dysfunction. Gastrointestinal side effects including diarrhea, nausea, and vomiting can also be present at these lower doses. With long-term use, neutropenia, neuropathy, and a vacuolar myopathy can develop. These side effects tend to resolve with discontinuation of the drug.

In view of the increasing complexity of the patients with gout flares, glucocorticoids are becoming more frequently used when NSAIDs or colchicine are contraindicated. When patients present with a confirmed mono- or oligoarticular gout flare, aspiration of synovial fluid followed by an intra-articular injection of a long-acting glucocorticoid may be all that is necessary to resolve the flare. It is very important to emphasize, however, that clinical judgment should be exercised in deciding which patients are good candidates for this approach, namely those in whom the clinical presentation, medical history, and laboratory studies make the possibility of septic arthritis minimal.

Oral courses of therapy are commonly done with prednisone or its glucocorticoid equivalent at doses of 30 to 60 mg/day. Tapering should be performed over the course of 10 to 14 days, a common mistake being to administer very short courses of glucocorticoids (7 days or less) with incomplete resolution or recurrence of the gout flare. Glucocorticoid-based regimens are equivalent in effectiveness to those based on NSAIDs, and possibly associated with fewer short-term adverse events (mainly fluid retention, hypertension, hyperglycemia, anxiety, and insomnia). The concern about adverse effects from glucocorticoids, albeit valid, is of less importance given the short-term courses the patients are supposed to receive. This is not the case in patients with recurrent acute flares or chronic gout managed with frequent doses of glucocorticoids.

Paradoxically, the injection of deposit glucocorticoids to relieve inflammation on rare occasion can induce an acute episode of severe pain, inflammation, and swelling secondary to crystallization of the glucocorticoid. The condition usually presents within 8 to 12 hours after the injection and has been described more frequently in association with triamcinolone hexacetonide preparations. The diagnosis can be supported by aspiration of synovial fluid and visualization of large, irregular, intensely birefringent, irregular crystals. The condition is self-limited, usually subsiding within 24 to 48 hours after the injection. Analgesics, NSAIDs, and ice packs could be used as symptomatic therapy.

Corticotropin (ACTH) shares the same profile of indications as systemic glucocorticoids, namely polyarticular flares in which NSAIDs are not effective or contraindicated. However, ACTH is costly compared with glucocorticoids and not widely available. Its mechanism of action seems to be through stimulation of endogenous adrenal hormones, but direct anti-inflammatory effects at the affected site could also be implicated. The drug is available for subcutaneous or intramuscular administration, and a single dose of 40 IU has been found to be rapid, efficient, and well tolerated even in patients that are taking moderate doses of glucocorticoids. Adverse effects include mild hypokalemia, fluid retention, hyperglycemia, and the development of rebound gout flares, the latter being controlled by the administration of other prophylactic therapy.

URATE-LOWERING THERAPY FOR HYPERURICEMIA AND GOUT

The decision of initiating chronic therapy for hyperuricemia causing gout should be individualized for each case as there is no evidence to this date regarding a benefit of treating asymptomatic hyperuricemia alone. However, patients need to understand that very high levels of serum urate place them at a very high risk for incident gout and possibly cardiovascular events, and at least lifestyle changes (reduction in alcohol intake, dietary changes, weight loss) should be considered. After an initial gout flare, urate-lowering therapy could be withheld given that joint damage is unlikely to occur in patients who remain asymptomatic, but such therapy is advocated in patients with two or more flares, one flare in the setting of very high serum urate (>8.0 mg/dL), or tophi.

The concomitant initiation of prophylactic therapy with colchicine, glucocorticoids, or NSAIDs along with urate-lowering therapy is strongly advocated to prevent flares. Prophylactic therapy should be maintained for a minimum of 6 months after urate-lowering therapy initiation or the occurrence of the last gout flare. Urate-lowering therapy should be intensified until the goal of a sub-saturation concentration of uric acid at 6 mg/dL is reached. More aggressive goals might be necessary for patients with large tissue deposits of urate, such as those with tophi or multiple radiographic erosions.

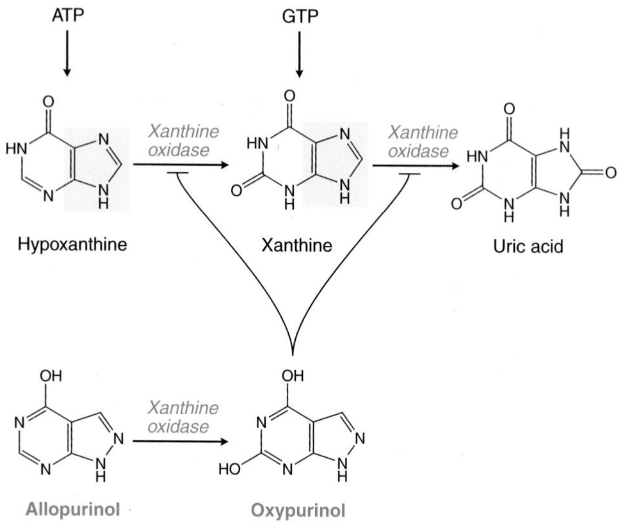

Figure 20.3 Xanthine oxidase inhibitors mechanism of action. Allopurinol is a structural analogue of hypoxanthine. (Similarity is highlighted in blue.) Oxidation of allopurinol yields oxypurinol, a noncompetitive inhibitor of xanthine oxidase. (At low doses, allopurinol is a competitive inhibitor of xanthine oxidase.) Inhibition of xanthine oxidase decreases the production of uric acid by inhibiting two steps in its synthesis. The increased plasma levels of xanthine and hypoxanthine are tolerated because these metabolites are more soluble than uric acid. (With permission from Golan DE, Tashjian AH, Armstrong EJ. *Principles of Pharmacology: The Pathophysiologic Basis of Drug Therapy.* 2nd ed. Baltimore: Wolters Kluwer Health; 2008.)

Allopurinol is the most widely used urate-lowering agent in view of its efficacy in overproducers and underexcretors of uric acid, easy dosing regimen, low cost, and acceptable safety profile. Allopurinol and its metabolite oxypurinol are substrates of xanthine oxidase, and act by inhibiting xanthine oxidase, blocking the conversion of hypoxanthine to xanthine and subsequently the latter to uric acid (Fig. 20.3). Initial doses of allopurinol range between 100 and 300 mg/day, with lower doses preferred because of a perceived lower incidence of flares and hypersensitivity reactions. Besides, some patients may reach serum urate goals with low doses of 100 to 200 mg/day. Even lower starting doses of 50 to 100 mg/day should be used in elderly patients and those with impaired kidney function. It is important to monitor serum urate levels every 2 to 4 weeks for dosage adjustments until the target concentration is reached. The most commonly used dosage of 300 mg/day achieves target serum urate concentrations in only half the patients and dosages as high as 900 mg/day are necessary in many patients, although this dose exceeds the FDA-approved daily dose of 800 mg/day. However, before escalating the dose to very high levels, adherence should be assessed because as many as 50% of patients are nonadherent with the medication, especially if they are having recurrent gout flares.

Adverse reactions from allopurinol are uncommon and mild. The most frequent toxicities are rash, gastrointestinal intolerance or diarrhea, headache, and leucopenia. Rashes can recur on reexposure to the drug and are an important cause of intolerance. Allopurinol desensitization protocols are available but infrequently used since alternatives to allopurinol are now available. The allopurinol hypersensitivity syndrome is an uncommon immune-mediated severe reaction with a mortality of up to 20%. It is characterized by fever, rash, acute renal insufficiency, eosinophilia, hepatic injury, and vasculitis. The most commonly identified risk factor for its occurrence is kidney dysfunction. Multiple drug interactions could be an additional limiting factor for the use of allopurinol; notable among these are increased levels of theophylline, warfarin, and azathioprine. Thiazide diuretics can inhibit the excretion of allopurinol and potentiate toxicity. Finally, a high incidence of skin rashes has been described with the combination of ampicillin or amoxicillin and allopurinol.

Febuxostat is an orally administered, nonpurine selective inhibitor of xanthine oxidase. The drug acts through a very stable and long-lived enzyme's inhibitory interaction with both the oxidized and reduced forms of the enzyme and a strong inhibition of substrate binding. Febuxostat, at approved doses ranging from 40 to 80 mg/day, is efficacious in reducing serum urate in patients with hyperuricemia and gout, comparing favorably with fixed doses of allopurinol in that respect (8). Early safety signals with respect to liver test abnormalities and cardiovascular outcomes have not been confirmed in recent large prospective trials, but need to be further monitored. Given cost considerations, febuxostat will likely find a niche in patients with gout who are unable to use allopurinol because of intolerances, adverse reactions, or drug–drug interactions. In addition, patients with tophaceous gout or with very high serum urate (SUA) levels (more than 10 mg/dL) may also benefit from the higher potency of febuxostat versus allopurinol at the fixed dosages tested. Patients with chronic kidney disease and organ transplantations are good febuxostat candidates.

However, allopurinol given its cost and experience with use will likely remain as the first-line drug for the management of gout in most patients.

Uricosuric drugs attempt to revert the most common physiologic abnormality in gout, which is underexcretion of uric acid. Probenecid and sulfinpyrazone are used internationally. Other drugs with mild uricosuric effects include losartan and fenofibrate. Most uricosuric agents act at the level of the transporter in the proximal tubule in a nonselective manner. When used on ideal candidates, probenecid and sulfinpyrazone allow a majority of patients to achieve serum urate goals. However, several limitations are encountered when trying to use uricosuric agents in practice. First, they rapidly lose effectiveness as the glomerular filtration rate (GFR) drops to less than 50 mL/minute. Second, their use is strongly discouraged in patients with history of renal calculi, as the uricosuric agents may further promote nephrolithiasis. Lastly, their use is not recommended in elderly patients, those on multiple medications (because of multiple drug interactions), and those who have trouble complying with multiple daily doses. For example, probenecid has known interactions with azathioprine, rifampin, salicylates, penicillins, indomethacin, and heparin. Probenecid is the most widely used uricosuric; usually initiated at a dose of 500 mg orally twice a day, the dosage can be slowly increased up to 3 g/day. Adverse effects include gastrointestinal intolerance, rash, hepatotoxicity, gout flares, nephrolithiasis, and nephrotic syndrome.

Urate oxidase (uricase) is a potent enzyme present in all mammals but higher primates and humans, which converts serum urate into more soluble allantoin. Nonrecombinant (obtained from *Aspergillus flavus*) and recombinant forms (obtained from *Saccharomyces cerevisiae*) have been used effectively as intravenous infusions in the prevention and treatment of tumor lysis syndrome. However, their complicated dosing schemes, severe adverse reactions, and secondary loss of efficacy severely restricted their use for treatment-refractory cases of gout.

A polyethylene glycol (PEG)–linked uricase (pegloticase) has been approved as second-line treatment for gout. The drug is administered as an intravenous infusion of 8 mg every 2 weeks, and requires premedication with antihistamines and glucocorticoids. In clinical trials it proved to be highly effective and potent in achieving marked serum urate reductions. It is important to note that about 40% of patients did not respond to the drug primarily or developed a secondary loss of response. Many patients had partial or complete resolution of their tophi burden. Use of the medication was limited by increase in the frequency of gout flares and infusion reactions (including cases of anaphylaxis). Its cardiovascular safety was called into question, but short-term clinical trials did not raise any clear safety signals. Clearly, postmarketing surveillance studies are necessary.

THERAPEUTIC APPROACHES IN DEVELOPMENT

The role of interleukin 1β (IL-1β) as an important product of inflammasome-mediated response to MSU led to the attempted use of blockers of this cytokine to treat gout flares. Anakinra, an IL-1β blocker approved for the treatment of rheumatoid arthritis only, was initially tested, and although effective, its local adverse reactions and high frequency of administration made it an inconvenient option. Longer acting IL-1β blockers (rilonacept and canakinumab) are in advanced stages of development and testing, showing promise for management of gout flares and prophylaxis of gout flares in patients receiving urate-lowering therapy.

SPECIAL THERAPEUTIC CONSIDERATIONS

Several observational studies have described an association between increased serum urate and hypertension, decreased GFR, and progression to end-stage renal disease. Experimental models of hyperuricemia in rats have shown that they develop renin-dependent hypertension, interstitial renal disease, glomerular hypertension, arteriolopathy, and an endothelial dysfunction partially reversible by the administration of allopurinol. In addition, allopurinol has been found to reverse hypertension in hyperuricemic and overweight adolescents with hypertension and to decrease the proportion of patients with deterioration of renal function in patients with hyperuricemia and chronic kidney disease. All these data suggest that asymptomatic hyperuricemia, which currently has no indication for treatment, may lead to adverse renal and cardiovascular outcomes (9).

Calcium Pyrophosphate Dihydrate Deposition Disease

Calcium pyrophosphate dihydrate deposition disease (CPPD) is the result of articular deposition of calcium pyrophosphate crystals. Overproduction of extracellular pyrophosphate leads to CPPD crystal formation and deposition, a process that is ubiquitous and essentially inevitable with aging. The condition has the characteristic of closely simulating other autoimmune and degenerative conditions, requiring a careful combined interpretation of clinical and radiologic data, along with microscopical analysis of synovial fluid for the characteristic crystals. Unfortunately, treatments do not aim at correcting the underlying metabolic defect, but at decreasing the pain, inflammation, and disability caused by the disease.

Increased production of pyrophosphate by articular chondrocytes in an environment enriched in extracellular calcium seems to be the necessary condition for the formation of CPPD crystals. These crystals elicit an inflammatory response through similar mechanisms as MSU crystals. The perpetuation of this inflammatory response leads to cell proliferation and generation of metalloproteinases that contribute to the structural collapse characteristic of joint degeneration.

The processes leading to CPPD are associated with different physiologic and pathogenic contributing factors (Table 20.5). The main associated factor is aging, with several autopsy and radiographic studies confirming an increased prevalence of chondrocalcinosis with advancing age. Well-known pathogenic associations include hemochromatosis, hyperparathyroidism, hypomagnesemia, hypophosphatemia, previous trauma, osteoarthritis, and gout. Other genetic and metabolic factors have also been postulated in association with the disease. Knowledge of these associations is important for two reasons: some of these conditions (e.g., hemochromatosis, hyperparathyroidism) could be suspected because of their presentation as CPPD, and correction of these conditions could slow the progression of CPPD.

Clinical Presentation

Calcium pyrophosphate dihydrate deposition disease can mimic several other rheumatologic conditions. The best known of these is the acute arthritis form known as *pseudogout*. Approximately 25% of patients present this way at some point in their disease, and as its name implies, clinically it closely resembles a gout flare. The most commonly affected joints are the knees, wrists, ankles, elbows, shoulders, and feet. It is important to emphasize that involvement of the first metatarsophalangeal joint does not rule out pseudogout, which can also affect this characteristic gout involvement site. As with gout, attacks of pseudogout are precipitated by trauma, surgery, hospitalizations, and acute illnesses. Notable among these predisposing

Table 20.5	**Conditions Predisposing to the Formation of Calcium Pyrophosphate Crystals**

PHYSIOLOGIC
- Aging

INJURY-RELATED
- Trauma
- Prior surgery to affected joint
- Postsurgical state[a]

RHEUMATOLOGIC
- Osteoarthritis
- Gout
- Neuropathic arthritis

ENDOCRINE
- Hyperparathyroidism[a]
- Hemochromatosis
- Hypothyroidism
- Acromegaly

METABOLIC
- Hypomagnesemia
- Hypophosphatemia

MISCELLANEOUS
- Wilson's disease
- Ochronosis

[a]Hyperparathyroidectomy surgery is a common predisposing factor.

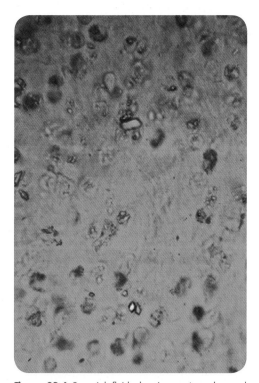

Figure 20.4 Synovial fluid showing rectangular and irregularly shaped calcium pyrophosphate dihydrate crystals at a magnification of 400×. (Courtesy of H. Ralph Schumacher, Jr., M.D., and Janet Dinnella, University of Pennsylvania (http://www.med.upenn.edu/synovium)).

factors, one precipitant is parathyroidectomy surgery. In addition to gout, the pseudogout form of CPPD needs to be differentiated from septic arthritis through synovial fluid analyses. Gout and pseudogout can coexist in the same joint.

Calcium pyrophosphate dihydrate deposition disease can also present with advanced degenerative joint disease, in a form known as *pseudo-osteoarthritis*. As with primary osteoarthritis, this form involves pain, progressive stiffness, and functional limitation. The pattern of joint involvement can be atypical for primary osteoarthritis, as it usually affects, in addition to the typical joints such as the knees, non–weight-bearing joints such as the wrists, elbows, and shoulders. A valgus knee deformity is highly suggestive of CPPD. The differentiation from primary osteoarthritis is often difficult.

A presentation closely resembling rheumatoid arthritis is known as *pseudorheumatoid arthritis*. It involves pain, stiffness, swelling, and mild elevation in inflammatory markers in a symmetric fashion and usually involving small joints. Mild synovial proliferation and erosions could make the differentiation with rheumatoid arthritis even more challenging. In elderly patients, polymyalgia rheumatica with peripheral arthritis can present in a similar way.

Additional presentations of CPPD include severe destructive arthritides resembling neuropathic arthropathies and axial skeleton disease with low back or neck pain. The latter could be acute and severe, even mimicking meningitis or inflammatory back pains.

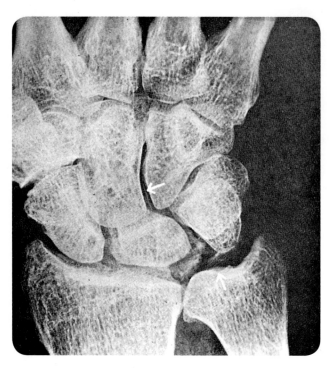

Figure 20.5 Anteroposterior radiograph of the wrist, showing calcification of the cartilaginous articular disc and a fine line of calcification parallel to the radiodensity of the underlying bone, indicative of articular cartilage calcification (*arrow*). (Reproduced with permission from Koopman WJ, Moreland LW, eds. *Arthritis and Allied Conditions: A Textbook of Rheumatology.* 15th ed. Philadelphia: Lippincott Williams & Wilkins; 2005.)

Studies

The diagnosis of CPPD can be reinforced when in the right clinical context, analysis of synovial fluid demonstrates the presence of small, weakly positive birefringent crystals on a polarizing light microscopic examination (blue when the larger axis of the crystal is parallel to the axis of the polarizer; see Fig. 20.4). These are usually rectangular, but could also be squared, oblong, or have other irregular shapes. An inflammatory synovial fluid also supports the role of the crystals in the inflammatory arthritis. An additional important reason to examine synovial fluid, mainly in patients with acute arthritis in which pseudogout is in the differential, is to rule out septic arthritis and gout. Limitations of synovial fluid analysis to establish a diagnosis of pseudogout include the technical challenges to identify the crystals (these are often small and can easily be missed) and the fact that calcium pyrophosphate crystals can be present in joints not affected by CPPD.

Another useful approach in the work-up of CPPD is through radiologic studies demonstrating the presence of chondrocalcinosis in suspicious joints. Chondrocalcinosis appears as a fine, punctate, discrete, or linear radio-opacity in cartilaginous areas (Fig. 20.5). Commonly involved are the knees, wrists, and hips at the levels of the symphysis pubis. Chondrocalcinosis is a common finding in radiologic studies in elderly individuals, so its finding should be interpreted as supportive of the diagnosis of CPPD in the right clinical context. Diagnostic criteria for CPPD have been published and are presented in Table 20.6.

Table 20.6 Diagnostic Criteria and Categories for Calcium Pyrophosphate Dihydrate Crystal Deposition Disease (Revised Version)

1. Demonstration of calcium pyrophosphate dihydrate crystals in tissue or synovial fluid by definitive means (e.g., characteristic x-ray diffraction of chemical analysis)

2. a. Identification of monoclinic or triclinic crystals showing weakly positive or no birefringence by compensated polarized light microscopy
   b. Presence of typical radiographic calcification

3. a. Acute arthritis, especially of knees or other large joints
   b. Chronic arthritis, especially of knee, hip, wrist, carpus, elbow, shoulder, or metacarpophalangeal joint, especially if accompanied by acute exacerbations. The following features help in differentiating from osteoarthritis:
      i. Uncommon site for primary osteoarthritis: wrist, metacarpophalangeal, elbow, and shoulder
      ii. Radiographic appearance; e.g., radiocarpal or isolated patellofemoral joint space narrowing
      iii. Subchondral cyst formation
      iv. Severe progressive degeneration, with subchondral bony collapse (microfractures), and fragmentation with formation of intra-articular radiodense bodies
      v. Variable and inconstant osteophyte formation
      vi. Tendon calcifications, especially of Achilles, triceps, and obturator tendons
      vii. Involvement of the axial skeleton and subchondral cysts of apophyseal and sacroiliac joints, multiple levels of disc calcification and vacuum phenomenon, and sacroiliac vacuum phenomenon

Categories

   A. Definite: Criteria 1 or 2(a) and 2(b) must be fulfilled
   B. Probable: Criteria 2(a) or 2(b) must be fulfilled
   C. Possible: Criteria 3(a) or 3(b) should alert the clinician to the possibility of underlying CPPD deposition

Treatment

The therapeutic approach to CPPD will depend on the specific presentation of the disease. The management is only symptomatic, as there is no way to remove calcium pyrophosphate deposits from synovial tissue. The identification and successful management of conditions that predispose to CPPD can prevent further deposition of calcium pyrophosphate in joints, but will not lead to resorption of existing calcium pyrophosphate deposits.

The management of acute attacks of pseudogout is similar to that of gout flares with NSAIDs, local or systemic glucocorticoids, and colchicine. Colchicine is regarded as effective in most cases of CPPD, but in reality, it is more effective relative to the acuity and inflammation of the presentation of CPPD (pseudogout > pseudorheumatoid > pseudo-osteoarthritis). Colchicine can also be used for prophylaxis of acute attacks in patients who suffer from those frequently. For CPPD associated only with joint degeneration, an approach similar to primary osteoarthritis (analgesic agents, physical therapy, bracing, localized injections) is preferred.

Clinical Course

Acute flares of gout and CPPD can be self-limited; use of anti-inflammatory agents can hasten recovery. A small number of patients with gout can continue to have some discomfort during the intercritical periods. The chronic form of gout can be deforming and cause significant disability. Unlike gout, CPPD can frequently present as a polyarticular arthropathy resembling rheumatoid arthritis and osteoarthritis respectively; these forms of CPPD tend to have a less erosive and destructive course than that of rheumatoid arthritis. Epidemiologic evidence linking hyperuricemia to an adverse cardiovascular outcomes is intriguing and merits further evaluation.

ICD9

716.9 **Arthritis, arthritic** *(acute) (chronic) (subacute)*
due to or associated with crystals
   275.49 [712.1] dicalcium phosphate
   275.49 [712.2] pyrophosphate
   275.49 [712.8] specified NEC
274.00 gouty
   274.01 acute

275.49 [712.3] **Chondrocalcinosis** *(articular) (crystal deposition) (dihydrate)*
due to
   275.49 [712.2] calcium pyrophosphate
   275.49 [712.1] dicalcium phosphate crystals
   275.49 [712.2] pyrophosphate crystals

274.9 **Gout**, *gouty*
274.00 arthritis
274.01 acute
274.00 arthropathy
274.01 acute
274.02 chronic (without mention of tophus (tophi))
   274.03 with tophus (tophi)
274.03 tophi
   274.81 ear
   274.82 specified site NEC

References

1. Lawrence RC, Felson DT, Helmick CG, et al. Estimates of the prevalence of arthritis and other rheumatic conditions in the United States. Part II. *Arthritis Rheum* 2008;5826–5835.
2. Campion EW, Glynn RJ, DeLabry LO. Asymptomatic hyperuricemia. Risks and consequences in the Normative Aging Study. *Am J Med* 1987;82:421–426.
3. Martinon F. Mechanisms of uric acid crystal-mediated autoinflammation. *Immunol Rev* 233:218–232.
4. Wallace SL, Robinson H, Masi AT, et al. Preliminary criteria for the classification of the acute arthritis of primary gout. *Arthritis Rheum* 1977;20:895–900.
5. Zhang W, Doherty M, Pascual E, et al. EULAR evidence based recommendations for gout. Part I: Diagnosis. Report of a task force of the Standing Committee for International Clinical Studies Including Therapeutics (ESCISIT). *Ann Rheum Dis* 2006;65:1301–1311.
6. Janssens HJ, Fransen J, van de Lisdonk EH, et al. A diagnostic rule for acute gouty arthritis in primary care without joint fluid analysis. *Arch Intern Med* 2010;170:1120–1126.
7. Terkeltaub RA, Furst DE, Bennett K, et al. High versus low dosing of oral colchicine for early acute gout flare: Twenty-four-hour outcome of the first multicenter, randomized, double-blind, placebo-controlled, parallel-group, dose-comparison colchicine study. *Arthritis Rheum* 2010;62:1060–1068.
8. Becker MA, Schumacher HR, Jr., Wortmann RL, et al. Febuxostat compared with allopurinol in patients with hyperuricemia and gout. *N Engl J Med* 2005;353:2450–2461.
9. Feig DI, Kang DH, Johnson RJ. Uric acid and cardiovascular risk. *N Engl J Med* 2008;359:1811–1821.

CHAPTER 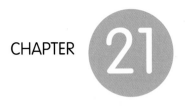 Osteopenic Bone Diseases and Osteonecrosis

Kenneth G. Saag, Gregory A. Clines, and Sarah L. Morgan

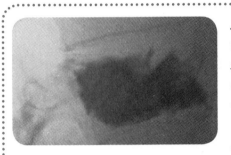

A 75-year-old male seen for compression fractures. He relates a strong family history of metabolic bone disease or fractures; his mother had severe osteoporosis, two sisters have osteoporosis, and his father had compression fractures, which complicated his emphysema. He presents with records documenting compressions fractures at thoracic vertebra 11 (T11), T12 and lumbar vertebra 4 (L4) and L5. He has undergone a kyphoplasty at L5. All compression fractures occurred without known trauma. He was initially treated with injectable calcitonin and has been on alendronate for approximately 10 years. He is referred because of concern for future fractures and worsening restrictive long disease in the setting of glucocorticoid-dependent obstructive lung disease.

He indicates that he has a history of infertility and problems with impotence. He has a long history of inhaled glucocorticoid use. There is no history of anabolic steroid use and no history of thyroid disease.

He grew up drinking milk, but currently drinks no milk and eats 2 oz of cheese per week. He consumes no calcium-fortified foods. He generally does not get any significant sun exposure. He consumes 15 glasses of wine per week and 2 oz of hard liquor per week.

His past medical history is remarkable for atherosclerotic heart disease, emphysema, hyperlipidemia, and osteoarthritis. His current medications include alendronate 70 mg/week, calcium carbonate plus vitamin D twice a day, ibuprofen two tablets daily for back pain, montelukast 10 mg orally daily, ipratropium bromide and albuterol sulfate inhaler two puffs four times a day, inhaled.

On physical examination, he is 68 in. tall (driver's license height is 74 in.), his weight is 238 lb, vital signs are normal. MP's posture is notable, head bowed forward with a slightly protuberant abdomen. He is wearing an extension brace. Eyes, no blue sclera. Mouth, no exposed bone. The thyroid is palpable without masses.

Lower thoracic kyphosis, no point pain to palpation. Chest, clear and cardiac examination murmur. Abdomen, no organomegaly or pain. Neurologic, nonfocal.

Laboratory data. Chemistry profile normal, calcium = 8.7, alkaline phosphatase = 99, PTH = 67 (nl 12 to 90). CBC, IFE, PSA all normal. Anti tissue transglutaminase (TTG) <5. 25-OH vitamin D total = 43. Calcium/creatinine ratio on a spot urine = 0.10.

The patient is started on teriparatide as an anabolic agent for his bone. There was no history of bone tumors, radiation therapy, and implantable radiation to pose an absolute contraindication. The baseline alkaline phosphates and baseline bone-specific alkaline phosphatase were normal.

Table 21.1 World Health Organization (WHO) Criteria for the Diagnosis of Osteopenic Bone Disease Based on T-score	
CATEGORY	**DEFINITION**
Normal	BMD better than 1 SD below the mean value of peak bone mass in young white women
Osteopenia (low bone mass)	BMD between 1.0 and 2.5 SD below the mean peak value
Osteoporosis	BMD more than 2.5 SD below the peak value
Severe osteoporosis	BMD criteria for osteoporosis and fracture

BMD, bone mineral density; SD, standard deviation.

Introduction

Osteoporosis is a systemic skeletal disease characterized by low bone mass and microarchitectural deterioration of bone tissue with a consequent increase in bone fragility and susceptibility to fracture. The World Health Organization (WHO) definitions of osteoporosis are based on epidemiologic data that relate fracture incidence to bone mineral density (BMD) in Caucasian women (Table 21.1).

By age 60 to 70 years, one of three non-Hispanic Caucasian women will have osteoporosis and the remainder, osteopenia (a state of low bone mass in between normal and osteoporotic BMD); by age 80 years, 70% will have osteoporosis. Figure 21.1 shows the prevalence of osteoporosis and osteopenia in American women both now and into the future.

The estimated number of fractures among North American women was >200,000 in 1990 and is estimated to increase to nearly 500,000 in 2025. The proportion of fractures attributable to osteoporosis is less for nonwhites than whites and less for men than women. The incidence rate for hip fractures is approximately 2 per 1,000 patient-years at age 65 to 69 in Caucasian and non-Caucasian women, and increases to about 26 per 1,000 patient-years at age 80 to 84. The incidence and prevalence of vertebral fractures is low prior to age 50 years and rises almost exponentially thereafter (Table 21.2). Among American women, the incidence of wrist fractures increases rapidly at the time of menopause and plateaus at about 700 per 100,000 person-years after age 60.

The lifetime risk of any fracture in the hip, spine, or distal forearm is about 50% in Caucasian women of age 50 and 20% in Caucasian men of similar age. There are special populations, such as a population of individuals with human

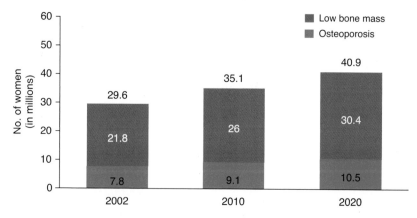

Figure 21.1 Prevalence of low bone mass and osteoporosis in women aged 50 years and older. (National Osteoporosis Foundation, available at: http://www.nof.org/advocacy/prevalence.)

CLINICAL POINTS

- Lifetime risk of osteoporotic fracture in Caucasian males is 20%.

- Obtain information of height loss over time from a driver's license.

- Unusual z-scores on DEXA scan can represent bone mineral disorder other than osteoporosis.

- Osteonecrosis of the jaw is a devastating complication from use of bisphosphonates and is associated with dental procedures.

- Diffuse bone pain can be a manifestation of osteomalacia.

- Osteonecrosis can be associated with alcohol abuse, prolonged use of corticosteroids, and many medical conditions including sickle cell disease and systemic lupus erythematosis (SLE).

Table 21.2 **Estimated Lifetime Fracture Risk in 50-Year-Old White Women and Men[a]**

SITE	WOMEN %, (95% CONFIDENCE INTERVAL[b])	MEN %, (95% CONFIDENCE INTERVAL[b])
Proximal femur	17.5 (16.8, 18.2)	6.0 (5.6, 6.5)
Vertebral fracture	15.6 (14.8, 16.3)	5.0 (4.6, 5.4)
Distal forearm fracture	16.0 (15.2, 16.7)	2.5 (2.2, 3.1)
Any fracture	39.7 (38.7, 40.6)	13.1 (12.4, 13.7)

[a]Age 50 years was chosen because this is about the average of menopause in women.
[b]Using incidence of clinically diagnosed fractures only.
From Melton LJ, Chrischilles EA, Cooper C, et al. How many women have osteoporosis? *J Bone Miner Res* 1992;7:1005–1010, with permission.

immunodeficiency virus (HIV) where a high prevalence and progression of osteoporosis or osteopenia has been documented. It is anticipated that the prevalence of osteoporosis and likely fractures will grow in this population.

Osteoporosis and consequent fractures are major public health concerns in the United States. The economic costs of osteoporotic fractures are large and somewhat difficult to assess because the total includes expenses for surgery and hospitalization, rehabilitation, long-term care costs, loss of productivity, and medications. Other burdens associated with fracture include poor resultant functional status, pain, a diminished quality of life, loss of independence, fear, and depression.

Hip fractures result in more than 7 million days of restricted activity and 6,000 admissions to nursing homes annually in the United States; nearly three quarters of all nursing home admissions are related to osteoporosis. For hip fractures, about half of the health care costs reflect nursing home expenses. There is an approximately 20% mortality within 1 year of hip fracture, and 50% of survivors never fully recover. The mortality associated with vertebral fractures is also greater than expected in the general population, whereas the mortality of patients with wrist fractures is similar.

Figure 21.2 shows the lifetime accrual and loss of BMD in men and women. Peak BMD is the maximum possible with normal growth and represents a genetically and environmentally determined apex from which future losses occur. Most skeletal density (both trabecular and cortical) is accumulated by age 18. In cortical bone, a slow phase of loss begins at age 40, ranging from 0.3 to 0.5% per year in men and women. At menopause in women not taking hormone replacement therapy, losses average about 1% per year, but may approach 3% to 5% per year. After this accelerated loss for about 8 to 10 years, the rate decreases in another slow phase. The cumulative lifetime losses of bone may be as much as 30% to 40% of peak BMD in women and 20% to 30% in men.

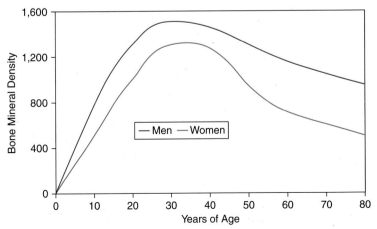

Figure 21.2 Age-related bone mineral density for men and women. From Christenson RH. Biochemical markers of bone metabolism: An overview. *Clin Biochem* 1997;30:573–593, with permission. (Reprinted in Saag KG, Morgan SL, Cao X, et al. Bone in health and disease. In: Koopman WJ, ed. *Arthritis and Allied Condition: A Textbook of Rheumatology.* 15th ed. Philadelphia: Lippincott Williams & Wilkins; 2005:2449–2541.)

Clinical Presentation

The clinical evaluation of osteoporosis should identify lifestyle risk factors and pertinent physical findings, and assess secondary causes of osteopenia. Table 21.3 provides conditions associated with osteopenia or osteoporosis.

Table 21.3 Diseases and Drug Therapies Associated with Osteopenia and Fracture

Unique to women
  Natural menopause
  Pregnancy
  Hypogonadism
    Agonist for gonadotropin-releasing hormone or
      Depo- Provera
    Gonadal dysgenesis (e.g., Turner's syndrome)
    Endometriosis

Unique to men
  Hypogonadism
    Constitutional delay of puberty
    Hemochromatosis (due to either infiltration
      of testes (hypergonadotropic) or pituitary
      (hypogonadotropic)
    Kallman's syndrome (isolated gonadotropin
      deficiency)
    Klinefelter's syndrome (genotype XXY)
    Orchitis, viral

Men and women
  Age-related bone loss
  Connective tissue diseases
    Ankylosing spondylitis
    Osteogenesis imperfecta
    Rheumatoid arthritis
    Spinal cord injury

Endocrine causes
  Acromegaly
  Adrenal trophy and Addison's disease
  Cushing's syndrome
  Diabetes mellitus type 1
  Glucocorticoid excess (endogenous and exogenous)
  Gonadotroph cell adenoma
  Hyperparathyroidism (primary and secondary)
  Hyperprolactinemia (as a cause of hypogonadism)
  Hyperthyroidism
  Hypercalcitoninemia?
  Hypogonadism (primary, secondary, or surgical)
  Panhypopituitarism
  Thyrotoxicosis

Gastrointestinal diseases
  Cholestatic liver disease (especially primary biliary
    cirrhosis)
  Gastrectomy
  Inflammatory bowel disease (especially regional
    enteritis)
  Postgastrectomy

Lifestyle/genetic factors
  Excessive alcohol
  Excessive caffeine?
  Excessive exercise (impairment of hypothalamic–
    pituitary axis)

Excessive protein intake
  Immobilization or microgravity
  Low calcium or vitamin D intake
  Sedentary lifestyle
  Smoking

Malignancy

  Lymphoproliferative and myeloproliferative
    diseases (lymphoma and leukemia)
  Multiple myeloma
  Systemic mastocytosis
  Tumor secretion of parathyroid hormone–related
    peptide

Nutritional disorders

Eating disorders, such as anorexia nervosa
  Osteomalacia
  Malabsorption syndromes
  Parenteral nutrition
  Pernicious anemia
  Bariatric surgery (especially Roux-en-Y bypass)

Other diseases
  Chronic obstructive pulmonary disease (often
    secondary to glucocorticoid usage)
  Chronic renal failure
  Congenital porphyria
  Hemochromatosis
  Hemophilia
  Homocystinuria
  Hypophosphatasia
  Thalassemia

Medications
  Aluminum
  Antiepileptics (some)
  Chemotherapeutic agents that cause chemical
    castration
  Cyclosporine A and tacrolimus
  Cytotoxic drugs
  Glucocorticoids and adrenocorticotropin
  Heparin (perhaps less severe with low-molecular-
    weight compounds)
  Lithium
  Methotrexate
  Tamoxifen (premenopausal use)
  Thyroid hormone (in excess)
  Selective serotonin reuptake inhibitors
  Proton pump inhibitors
  Thioglitazones

From Morgan SL, Saag KG, Cao X, et al. Bone in health and disease. In: Koopman WJ, ed. *Arthritis and Allied Condition: A Textbook of Rheumatology.*
15th ed. Philadelphia: Lippincott Williams & Wilkins; 2005:2449–2541.

A careful evaluation of osteoporosis includes *identification* of a family history of metabolic bone disease, lifestyle risk factors, history of change in height and weight, history of previous fractures, reproductive history (evidence of hypogonadism), endocrine history, dietary factors (including lifetime and current consumption of calcium, vitamin D, sodium, and caffeine), a smoking history, alcohol intake, exercise, history of renal or hepatic failure, and past and current medications and supplements. In addition, factors that increase the risk of falls, such as neuromuscular disease and unsafe living conditions, should also be sought. A history of bone pain is useful; however, osteoporosis is not painful unless fractures develop. Further, a large proportion of vertebral fractures may occur without overt symptoms.

Examination

Height measurement is a vital part of the physical examination at each visit. Comparison of current height with that on a driver's license is helpful in uncovering height loss. Loss of 2 in. or more is a fairly sensitive indicator of vertebral compression. The spine should be examined for conformation and spinal and paraspinous tenderness. If kyphosis is present, the possibility of pulmonary compromise should be considered. A "buffalo hump," easy bruisability, and striae suggest Cushing's syndrome. Blue sclerae may indicate osteogenesis imperfecta. The number of missing teeth has been correlated to the severity of loss in BMD. A joint assessment may suggest rheumatologic causes of low BMD. The neurologic examination is important because muscular weakness predisposes to falls and an underlying neurologic problem may be discovered.

Studies

LABORATORY EVALUATION

Routine Laboratory Testing
The laboratory assessment seeks possible secondary causes of loss of BMD. Table 21.4 provides tests that may be appropriate. Many are not cost-effective if obtained for every patient. Intact PTH concentration, for example, should be

Table 21.4 Laboratory Evaluation of Decreased Bone Mass

TEST	DIAGNOSIS RULED IN OR RULED OUT
Serum protein electrophoresis/complete blood count	Multiple myeloma
Serum calcium and phosphorus	Hyperparathyroidism
Serum intact parathyroid hormone	Hyperparathyroidism
Serum creatinine	Renal failure
Liver enzymes	Liver failure
24-hour urine-free cortisol or dexamethasone suppression test	Cushing's syndrome
Thyroid-stimulating hormone	Hyperthyroidism
Follicle-stimulating hormone	Menopause
Free testosterone	Male hypogonadism
Urine calcium/creatinine ratio	Hypercalciuria
25-monohydroxy vitamin D_3 and alkaline phosphatase	Vitamin D deficiency or osteomalacia

Table 21.5 Biochemical Markers of Bone Turnover

FORMATION	RESORPTION
From osteoblasts, in serum	*From osteoclasts*
Bone alkaline phosphatase	Tartrate-resistant acid phosphatase
Osteocalcin	
From bone matrix, in serum	
Procollagen I C-terminal propeptide	N-terminal telopeptide of type I collagen
Procollagen I N-terminal propeptide	C-terminal telopeptide of type I collagen
From bone matrix, in urine	
	Pyridinoline and deoxypyridinoline cross-links
	N-terminal telopeptide of type I collagen
	Hydroxyproline from collagen degradation

From Rosalki SB. Biochemical markers of bone turnover. *Int J Clin Pract* 1998;52:256, with permission.

measured if the calcium concentration is elevated and the phosphorus concentration is low or if clinical suspicion is high for hyperparathyroidism.

Specific Bone Turnover Markers

Biochemical markers of bone turnover are sometimes used in the management of osteoporosis. While bone formation and resorption are usually "coupled," net imbalances can be evaluated with these assays. Table 21.5 provides bone turnover markers that can be classified as indices of bone formation or resorption. "Bone balance" is the net difference between formation and resorption.

Imaging

Dual-energy x-ray absorptiometry (DXA) is currently the "gold standard" for patient care and clinical investigation for osteoporosis. On DXA, bone mass is reported as an absolute value in g/cm^2, a comparison to age- and sex-matched reference range (the Z-score), and a comparison to mean bone mass of young adult normal individuals (the T-score or young-adult Z-score; see Fig. 21.3). T-scores are used to predict fracture risk and classify disease status. A change of one standard deviation in the T- or Z-score correlates to a change of approximately $0.06 \ g/cm^2$, or about 10% of BMD. Although the Z-score is of less clinical value than the T-score, Z-scores significantly deviating from normal may indicate alternative causes of metabolic bone disease. Dual-energy x-ray absorptiometry scans also produce a density-based image useful in interpreting scan quality (see Fig. 21.3 and below). These readings are compared to the National Health and Nutrition Examination Survey (NHANES) III database.

Dual-energy x-ray absorptiometry measures BMD at central and peripheral sites. The choice of site(s) scanned should depend on the anticipated rates of change in bone mass within these skeletal locations and precision of the testing device at these sites. The central DXA sites of the hip and spine, followed by peripheral sites of the wrist and heel, are the most desired imaging locations. Central DXA of the spine and hip has excellent precision and good accuracy. Central DXA is generally preferred because the quantity of cancellous bone of central sites is highly indicative of the osteoporosis burden and fracture risk. In osteoporosis, the earliest bone loss begins in cancellous bone. A higher proportion of early postmenopausal women have lower cancellous BMD

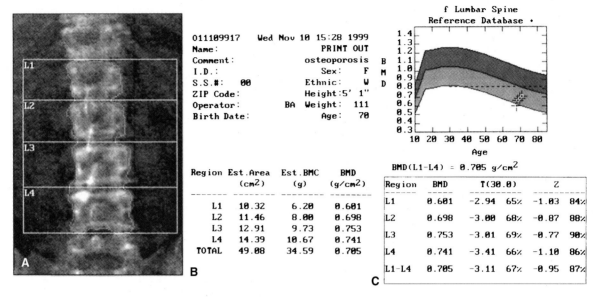

Figure 21.3 Dual-energy x-ray absorptiometry (DXA) printout. For a 70-year-old white woman. **A:** DXA of this patient's lumbar spine showing imaging windows for vertebrae L1 to L4. Estimated vertebral areas, bone mineral content (BMC), and bone mineral density (BMD) are shown (*middle*). Bone mineral density is plotted against a lumbar spine reference database showing the patient's current value as well as previous readings indicated by crosses (*right, top*). The dark (*top*) bar of the graph indicated 2 standard deviations above normal and the *lighter* (*bottom*) bar 2 standard deviations below peak bone mass. *T-scores* (peak bone mass matched) show that the patient is well below the World Health Organization's definition of osteoporosis (*T-score* <−2.5) at each vertebral level and for the lumbar spine overall. The *Z*-score is an age-matched measurement. **B:** Similar parameters are shown for the left hip, and based on *T-scores*, there is osteoporosis at both the femoral neck and the total hip. **C:** At both the hip and lumbar spine, there has been significant 3-year improvement in BMD. The serial plot (*left*) and table show a nearly 12% increase at the left hip. The *asterisk* signifies a significant increase of decline between two values. An 18.4% increase in BMD was also seen at the lumbar spine (data not shown). (From Saag KG, Morgan SL, Cao X, et al. Bone in health and disease. In: Koopman WJ, ed. *Arthritis and Allied Condition: A Textbook of Rheumatology*. 15th ed. Philadelphia: Lippincott Williams & Wilkins; 2005:2449–2541.)

than cortical BMD. Approximately a third of the spongy trabecular bone of the hip and spine remodels each year as opposed to only 3% turnover of compact cortical bone comprising a greater proportion of peripheral skeleton. At the spine, DXA reports measurements of an individual vertebra as well as average BMD of the L1 to L4 (see Fig. 21.3). At the hip, femoral neck, and the total hip are the three measurement sites of greatest clinical interest. Central measurements are used to diagnose osteoporosis, assess fracture risk, and follow up the response to antiosteoporotic therapies.

Peripheral DXA of the forearm is moderately correlated with central DXA results and can, thus, be used as an alternative to predict fracture risk. Heel DXA correlates well with other heel imaging technologies and adequately discriminates osteoporotic from normal young subjects. However, the much slower rate of bone remodeling at sites such as the heel limits this technology for monitoring the response to therapy. The enhanced portability of dedicated peripheral bone mass measurement instruments and their lower cost renders them increasingly attractive for community osteoporosis screening.

Vertebral fracture analysis (VFA) is a point of service examination that can be performed on many DXA scanners. Vertebral fracture analysis concentrates on the morphometry of individual vertebral bodies for the purpose of identifying vertebral compression fractures.

Bone mineral density measured by DXA is a good predictor of the risk of hip and spinal fractures. Spinal fracture is inversely proportional to bone mineral content. For each decline of about 1 standard deviation of bone mass, there is a 1.3- to 2.5-fold increase in fracture risk of any site. Although fracture risk at any site can be accurately assessed using a variety of noninvasive bone mass measurements done at any site, BMD at the femoral neck is better than BMD at

SECTION 4 Osteoarthritis and Metabolic Bone

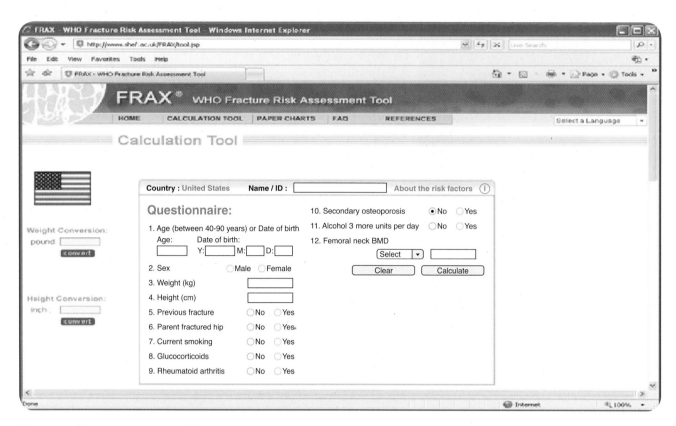

Figure 21.4 The FRAX WHO Fracture Risk Assessment Tool. Calculates the 10-year probability of hip and major osteoporotic* fracture in previously untreated patients. Major osteoporotic fracture is defined as vertebral, hip, forearm, or humerus fracture. (National Osteoporosis Foundation. *Clinician's Guide to Prevention and Treatment of Osteoporosis.* Washington, DC: National Osteoporosis Foundation; 2008. FRAX® WHO Fracture Risk Assessment Tool. Available at: www.shef.ac.uk/FRAX/tool.jsp.)

the spine, radius, and calcaneus to predict hip fracture. Decreases of 2 standard deviations in radial and calcaneal bone mass are associated with 4- to 6-fold increases in risk for vertebral fracture. Increasing age and decreasing BMD of the radius predict subsequent nonspinal fractures. It is estimated that a 50-year-old woman has a 19% lifetime risk of fracture if radial bone mass is in the 10th percentile compared with an 11% lifetime risk if the measurement is in the 90th percentile. Absolute fracture risk for the next 10 years can be calculated by incorporating clinical information on fracture risk with BMD and using the FRAX tool available on the Web (http://www.sheffield.ac.uk/FRAX/; see Fig. 21.4).

Prevention and Therapy

Although decrements in BMD may accurately predict fracture risk, when evaluating prevention and treatment studies, the effect of an intervention on fracture incidence is the most critical outcome.

Numerous general medical and specialty societies have promulgated guidelines for osteoporosis prevention and treatment. In 2009 the National Osteoporosis Foundation (NOF) issued guidelines in collaboration with 10 medical organizations. These recommendations are based on age, BMD T-score, and whether or not there are accompanying risk factors. The NOF guidelines advocate pharmacologic intervention to reduce the risk of fractures in:

- a hip or vertebral (clinical or morphometric) fracture;
- T-score ≤–2.5 at the femoral neck or spine after appropriate evaluation to exclude secondary causes;

- low bone mass (T-score between –1.0 and –2.5 at the femoral neck or spine) *and* a 10-year probability of a hip fracture ≥3% *or* a 10-year probability of a major osteoporosis-related fracture ≥20% using the US-adapted WHO algorithm (see FRAX, Fig. 21.2);
- Clinician's judgment and/or patient preferences may indicate treatment for people with 10-year fracture probabilities above or below these levels.

NONPHARMACOLOGIC PREVENTION

Exercise

Moderate to intensive weight-bearing exercise can lead to modest increases of about 1% to 3% in BMD. For an exercise to be effective in altering BMD, it must strain the skeletal site being evaluated. For example, bone mass gains are particularly notable in the tibia in runners and in the spine among weight lifters. Older women may demonstrate lumbar BMD gains with regular vigorous weight-bearing exercise performed multiple times per week. Continued physical activity is required to maintain observed BMD gains. Spinal extension exercises are preferred over flexion maneuvers, which may lead to spinal compression deformities.

Hip Protectors

Protective hip pads worn in specialized undergarments have effectively reduced fracture rates in nursing home patients in some studies. Adherence to these devices is problematic and other studies have not been supportive of their efficacy.

PHARMACOLOGIC PREVENTION

Calcium and Vitamin D

Calcium alone may somewhat reduce, but not fully prevent, bone loss early after menopause. In postmenopausal women, sufficient calcium provided through dietary and exogenous sources decreases appendicular skeletal bone loss by 1% to 3% compared to women who do not consume adequate calcium. Calcium may be most beneficial for women later after menopause. However, even among younger women and men, calcium supplementation prevents bone loss at various skeletal sites.

Varying amounts of elemental calcium are found in different food groups and nutritional supplements. Calcium is equally well absorbed (25% to 30%) from either milk products or calcium carbonate. Although some studies suggest that calcium citrate has slightly higher absorption than other preparations, other investigations indicate that they are equally well absorbed.

One area of controversy concerns the use of calcium supplements in patients with a history of nephrolithiasis. High intake of dietary calcium appears to decrease the risk of stones, whereas intake of high doses of supplemental calcium may modestly increase risk. Dietary calcium may beneficially bind oxalate, the primary component in most renal stones.

Although calcium supplements are well tolerated by many, constipation (in about 10% of users) and dyspepsia limit long-term adherence. Individual trials of different preparations and times of administration may maximize patient satisfaction. Institute of Medicine 2010 Consensus recommendations for daily doses of elemental calcium are provided in Table 21.6. The increasing varieties of food and beverage products available in the United States that are calcium fortified have reduced the reliance on exogenous calcium salt supplements to achieve daily requirements. There is evidence from some, but not other, studies that excessive calcium supplementation may increase cardiovascular events, such as myocardial infarction, in certain populations.

Vitamin D is a group of fat-soluble sterols that includes ergocalciferol (vitamin D_2) and cholecalciferol (vitamin D_3); vitamin D_3 is more potent than vitamin D_2. These inactive prohormones are hydroxylated in the liver and kidney

Table 21.6 Calcium and Vitamin D Recommended Daily Allowances from the Institute of Medicine		
AGE RANGE (YEARS)	**CALCIUM (MG/DAY)**	**VITAMIN D (IU/DAY)**
9–18	1,300	600
19–50	1,000	600
51–70 (men)		
51–70 (women)	1,200	600
>70	1,200	800

to produce the active vitamin D metabolite calcitriol or 1,25-dihydroxyvitamin D. Calcitriol increases calcium absorption and may prevent spinal bone loss, particularly among older women. Despite BMD gains, several studies have not shown a beneficial effect of active vitamin D metabolites on fracture rate. Recent evidence suggests that the important biological effects of vitamin D in bone are not dependent on circulating calcitriol, but on local concentrations of this active hormone generated through conversion from the inactive vitamin D. The potential for hypercalciuria and hypercalcemia with active vitamin D preparations limits their routine use and requires careful serum and urine monitoring. If calcitriol is used, it is important to moderate calcium supplementation.

Inactivated vitamin D analogues also have beneficial effects on bone. Vitamin D lowers the risk of hip and other nonvertebral fractures among older women and men in some, but not all, studies. Vitamin D may also lower fall risk. Table 21.6 provides guidelines for vitamin D daily requirements of older adults. In individuals with documented vitamin D deficiency or calcium malabsorption, more vitamin D supplementation is needed.

Estrogen

Because of the accelerated rate of bone loss at menopause, estrogen replacement therapy (ERT) has been used in postmenopausal women for osteoporosis prevention. Estrogen replacement therapy is most effective in decreasing bone mass when initiated soon after menopause and used continuously. Estrogen in combination with progestin significantly reduced the risk of hip fractures on the basis of the large Women's Health Initiative (WHI). However, this combination in WHI was also associated with an increase in cardiovascular adverse outcomes and breast cancer incidence. Venous thromboembolic events are three to four times more common among estrogen users than nonusers. Daily administration of estrogen with continuous low-dose progestin (e.g., medroxyprogesterone 2.5 mg/day) is generally well tolerated with rare breakthrough bleeding and no documented increase in the endometrial thickness. Lower doses administered through transdermal preparations have benefits in bone without producing excessive thromboembolic risk.

Ultimately, the decision to initiate ERT needs to be individualized and is based on a balanced assessment of risk and benefits by the physician and patient. The presence of definitive fracture risk reduction data, a small increased risk for breast cancer, potential for hypercoagulability, an increasing concern about an cardiovascular risk, and the use of alternative bone-protective agents have attenuated enthusiasm for estrogens as antiosteoporotic agents, beyond the period immediately following menopause.

Selective Estrogen Receptor Modulators

Selective estrogen receptor modulators (SERMs) are nonsteroidal synthetic compounds that have estrogen-like properties in the bone and cardiovascular systems, yet are estrogen antagonists to the breast and, in some cases, the endometrium. Raloxifene is the only SERM currently licensed in the United States for osteoporosis. It significantly lowers biochemical markers of bone remodeling to levels equivalent to conjugated estrogens. In postmenopausal women, after 6 months of raloxifene 60 mg/day, bone mass in the lumbar spine and at the total hip increased significantly. Low-density lipoproteins, total cholesterol, and triglycerides all declined and high-density lipoproteins increased. In a large multicenter trial, raloxifene slightly but significantly increased BMD of the spine and femoral neck BMD, and reduced vertebral fracture risk by 30%. It has not been proved to prevent fractures at nonvertebral sites. The risk of invasive breast cancer also was decreased by raloxifene. In contrast to estrogen, hot flashes and other menopausal symptoms may recur with raloxifene. Similar to estrogen, with raloxifene there is an increase in lower extremity edema and a threefold increased risk of deep venous thrombosis.

Calcitonin

When used for prevention or treatment of osteoporosis, synthetic calcitonin (derived from salmon) is administered either subcutaneously (up to 100 IU daily for osteoporosis) or more commonly intranasally (200 IU daily). Calcitonin should be given with adequate calcium (at least 1 g) and vitamin D (400 IU daily). Randomized controlled trials of injectable and intranasal calcitonin for treatment of established postmenopausal osteoporosis have consistently shown either stabilization of BMD or small, but significant, increases in vertebral BMD. Beneficial BMD effects at the hip have not yet been reported. A 5-year multicenter study of calcitonin nasal spray showed a 36% reduction in vertebral fractures in the 200 IU, but not in the 100 or 400 IU groups. Interpretation of study was limited by an approximately 50% dropout rate. Nasal calcitonin is generally well tolerated, other than occasional rhinitis minimized by alternating nostrils each day. Headache, flushing, nausea, and diarrhea have been reported more commonly with subcutaneous than with intranasal calcitonin. On the basis of its weak antiresorptive effects and the availability of a growing armamentarium of other antiosteoporosis agents, the use of calcitonin has declined over time and is currently relegated to a second- or third-line option.

Bisphosphonates

Bisphosphonates comprise a class of antiresorptive agents characterized by a phosphorus–carbon–phosphorus bond. They are recognized as potent inhibitors of bone resorption and reduce risks for fractures when administered orally or by intravenous infusion. Variations in the structure of their amino side chains alter the pharmacologic activity. Bisphosphonates variably suppress osteoclasts and/or lead to premature death of osteoclasts as their primary mechanism of action. Oral bisphosphonates are poorly absorbed with bioavailability of less than 1% and are bound by divalent cations. Thus, with the exception of one preparation of risedronate that is deemed acceptable to take with food, they should be taken on an empty stomach to maximize absorption. Bisphosphonates tightly bind to hydroxyapatite crystals in the resorption lacunae of bone where they have a long skeletal retention (about 10 years for alendronate). This property results in protracted partial suppression of bone remodeling for months to years after the medications are discontinued.

Four bisphosphonates alendronate, risedronate, ibandronate, and zoledronic acid are licensed in the United States for treatment of osteoporosis. Potential modes of administration of these agents vary somewhat as given in Table 21.7.

Alendronate inhibits bone resorption without detrimental effects on mineralization over the short to moderate term. Studies of postmenopausal women receiving 10 mg/day showed that lumbar spine BMD increased up to 9% over a 2-year period. In a large US study of older women with at least one prior vertebral fracture and low femoral neck BMD, alendronate significantly reduced vertebral and hip fractures by 47% and 51%, respectively. In subjects without prevalent

Table 21.7 Prescription Drug Therapy for Osteoporosis

AGENT	MOST COMMON DOSE	ROUTE	FREQUENCY	EFFECT ON FRACTURE RISK		
				VERTEBRAL	NONVERTEBRAL	HIP
Estrogen	Variable	Pill/patch	Daily/weekly			
Raloxifene	60 mg	Pill	Daily	√	—	—
Calcitonin	200 IU	Nasal spray	Daily	√	—	—
Alendronate	70 mg	Pill	Weekly	√	√	√
Risedronate	35 mg/140 mg	Pill	Weekly/monthly	√	√	√
Ibandronate	150 mg/3 mg	Pill/IV	Monthly/3 months	√	—	—
Zoledronic acid	5 mg	IV	Yearly	√	√	√
Denosumab	60 mg	Subc injection	6 months	√	√	√
Teriparatide	20 µg	Subc injection	Daily	√	√	—

IV, intravenous; Subc, subcutaneous.

vertebral fractures, alendronate 10 mg/day decreased radiographic vertebral fractures by 44%. A similar multinational study of alendronate similarly identified a 47% risk reduction for nonvertebral fractures. Long-term extensions to this original study suggest that alendronate effects on BMD persist for up to 10 years and BMD gains are only modestly lost, at the hip sites more so than the spine, when the medicine is withdrawn. On the basis of convenience and potentially better adherence, coupled with near-equivalent BMD data compared to daily administration, alendronate is almost exclusively given as a weekly preparation.

Treatment with 5 mg/day of risedronate significantly lowered the risk of new vertebral (41% reduction) and nonvertebral (39% reduction) over a 3-year period in women with at least one prior vertebral fracture. A beneficial effect of each treatment on hip fractures among women with very low bone mass has also been demonstrated. Risedronate is generally well tolerated with no significant differences in upper gastrointestinal (GI) adverse events compared to those receiving placebo.

In large clinical trials of ibandronate, BMD at both the spine and the hip were increased significantly above placebo and fracture risk reduction was 52% at the spine. Ibandronate is the only bisphosphonate in the United States that can be administered either orally or intravenously.

Zoledronic acid is a once-yearly intravenous bisphosphonate. In phase III clinical trials it significantly increased BMD at the spine and hip and resulted in a significant reduction in spine (70%) and vertebral fractures (25%). Another large clinical trial demonstrated that among men and women with prior hip fractures, it significantly reduced their risk of a subsequent clinical fracture by 35%. An unexplained reduction in all-cause mortality was also observed in that study.

Oral bisphosphonates may cause GI intolerance, particularly at low gastric pH. Recommendations to reduce GI and maximize absorption include ingesting pills with 8 oz water, remaining upright for at least 30 minutes after swallowing the tablet, and having nothing to eat or drink for 30 to 60 minutes before and after ingesting each pill. Achalasia and esophageal strictures are contraindications to oral bisphosphonate therapy. While most GI toxicity of bisphosphonates is a nonserious side effect, there have been rare reports of severe esophagitis. Some studies suggest that GI safety may be better for particular agents. Esophageal cancer has been associated with chronic bisphosphonate administration in one report.

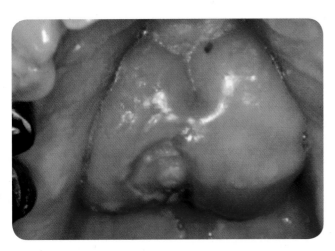

Figure 21.5 Osteonecrosis of the palatal torus in patients with osteoporosis taking alendronate. (Woo SB, Hellstein JW, kalmar JR. Systematic review: bisphosphonates and osteonecrosis of the jaws. *Ann Intern Med* 2006;144:753–761.)

Intravenous bisphosphates, particularly zoledronic acid, can lead to an acute-phase reaction, with arthralgias and flulike symptoms in up to 15% of persons. These symptoms are attenuated with coadministration of acetaminophen and less frequent with repeated intravenous administration or among prior users of oral bisphosphonates. Intravenous bisphosphonates may also at least transiently compromise renal function. All bisphosphonates, particularly intravenous preparations, require a creatinine clearance in excess of 30 mL/minute to minimize renal risk and also to help assure that the bone disease being treated is actually osteoporosis and not a form of metabolic bone disease associated with chronic kidney disease. An additional potential safety signal with intravenous zoledronic acid was the report of clinically relevant atrial fibrillation in one of the large clinical trials. This outcome was not observed in other large zoledronic acid studies or with other bisphosphonates.

While bisphosphonate safety overall has been acceptable in clinical trials, beyond clinical trials, there have been numerous case reports linking alendronate, and to a lesser degree, other bisphosphonates with a variety of adverse effects that could potentially result from prolonged or significant suppression of bone remodeling.

Osteonecrosis of the jaw (ONJ) has been associated with bisphosphonate exposure and is defined as an area of bare alveolar bone occurring anywhere in the mouth (see Fig. 21.5). It occurs most commonly following dental manipulation such as tooth extraction. Osteonecrosis of the jaw has been reported in up to 10% of persons who receive high-dose bisphosphonates (predominately intravenously) for the treatment of malignant conditions. The incidence in persons with osteoporosis taking bisphosphonates appears to be much lower, although exact rates are unknown.

A newer concern is the development of atypical fractures in the subtrochanteric (see Fig. 21.6A) and more distal regions of the hip and femur that are

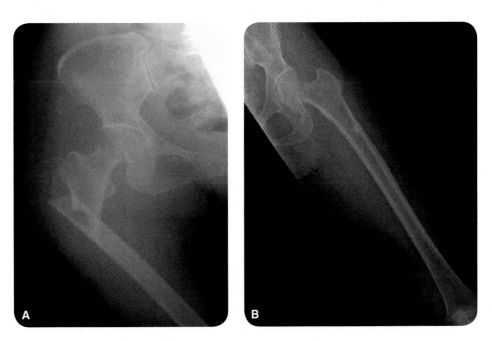

Figure 21.6 Radiographs of atypical femoral fractures. **A:** Fracture demonstrating characteristic transverse pattern in subtrochanteric region with medial bone "beaking." **B:** Contralateral femur showing area of stress reaction over later femoral cortex. This pattern is commonly associated with hip pain.

experienced without trauma and are often preceded by a hip pain syndrome associated with a radiographic stress reaction over the outer cortex of bone (see Fig. 21.6B). Observational studies to date have not established a positive link with bisphosphonate, but consensus statements of expert groups suggest this issue merits attention. This may be relevant particularly for long-term bisphosphonate users, those on glucocorticoids, and those receiving bisphosphonates with a state of lower bone turnover.

An overarching issue with all bisphosphonate therapies is how long to treat and whether there is a rationale for an eventual "drug holiday." On the basis of the protracted suppression of bone turnover by bisphosphonates along with emerging potential safety concerns that may relate to prolonged bisphosphonate exposure, it may be prudent to stop bisphosphonate therapy for a year or more in persons who have had a significant BMD response, are at relatively low risk for femoral neck fracture, and have had 5 years or more of oral therapy or several years or more of intravenous therapy. Monitoring bone turnover for "escape" during this time may prove as or more useful than BMD changes in determining when to reinitiate bisphosphonate or alternate therapies.

Teriparatide (Recombinant Parathyroid Hormone 1–34)

Teriparatide is an osteoporosis anabolic therapy approved for use in postmenopausal and male osteoporosis in the United States. In contrast to bisphosphonates, which block bone resorption, teriparatide predominately stimulates the osteoblast to form new bone. Large clinical trials support its efficacy on increasing BMD and reducing vertebral (65% risk reduction) as well as significantly reducing nonvertebral fractures. There is no specific data on hip fracture risk reduction. In contrast to antiresorptive agents such as bisphosphonates and denosumab, markers of bone formation and, to a lesser degree, bone resorption are increased. In early phase investigations with teriparatide, a Fisher rat model developed osteosarcoma. While this toxicity concern was not replicated in other animal models and the reports of osteosarcoma through passive surveillance appear roughly commensurate with the background rate in the general population, this is an issue that should be discussed with patients and that mandates only a 2-year period of use. Along with injection site reactions, arthralgias, myalgias, and flushing may follow the daily injections of this compound. Hypercalcemia is also seen but rarely exceeds 1 mg/dL increase in overall calcium level.

Denosumab

Denosumab is a monoclonal antibody that is soluble receptor that binds and inhibits RANKL. RANKL is a signaling molecule produced by osteoblasts that are responsible for differentiation and activation of osteoclasts and their precursors. Denosumab is potent inhibitor of bone resorption with a very rapid onset and an equally quick offset of action, resembling the degree of changes in bone turnover seem with sex steroid administration and discontinuation. Multisite clinical trials demonstrated its significant impact on bone density and its 68% and 40% reduction in spine and hip fractures, respectively. A small increase in infections has been seen with denosumab in some, but not in all, clinical trials. It is uncertain if its powerful antiresorptive effects will be associated in the future with jaw osteonecrosis or atypical fractures that have been putatively linked with the bisphosphonates.

SURGICAL AND OTHER INTERVENTIONAL APPROACHES

Percutaneous vertebroplasty and kyphoplasty, procedures that typically inject poly(methyl methacrylate) into the vertebral body, are used for the treatment of painful vertebral compression deformities. Some, but not all, studies have demonstrated short-term pain relief and an improvement in acute function. The mechanism of pain relief of this proposed technique is not well understood and it is also unclear what advantage one procedure (vertebroplasty vs. kyphoplasty) may have over the other. Kyphoplasty traditionally requires general anesthesia but uses an inflatable balloon to expand the vertebral space prior to injection of the bone cement. One concern with introducing a very rigid fixation into a very osteoporotic spine is the potential for an acceleration of fractures above and below the spinal level being treated.

Glucocorticoid-induced Osteoporosis

INTRODUCTION

Osteoporosis is a well-recognized complication of supraphysiologic levels of glucocorticoids. Glucocorticoid-induced osteoporosis (GIOP) is second in frequency only to the osteoporosis after menopause and is the most common form of drug-induced osteoporosis. During the first 6 to 12 months of glucocorticoid therapy, there is an initial rapid loss of 3% to 27% of BMD. Trabecular bone is preferentially affected, followed ultimately by losses in cortical bone. Cumulative steroid dose is the primary predictor of bone loss. Following approximately 2 years of glucocorticoid therapy, rate of bone loss slows in many patients. However, BMD continues to be lost at a rate higher than that with normal aging. Studies of steroid-dose effects are confounded by the variable timing of glucocorticoid administration, differing disease processes, variable alternative osteoporosis risk factors (independent of glucocorticoid use), and the fact that fracture risk is ultimately determined by factors other than only BMD. Glucocorticoids increase the risk of fractures roughly by twofold, independent of age, gender, and rheumatoid arthritis (RA). Women with RA taking low-dose prednisone have a nearly 33% chance of self-reporting a clinical fracture after 5 years. Although safer for bone than oral or enteral glucocorticoids, even nonsystemically administered glucocorticoids may have biological effects on bone.

The etiology of GIOP is multifactorial and occurs, in many cases, concomitantly with normal age- and menopause-associated bone loss. There are two major pathways by which patients on glucocorticoids develop abnormalities in bone metabolism: reduced bone formation and increased bone resorption. While acceleration of bone resorption is clearly an important pathway, the predominant problem in glucocorticoid-induced osteoporosis may be suppression of bone formation via a direct toxic effect on osteoblasts and osteocytes in bone.

HISTORY AND PHYSICAL EXAMINATION

There should be a high suspicion for potential bone loss among all patients initiating or chronically using glucocorticoids. A partially effective way to determine a glucocorticoid user's risk for future bone loss is to assess BMD by DXA. Most guidelines suggest assessing BMD if the patient receives ≥7.5 mg prednisone or its equivalent for at least 1 to 6 months. Bone mineral density underestimates the effects of glucocorticoids on bone; persons fracture at a better BMD threshold. This should be considered when making risk stratification decisions on the basis of bone mass measurement.

PREVENTION AND TREATMENT

The most effective intervention to prevent bone loss and fractures among glucocorticoid users is discontinuation of treatment or, at a minimum, reducing the dose. Practically, this is not always possible because of the severity of many chronic inflammatory diseases.

Calcium and Vitamin D

Supplements of elemental calcium 1,200 to 1,500 mg/day are necessary, although generally not sufficient as a sole therapy, for most patients on glucocorticoids. Vitamin D can be administered in a variety of formulations that have been investigated for GIOP prevention and treatment. Subjects who received a combination containing calcitriol, calcium, and calcitonin experienced significantly less bone loss in the spine than those receiving calcium alone. Inactivated vitamin D preparations also have merit. Because of impairment in calcium absorption mediated by glucocorticoids and the common occurrence of vitamin D deficiency among housebound patients suffering with chronic inflammatory conditions, vitamin D should be prescribed for all glucocorticoid users. This can be accomplished with 800 IU/day vitamin D_3, available in many multivitamins and vitamin D–supplemented calcium preparations. With careful use of exogenous calcium and monitoring of urine and serum calcium, vitamin D can be administered alternatively as calcitriol.

Bisphosphonates and Teriparatide

Similar to postmenopausal and male osteoporosis, bisphosphonates constitute the predominant therapy for those with or at risk for steroid-associated bone loss and fracture. When administered over 1 or 2 years to patients on glucocorticoids for a variety of chronic inflammatory disorders, alendronate, risedronate, and zoledronic acid prevent and/or reverse bone loss at the spine and of the hip. The magnitude of vertebral fracture risk reduction seen for bisphosphonate in persons on glucocorticoids is very similar to that observed for postmenopausal women. Teriparatide also increases BMD in persons at high risk for glucocorticoid-associated osteoporosis and lowered vertebral fracture risk compared to alendronate.

Treatment Algorithm

A treatment algorithm is proposed in Figure 21.7. Given the accumulating data on the efficacy of bisphosphonates and teriparatide for preventing and treating GIOP, initial administration of a bisphosphonate should be strongly considered in many persons on chronic glucocorticoids and teriparatide given to those at highest risk. While this algorithm represents a rational approach, GIOP management is rapidly changing and will be further refined, based on emerging literature as well as societal cost-effectiveness considerations.

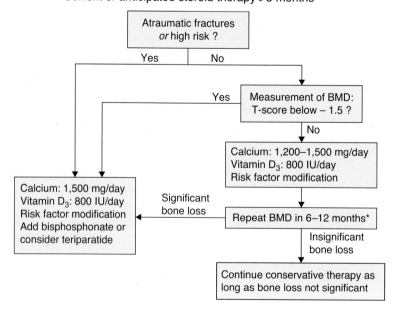

Figure 21.7 Treatment algorithm for the management of glucocorticoid-associated bone disease. Asterisks indicate during the first 2 years of therapy and then less regularly. (Adapted from Rosen HN, Rosenblatt M. Prevention and treatment of glucocorticoid-induced osteoporosis. In: Rose B, ed. *UptoDate*. Vol. 6, No. 3. Wellesley, MA: UpToDate. Reprinted in, Saag KG, Morgan SL, Cao X, et al. Bone in health and disease In: Koopman WJ, ed. *Arthritis and Allied Condition: A Textbook of Rheumatology*. 15th ed. Philadelphia: Lippincott Williams & Wilkins; 2005:2449–2541.)

Male Osteoporosis

INTRODUCTION

Osteoporosis in men is common: about 20% of all osteoporotic fractures occur in men. As the population ages, osteoporosis in men is becoming an even greater public health problem.

In North America, men aged 50 years have an approximate 13% lifetime risk for fracture of the hip, spine, or forearm. In the United States, the incidence of hip fracture in men older than 65 years is 4 to 5 in 1,000; about half that in women of similar age. Incidence of hip fracture in men differs between different ethnic groups. African-American men have a rate about half that of Caucasians, and Japanese men living in Japan or Hawaii may have a lower frequency than Caucasian American men. Osteoporotic vertebral fractures in men are more common in the low thoracic region, but may occur at any level. Elderly men less often fracture more than one vertebral body. Most fractures are the anterior compression type; crush fractures occur less commonly than in women, thereby accounting for less kyphosis in men.

The greater bone mass in men than in women is mostly related to body size, with the exception of a few sites such as the radius. After attaining peak bone mass, men maintain a stable BMD during middle age and then lose bone at an accelerating rate into old age. This rate may reach 5% to 10% per decade, and is greater in trabecular than cortical bone. As many as 20% to 40% of men with an osteoporotic fracture have no identifiable medical condition or risk factor associated with osteoporosis; they are designated as having primary osteoporosis to distinguish them from men who have lost substantial bone mass secondary to any of various conditions.

HISTORY AND PHYSICAL EXAMINATION

In men with clinical features or findings suggestive of metabolic bone disease (such as radiographic osteopenia, low-trauma fractures, or disorders associated with bone loss), measurement of BMD should be considered. These measurements may be used to confirm low bone mass, gauge its severity, and serve as a baseline to assess the progression of disease or therapeutic response. Criteria to define osteoporosis in men are not as clear as for women. Estimates of fracture risk derived from measurements of women may not apply to men. Lower bone density is associated with an increased risk for fracture and measurements can be used to monitor serial changes in bone mass.

The initial history and physical examination should be undertaken with knowledge of conditions associated with osteoporosis. Special attention should be given to signs of genetic, nutritional, and lifestyle factors (alcohol or tobacco), systemic illness, and medication usage. If the cause of osteoporosis remains undefined, measurement of serum thyroid-stimulating hormone, and 24-hour urinary calcium and cortisol should be considered.

TREATMENT

To achieve maximal adult bone mass, adolescent boys should be encouraged to ingest 1,300 mg calcium daily in their diets, participate in regular weight-bearing exercise, maintain ideal body weight, and avoid use of tobacco and excessive alcohol. Extending this approach into adulthood, it is recommended that men aged 19 to 50 consume 1,000 mg calcium daily and that men older than 50 years consume 1,000 to 1,200 mg daily (see Table 21.6).

Testosterone increases BMD in hypogonadal men or those on glucocorticoid therapy, and has been used empirically in eugonadal men, albeit in short-term trials. The goal of therapy is a physiologic testosterone profile. Side effects generally are not serious, although long-term safety is not well established.

Excessive libido is uncommon. Weight may increase because of anabolic effects on lean mass or salt and water retention, particularly in men with cardiac disease, cirrhosis, or nephrotic syndrome. Urinary retention is uncommon in the absence of prostatic cancer, and there is generally no significant effect on serum prostatic-specific antigen or prostatic volume. Whether the likelihood for prostatic cancer increases must await large clinical trials. Some men develop erythrocytosis because of augmented erythropoiesis. Levels of total and HDL cholesterol frequently decrease. Gynecomastia may develop. 17α-alkylated androgens should be avoided because of greater risks for increased liver enzymes, cholestasis, and liver tumors. Contraindications to androgen therapy include prostatic cancer, prostatic hypertrophy, and sleep apnea.

Among other therapies, bisphosphonates currently offer substantial promise along with teriparatide and denosumab. Correction of hypercalciuria with hydrochlorothiazide 25 mg twice daily can significantly increase bone mass. Supplementation with vitamin D and calcium should be encouraged, since they are relatively inexpensive and safe, may have modest independent benefits to bone, and may potentiate other therapeutic interventions.

Osteomalacia

INTRODUCTION

Normal bone growth and mineralization require adequate vitamin D, calcium, and phosphorus. A prolonged deficiency of any of these leads to accumulation of unmineralized bone matrix, or osteoid, and slow bone formation. Decreased mineralization in young patients causes rickets because of damage of growth plates (epiphyses) and newly formed trabecular and cortical bone. Strength of the bone matrix is decreased, leading to structural deformities in weight-bearing bones, such as bowing. In older individuals in whom epiphyses have closed and only bone is affected, this defective mineralization is called osteomalacia.

Causes 0f Osteomalacia

Vitamin D-related
  Low dietary intake
  Low sunlight exposure
  Malabsorption
    Biliary disease
    Celiac disease
    Bariatric surgery
    Bile acid-binding resins
  Increased renal clearance
    Nephrotic syndrome
  Increased catabolism
    Phenytoin
    Barbiturates
    Rifampin
  Pseudovitamin D-deficient rickets
  Hereditary vitamin D-resistant rickets

Hypophosphatemia
  Tumor induced osteomalacia
  Genetic Hypophosphatemic rickets syndromes
  Fanconi's syndrome
  Renal tubular acidosis (type 2)

Miscellaneous
  Hypophosphatasia
  Aluminum intoxication
  Fluorosis
  Bisphosphonate overdose

HISTORY AND PHYSICAL EXAMINATION

Clinical manifestations of osteomalacia may mimic rheumatic disorders with generalized aching bone pain, easy fatigue, proximal weakness, and periarticular tenderness. These symptoms promptly resolve with treatment to correct the mineralization defect. Radiographs of patients with rickets may show general demineralization with thinning of cortical surfaces of long bones, widening, fraying, and cupping of distal ends of the shaft, and loss of the zone of provisional cartilaginous calcification. Some patients with osteomalacia exhibit thin cortical radiolucent lines (stress fractures) perpendicular to the bone shaft that are often symmetrical and bilateral (called Looser's zones); other patients may have multiple old rib fractures with poor callus formation.

STUDIES

Laboratory features of vitamin D–deficiency osteomalacia are low or normal serum calcium level, hypophosphatemia, increased serum alkaline phosphatase level, and a low serum 25-hydroxyvitamin D. Secondary hyperaparathyroidism ensues to raise serum calcium to near normal. Hypophosphatemia is the result of phosphate wasting because of elevated PTH as well as reduced gut absorption from vitamin D deficiency. Individually, elevated PTH and hypophosphatemia stimulate renal synthesis of 1,25-dihydroxyvitamin D to maintain normal serum levels. Urine calcium is also expectedly low. Calcium-deficiency osteomalacia is associated with similar laboratory findings except that vitamin D and serum phosphorus are often normal.

In osteomalacia because of hypophosphatemic states associated with hyperphosphaturia, serum calcium, PTH, and 25-hydroxyvitamin D are normal, serum alkaline phosphatase levels are usually increased, serum phosphorus and 1,25-dihydroxyvitamin D levels are low, and urinary phosphorus excretion is very high. Patients with type II renal tubular acidosis have defective reabsorption of bicarbonate and manifest hyperchloremic hypokalemic acidosis with hypophosphatemia because of augmented phosphaturia. Low serum 1,25-dihydroxyvitamin D levels in some patients may be the consequence of abnormal proximal tubular metabolism. Hypophosphatasia is a rare autosomal-dominant disorder with decreased serum bone alkaline phosphatase level; serum calcium, phosphorus, 25-hydroxyvitamin D, and 1,25-dihydroxyvitamin D levels are not reduced.

TREATMENT

Treatment is based on the underlying disorder. Vitamin D–deficient osteomalacia requires high doses of vitamin D to restore proper bone mineralization. Ergocalciferol, or vitamin D_2, should be administered at a dose of 50,000 IU twice a week for at least 8 weeks before reassessment of serum calcium and vitamin D. Vitamin D levels greater than 30 ng/mL have been proposed to be associated with optimal bone health. Once that level has been achieved, several vitamin D maintenance regimens are available, including cholecalciferol (vitamin D_3) 1,000 to 2,000 IU daily or ergocalciferol 50,000 IU every 2 to 4 weeks. In patients with gut malabsorption, even higher doses may be required. Generally, the active form of vitamin D (1,25-dihydroxyvitamin D) should be avoided as it has a short half-life and is associated with a higher risk of hypercalcemia. Sunlight is another method to maintain vitamin D stores in patients who are not prone to sunburn or skin cancer. Supplemental calcium, 1,000 to 2,000 mg/day, is necessary for both vitamin D– and calcium-deficient osteomalacia.

In patients with renal tubular acidosis, restoration of the serum bicarbonate level to normal using sodium or potassium citrate supplements reverses bone resorption and hypercalciuria. Patients with osteomalacia because of hyperphosphaturia require oral phosphate supplements, generally 1 to

4 g/day divided in four to six doses and 1,25-dihydroxyvitamin D, 0.5 to 1.5 μg/day. Calcium supplements may be necessary to avoid symptomatic hypocalcemia, but should not be taken concomitantly with a phosphorus supplement. Once the bone disease has healed, the 1,25-dihydroxyvitamin D can be discontinued.

Primary Hyperparathyroidism

INTRODUCTION

Primary hyperparathyroidism and malignancy are the two most common causes of hypercalcemia, accounting for more than 90% of patients with hypercalcemia. The prevalence of primary hyperparathyroidism ranges from 1 in 400 to 1 in 1,000, and has increased several-fold in the last 25 years because of more routine serum calcium measurements. Most individuals are between 40 and 60 years and the female/male ratio is about 3:1. A parathyroid adenoma is the cause in about 80% of patients, whereas hyperplasia of all glands is found in about 15% to 20% of patients and parathyroid carcinoma in less than 0.5%. If the disorder appears in childhood, a familial hyperparathyroid syndrome such as a multiple endocrine neoplasia should be considered.

HISTORY AND PHYSICAL EXAMINATION

Oversecretion of PTH primarily affects the skeleton and kidneys. Pronounced osseous manifestations, such as subperiosteal resorption of the middle phalanges and distal clavicle, "salt-and-pepper" skull, and bone cysts are now relatively uncommon. More frequent is loss of bone mass, preferentially in sites rich in cortical bone, such as the distal third of the forearm or femoral neck. Nephrolithiasis develops in about 5% of patients. Diffuse deposition of calcium–phosphate complexes may cause nephrocalcinosis that can lead to interstitial fibrosis and reduce renal clearance. About 25% to 30% of patients have hypercalciuria. Complications because of severe hypercalcemia, such as proximal weakness in the legs, weight loss, nausea, constipation, pancreatitis, and band keratopathy, are now rare.

STUDIES

The diagnosis is generally established by an increased serum intact PTH concentration in a patient with hypercalcemia. The serum phosphorus concentration is low normal or low, and some patients exhibit a mild nongap hyperchloremic metabolic acidosis. Patients with significant bone disease may have increased levels of markers of bone formation. Primary hyperparathyroidism should be distinguished from the less common familial hypocalciuric hypercalcemia (FHH). This autosomal-dominant genetic condition is caused by mutations in the calcium-sensing receptor. A low urine calcium/creatinine clearance ratio of less than 0.01 is characteristic of FHH. This condition does not require specific treatment, and patients and other affected family members should be counseled that surgical parathyroidectomy is not required.

TREATMENT

The cure for primary hyperparathyroidism is surgical removal of the parathyroid adenoma or carcinoma, or most of the hyperplastic tissue, after which bone mass often increases for several years. The general guidelines for recommending surgery in patients without carcinoma are a serum calcium concentration greater than 1 mg/dL above the upper limit of normal, a creatinine clearance less than 60 mL/minute, a DXA T-score equal to or less than −2.5 in the hip, spine, or distal radius and age less than 50. Rarely, postoperative hypocalcemia, hypophosphatemia, and hypomagnesemia, or "hungry bone" syndrome, can occur especially in patients with extremely low vitamin D stores. Other risk factors include resection of large adenomas and older age.

For preoperative management or patients deemed unable to undergo parathyroid surgery, medical management includes adequate hydration and moderate intake of calcium, avoidance of thiazide diuretics that may increase serum calcium concentrations, and regular ambulatory exercise. Medications prescribed for osteoporosis that reduces bone resorption such as estrogen–progestin, raloxifene, and bisphosphonates reduce bone loss, but they are minimally effective at lowering serum calcium. Recent evidence suggests benefit in reducing serum calcium in primary hyperparathyroidism, but is not FDA approved for this indication.

Secondary Hyperparathyroidism

Secondary hyperparathyroidism is relatively common and may cause enough bone loss to contribute to the genesis of osteoporosis. Vitamin D deficiency, low dietary calcium, glucocorticoid therapy, fat malabsorption, loop diuretic therapy, and renal insufficiency may cause secondary hyperparathyroidism. Treatment includes calcium supplements and vitamin D replacement. In chronic kidney disease, conversion of vitamin D to the active 1,25-dihydroxyvitamin D is impaired, so replacement with the active vitamin D is indicated. The calcimimetic agent cinacalcet is effective in managing secondary hyperparathyroidism because of chronic kidney disease.

Osteogenesis Imperfecta

Occasionally an adult with multiple fractures, especially in the long bones of the legs, and radiographic osteopenia has osteogenesis imperfecta. A genetically determined inability to form quantitatively or qualitatively normal collagen characterizes this group of disorders. Several mutations in the gene for type 1 procollagen have been identified; all result in formation of unstable collagen helices. Most patients develop fractures in childhood. Some individuals are deaf or have blue sclera, but others have only osseous manifestations.

If no phenotypic characteristic of osteogenesis imperfecta is present except for fragile bones, diagnosis can be difficult. A positive family history and a history of multiple fractures in childhood are suggestive. Radiographs show thinning of cortical and trabecular areas of bones, especially metacarpals and metatarsals. Platybasia of the skull and bone islands in the cranium suggest osteogenesis imperfecta. Bone biopsy shows diminished quantities of osteoid and excessive osteocyte numbers. Therapy with gonadal hormones, bisphosphonates, and anecdotal use of teriparatide has been advocated. Bisphosphonates may reduce the subsequent fracture rates.

Hyperthyroidism

Bone disease of hyperthyroidism (either organic or iatrogenic from overzealous use of thyroid supplements) is a type of high-turnover osteoporosis. Serum triiodothyronine levels inversely correlate with bone mass. Patients may have bone pain and fracture, in addition to other features of hyperthyroidism. Radiographs may show diffuse osteopenia; abnormal striations of cortical bone are observed occasionally. Biochemical parameters usually include normal or mildly increased serum calcium levels and increased serum alkaline phosphatase levels. Urinary excretion of calcium and collagen breakdown fragments is often increased. Correction of the hyperthyroid state often restores bone mass. Estrogen for women or bisphosphonates may be considered if an accelerated rate of bone loss or decreased bone mass is present.

Metabolic Bone Manifestations of GI Diseases

Patients afflicted with GI disorders may develop a spectrum of bone disease, ranging from osteoporosis to osteomalacia. Several pathogenic mechanisms contribute (a) calcium malabsorption, alone or combined with malabsorption of vitamin D, leading to secondary hyperparathyroidism; (b) impaired absorption of vitamin D, altered metabolism of vitamin D, or reduced enterohepatic circulation of vitamin D metabolites; and (c) glucocorticoid treatment of inflammatory bowel disease. Although early reports suggested that the bone disorder in patients with primary biliary cirrhosis was predominantly osteomalacia, subsequent histomorphometric studies showed that osteoporosis was more common. Bone disease after gastrectomy is also more commonly osteoporosis than osteomalacia. Calcium malabsorption is more likely due to loss of duodenal absorptive surface than achlorhydria. Celiac sprue has long been known to cause rickets in children and osteomalacia in adults. These skeletal complications develop even without steatorrhea or frequent bowel movements. Patients with inflammatory bowel disease may have decreased BMD because of osteomalacia or osteoporosis, and the risk is greater for Crohn's disease than ulcerative colitis.

Osteonecrosis

INTRODUCTION

Osteonecrosis, also commonly referred to as avascular necrosis, is an insidious disorder leading to destruction of viable periarticular epiphyseal and subchondral bone. Osteonecrosis leads to a change in joint contour and a secondary painful destructive arthropathy. It predominately affects weight-bearing joints, most commonly the femoral head, leading to joint motion-induced pain. It is estimated to effect up to 20,000 persons a year and leads to an estimate of 10% of all total knee arthroplasties. There is a strong male predominance. A related condition, predominately affecting children, is osteochondrosis. This condition is a degeneration followed by reossification of nonfused epiphyses. Osgood–Schlatter disease of the tibial tuberosity is the best-known variant of osteochondrosis, but other types are well described and may occur in adults.

There are a variety of risk factors for osteonecrosis, with trauma being the most common. A classic presentation is the development of femoral head osteonecrosis months to years after open reduction and internal fixation of a femoral neck fracture. This is thought to occur secondary to a compromise of the tenuous blood supply to the femoral head. The less common nontraumatic causes are predominantly by glucocorticoids and alcohol abuse. Osteonecrosis of the hips, knees, or humeral heads is detectable by magnetic resonance

Table 21.8 Potential Etiologic Factors for Osteonecrosis

TRAUMATIC	
NONTRAUMATIC (LESS RARE)	**NONTRAUMATIC (RARE)**
Steroids	Coagulopathy
Alcohol	Pancreatitis
Systemic lupus erythematosis	Gaucher's disease
Organ transplant	Chronic kidney disease
Sickle cell disease	Pregnancy
	Hyperlipidemia
	Caisson's disease

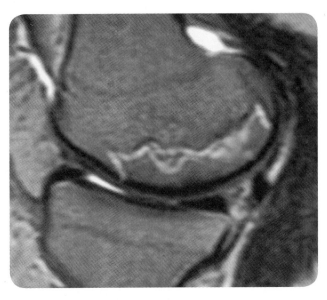

Figure 21.9 Osteonecrosis on magnetic resonance imaging. "Double-line sign" on T_2 images with peripheral margin dark surrounding bright inner line. (Mitchell DG, Rao VM, Dalinka MK, et al: Femoral head avascular necrosis: correlation of MR imaging, radiographic staging, radionuclide imaging, and clinical findings. *Radiology* 1987;162:709–715.)

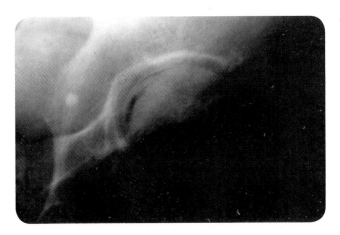

Figure 21.8 Hip radiograph demonstrating crescent sign. Area of collapse of subchondral bone with accompanying radiolucency.

imaging (MRI) in 5% to 10% of renal transplant recipients within 3 to 6 months of engraftment. Osteonecrosis may accompany HIV disease, particularly in these setting of lipodystrophy. Other somewhat common and less common factors etiologically associated with osteonecrosis are provided in Table 21.8.

There are multiple pathogenic mechanisms that may contribute to osteonecrosis, including compromise of the boney vasculature (most common with trauma) and as programmed cell death (apoptosis) of the osteoblasts and osteocytes. The latter mechanism may predominate in glucocorticoid-mediated osteonecrosis.

STUDIES/IMAGING

Plain radiographs can yield clues, but suffer from poor sensitivity for early lesions. Characteristic radiographic appearances of bone collapse and subchondral fracture are seen in later stage disease (see Fig. 21.8). Bone scintigraphy (bone scans) is useful in the early diagnosis and demonstrates decreased or absent radiotracer activity surrounded by increased activity ("donut lesion") because of revascularization. While bone scan has considerable sensitivity, it has low specificity for differentiating osteonecrosis from infection, myeloma, and metastatic disease. Magnetic resonance imaging is the most sensitive modality for early diagnosis and staging. A "double-line" sign is evident, and inversion recovery proton density imaging may provide a sensitive means to detect early lesions (see Fig. 21.9).

A similar appearing, but self-limiting, entity is transient regional osteoporosis (TRO) of the hip. Magnetic resonance images for TRO are very similar to osteonecrosis, but this condition commonly resolves in 6 to 12 months. It most commonly follows pregnancy, but is also observed in middle-aged men.

TREATMENT

There is no proven standard therapy for effectively managing osteonecrosis once it develops. Many patients go on to boney collapse and require total joint replacement, in joints where this is possible. Withdrawal of any inciting agents

SECTION 4 Osteoarthritis and Metabolic Bone

WHEN TO REFER

- Osteoporosis that is progressing in spite of appropriate calcium and vitamin D supplementation as well as use of bisphosphonates.

- Patients with osteoporosis intolerant to bisphosphonates.

- Evaluation of osteomalacia.

- Evaluation of young patients with multiple fractures.

coupled with a period on limited or non–weight bearing may circumvent surgery and lead to gradual self-limited healing. Surgical approaches to this problem, short of eventual total joints, include core decompression with or without a central bone graft. The evidence surrounding the optimal timing and effectiveness of these approaches is equivocal. Joint realignment and partial or total joint arthroplasty are generally best tolerated and associated with the best pain and function outcomes. Options for medical management of osteonecrosis are also rather limited. Most small studies are mostly anecdotal, but at least one open-label randomized, but nonblinded, study suggests a potential role for bisphosphonates.

ICD9

756.51 **Osteogenesis imperfecta**
268.2 **Osteomalacia, unspecified**
733.00 **Osteoporosis** *(generalized)*
737.30 **Scoliosis** *(acquired) (postural)*
733.00 [737.43] due to or associated with osteoporosis

Suggested Readings

Bilezikian JP, Khan AA, Potts JT, Jr. Guidelines for the management of asymptomatic primary hyperparathyroidism: Summary statement from the third international workshop. *J Clin Endocrinol Metab* 2009;94(2): 335–339.

Black DM, Delmas PD, Eastell R, et al. Once-yearly zoledronic acid for treatment of postmenopausal osteoporosis. *N Engl J Med* 2007;356(18):1809–1822.

Bonnick SL. *Bone Densitometry in Clinical Practice.* Totowoa, NJ: Humana; 1998.

Cauley JA, Robbins J, Chen Z, et al. Effects of estrogen plus progestin on risk of fracture and bone mineral density: the Women's Health Initiative randomized trial. *JAMA* 2003;290(13):1729–1738.

Chesnut CH, III, Silverman S, Andriano K, et al. A randomized trial of nasal spray salmon calcitonin in postmenopausal women with established osteoporosis: The prevent recurrence of osteoporotic fractures study. PROOF Study Group. *Am J Med* 2000;109(4):267–276.

Chesnut CH, III, Skag A, Christiansen C, et al. Effects of oral ibandronate administered daily or intermittently on fracture risk in postmenopausal osteoporosis. *J Bone Miner Res* 2004;19(8):1241–1249. Epub March 29, 2004.

Cummings SR, Black DM, Thompson DE, et al. Effect of alendronate on risk of fracture in women with low bone density but without vertebral fractures: Results from the Fracture Intervention Trial. *JAMA* 1998;280(24):2077–2082.

Ettinger B, Black DM, Mitlak BH, et al. Reduction of vertebral fracture risk in postmenopausal women with osteoporosis treated with raloxifene: Results from a 3-year randomized clinical trial. Multiple Outcomes of Raloxifene Evaluation (MORE) Investigators. *JAMA* 1999;282(7):637–645.

Harris ST, Watts NB, Genant HK, et al. Effects of risedronate treatment on vertebral and nonvertebral fractures in women with postmenopausal osteoporosis: a randomized controlled trial. Vertebral Efficacy With Risedronate Therapy (VERT) Study Group. *JAMA* 1999;282(14):1344–1352.

Institute of Medicine of the National Academies. *Dietary Reference Intakes for Calcium and Vitamin D.* November 30, 2010, Consensus Report.

Orwoll ES. Osteoporosis in men. *Endocrinol Metab Clin North Am* 1998;27(2):349–367.

National Osteoporosis Foundation. *Clinician's Guide to Prevention and Treatment of Osteoporosis.* Washington, DC: National Osteoporosis Foundation; 2010.

Primer on the Metabolic Bone Diseases and Disorders of Mineral Metabolism. Rosen, CJ (Ed.) 7th ed. Washington, DC: The American Society for Bone and Mineral Research.; 2008.

Riggs BL, Khosla S, Melton LJ, III. A unitary model for involutional osteoporosis: Estrogen deficiency causes both type I and type II osteoporosis in postmenopausal women and contributes to bone loss in aging men. *J Bone Miner Res* 1998;13(5):763–773.

Writing Group for the Women's Health Initiative Investigators. *JAMA* 2002;288:321.

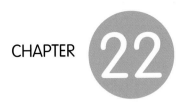

CHAPTER 22 Arthropathies Associated with Systemic Diseases

Leann Maska and Amy C. Cannella

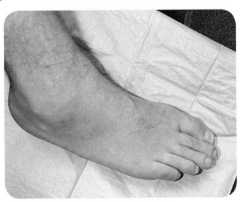

A 60-year-old Caucasian gentleman with long-standing poorly controlled type 2 diabetes mellitus presents to your office with symptoms of swelling and moderate pain in his right midfoot over the past 3 weeks. He is unable to recall any specific trau-matic event. On examination, the foot is warm, swollen, tender, and erythematous (Fig. 22.1). Your differential includes cellulitis, acute gouty arthritis, osteomyelitis, and fracture. An important addition to this differential is consideration of acute Charcot neuroarthropathy (CN). To rule out underlying infection, the best imaging study is combination of a three-phase bone scan with a labeled white blood cell (WBC) scan.

Joint pain is one of the most common reasons for a patient to see his or her primary care provider. Office visits in the United States for musculoskeletal pain in 2000 accounted for 280 visits per 1,000 people, and were evenly divided between acute and chronic symptoms (1). Although not inclusive, this chapter aims to cover associations between a variety of systemic diseases and their related musculoskeletal manifestations.

Endocrine Diseases with Associated Arthropathies

DIABETES MELLITUS

Diabetes is an increasingly common medical condition in the United States, with a prevalence of more than 23 million people, including both diagnosed and undiagnosed cases, or one in ten adults (2). Health care providers must be familiar with the myriad of extraglandular complications of the disease. It is thought that the associated arthropathies are due to complications of diabetes, including neuropathy and microvascular disease. Furthermore, a high-glucose and insulin environment has been shown to have pathologic effects on many key cells and matrix components of connective tissues (3). Although relatively uncommon, charcot neuroarthropathy is an important problem to recognize as it leads to significant deformity and joint destruction. Conversely, adhesive capsulitis of the shoulder is quite common, but often improves with conservative management. Both are discussed in more detail below. Other notable arthropathies associated with diabetes mellitus include diffuse idiopathic skeletal hyperostosis (DISH), carpal tunnel syndrome, and osteoarthritis.

SECTION 4 Osteoarthritis and Metabolic Bone

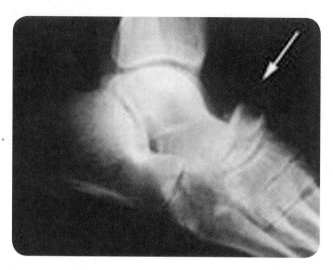

Figure 22.1 Subluxation of the navicular and soft tissue swelling as an early manifestation of a neuropathic joint (Courtesy of Gerald F. Moore, MD.)

CHARCOT NEUROARTHROPATHY

Clinical Presentation

The incidence of CN is reported at approximately 1 in 333 patients with diabetes (4). The exact pathogenic mechanism of CN is incompletely understood; however, a combination of both neurovascular and neurotraumatic theories is generally accepted (4). Current hypothesis suggests that somatic and autonomic neuropathy leads to increased blood flow to the joint, resulting in bone resorption and susceptibility to minor trauma. Continued mechanical stress occurs because of loss of protective pain sensation, and major destructive changes result in fractures and deformities.

Patients with CN can present with an acute or chronic process. In acute CN, the earliest symptoms are persistent swelling and pain, although sensory deficits may preclude associated discomfort. A history of trauma may be present, although one study showed that nearly 75% of patients did not recall any precipitating event. Progression from acute to chronic neuroarthropathy can be rapid, with irreversible damage seen in less than 6 months. Patients with chronic CN can present with established deformity and may complain of associated difficulties with ambulation.

Examination

On physical examination, a foot with acute CN is typically warm, swollen, and tender. Moderate-to-marked erythema may also be present (4). The midfoot is most commonly involved and has a better prognosis than hindfoot involvement because of weight distribution effects. Typical deformities include a collapsed arch and rocker-bottom foot with callus formation and possible ulcerations.

Studies

Diagnosis is primarily made by clinical history and examination. Plain radiographs are inexpensive and can show anatomic bony deformities, demineralization, and periosteal reaction. When severe, CN can result in fragmentation of the metatarsal heads, or even "pencil and cup" deformities of the MTP joints. Radiographic progression can occur rapidly, oftentimes within several weeks of a normal x-ray (Fig. 22.2) (4).

It is critical to rule out infection in the diagnostic work-up of CN. Radiographs are neither sensitive nor specific for differentiating infection from CN. The combination of a three-phase bone scan with a tagged WBC scan has a sensitivity and specificity of 80% to 90%. In acute CN, a three-phase bone scan should be positive in all three phases, reflecting increased bone turnover, and a tagged WBC scan should be negative in the absence of infection. However, false positive WBC scans can occur in the setting of very rapidly advancing CN. Further imaging can be done with complementary marrow scanning, which if positive in the same area, indicates acute neuroarthropathic changes and not infection (4). Although magnetic resonance imaging (MRI) does not differentiate CN from infection, it gives excellent anatomic definition, does not require gadolinium to see edematous changes, and may be useful for monitoring progression of disease (4).

Treatment

The management of CN is limited and mainly consists of reduction in weight-bearing activity. Plaster casting for several weeks to allow the acute phase to resolve, followed by total-contact cast applications that allow for better ambulation, is commonly utilized. Other specialized footwear for acute CN applications include Charcot restraint orthotic walkers,

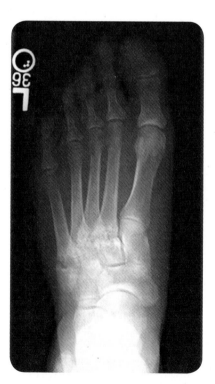

Figure 22.2 Destruction of midfoot joints in Charcot neuroarthropathy. (Courtesy of Gerald F. Moore, MD.)

patellar tendon-bearing braces, total-contact bivalve ankle-foot orthoses, and pneumatic walking braces that allow earlier mobilization with relative joint immobility (4). Treatment of chronic CN centers on reducing plantar pressures and preserving skin integrity to prevent ulcerations. Orthotic consultation can be very helpful in managing and treating chronic deformities. Routine surgery is not advocated, as potential risks include long-term worsening of the condition, possible nonunion, infection, and general risk of surgery and anesthesia.

Clinical Course
Early diagnosis of CN can potentially prevent complications including severe deformity, ulcerations, and even limb amputation. Because CN is a relatively uncommon condition, referral to a specialist with a multidisciplinary team approach is preferred.

ADHESIVE CAPSULITIS
Clinical Presentation
Compared to 2% to 5% of the general population, approximately 20% of people with diabetes are affected at some time by adhesive capsulitis of the shoulder. This relatively common condition is defined as the insidious onset of shoulder pain with a gradual loss of both active and passive range of motion (ROM) (5).

The natural history of adhesive capsulitis is a progression through four sequential and descriptive stages: (a) preadhesive stage (diffuse glenohumeral synovitis seen on arthroscopy); (b) freezing stage (hypertrophic and hypervascular synovitis with capsular fibroplasia and scar formation); (c) frozen stage (significant hypertrophy and hypervascularity with dense capsular scar); (d) thawing phase (apparent remodeling without synovitis) (5). Pain is initially severe and improves with decreasing synovitis in later stages. A progressive decline in ROM is notable until stage 4, or thawing occurs.

Sleep-disturbing pain is often a motivating factor for patients to seek medical attention. Certain elements of the history can help determine where each patient resides on the continuum (Table 22.1). For example, a patient who is unable to sleep through the night, has significant limitations in ROM, and suffers from ongoing pain is likely in stage 2, or active freezing.

Examination
Significant limitation of both active and passive abduction of the shoulder exist; however, the extent of restriction is stage dependent. Active ROM that is accompanied by scapular movement is a clue to diagnosis. Patients often display transient severe pain with abrupt or end-range movements. Although normal strength has been considered a classic finding, recent studies using handheld dynamometry have demonstrated weakness in the internal and external rotators, abductors, and elevators (5).

Table 22.1 Stages of Adhesive Capsulitis

STAGE	DURATION (MONTHS)	PAIN	SLEEP DISRUPTION	STIFFNESS
Preadhesive	0–3	+++	+	+
Freezing	3–9	+++	++	++
Frozen	9–15	+	−	+++
Thawing	15–24	−	−	±

SECTION 4 Osteoarthritis and Metabolic Bone

Studies

History and physical examination alone are often adequate to diagnose adhesive capsulitis. However, imaging studies can help rule out other pathology. Plain radiographs are limited to finding bony pathology. Magnetic resonance imaging can differentiate soft-tissue abnormalities of the rotator cuff and labrum. Ultrasonography has also proved to be useful in deciphering adhesive capsulitis from rotator cuff tendinopathy (5).

Treatment

Discussions with the patient should include education regarding the natural history of adhesive capsulitis, preparation for an extended recovery, and alleviation of fear of a more serious disease. A home exercise program outlined by a physical therapist can be effective in relieving symptoms, and also places the patient in an active role. Glenohumeral corticosteroid injection, exercise, and joint mobilization all lead to improved short- and long-term outcomes. Corticosteroid injections have been shown to result in more rapid improvements at 4- to 6-week intervals and are therefore a reasonable option for patients with more severe symptoms, who have not responded well to rehabilitation (5). However, there is concern for potentially elevated serum glucose levels in patients with diabetes who receive intra-articular corticosteroids. If conservative management is unsuccessful, obstinate frozen shoulder may be further managed with manipulation under anesthesia or surgical capsular release.

Clinical Course

Adhesive capsulitis is usually self-limited, lasting 12 to 24 months. However, mild symptoms can persist for years, depending on the extent of fibroplasias. Some studies report that up to half of patients have limited ROM more than 3 years after symptom onset.

HYPOTHYROIDISM

Symmetrical arthropathy with stiffness of the hands and knees is a common initial presentation of patients with hypothyroidism. Examination including palpation of involved joints may reveal synovitis. Synovial fluid is typically noninflammatory with high levels of hyaluronic acid.

Hypothyroidism is also associated with calcium pyrophosphate deposition (CPPD), which would result in an inflammatory synovial fluid with weakly positively birefringent rhomboidal crystals seen under polarized light microscopy (Fig. 22.3). Indeed, multiple systemic diseases are associated with CPPD arthropathy (Table 22.2). Carpal tunnel syndrome can also be an initial presentation in up to 7% of patients with hypothyroidism.

Chronic autoimmune thyroiditis, or Hashimoto's thyroiditis, has a variety of associated rheumatic manifestations, such as mild nonerosive arthritis, polyarthralgia, myalgia, and sicca syndrome. Most manifestations are secondary to hypothyroidism and do not resolve until a euthyroid state is achieved. However, in treated or euthyroid Hashimoto's thyroiditis, arthropathies may be due to an associated autoimmune etiology, such as Sjogren's syndrome, rheumatoid arthritis, or systemic lupus erythematosus.

HYPERTHYROIDISM

Hyperthyroidism, including Grave's disease, can present as pretibial myxedema and ophthalmopathy. Digital soft-tissue swelling with periostitis of metacarpophalangeal

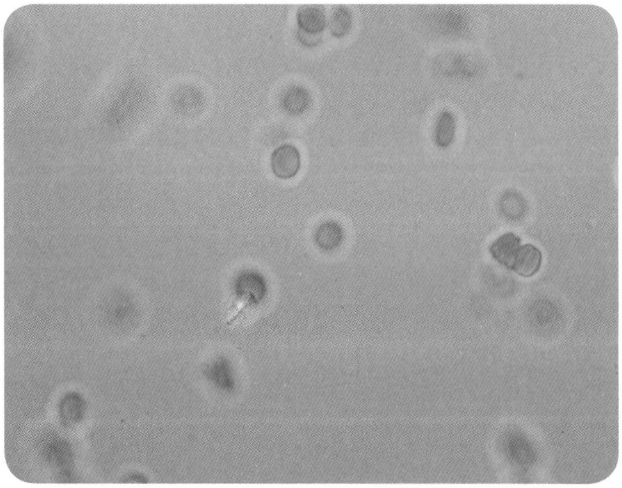

Figure 22.3 Calcium pyrophosphate deposition crystal. (Courtesy of Gerald F. Moore, MD.)

Table 22.2 Systemic Diseases Associated with Calcium Pyrophosphate Deposition Arthropathy

Hyperparathyroidism

Hypothyroidism

Hemochromatosis

Hypophosphatemia

Hypomagnesemia

(MCP) joints also occurs. Nail changes include onycholysis and clubbing (thyroid acropachy).

Osteoporosis is a relatively common and serious manifestation of hyperthyroidism that should not be missed. Iatrogenic overreplacement of thyroxine can also lead to osteoporosis. Treatment goals include normalization of thyroid-stimulating hormone and improvement in bone mineral density as measured by densitometry.

HYPERPARATHYROIDISM AND HYPOVITAMINOSIS D

Calcium homeostasis with bone metabolism and remodeling are intricately controlled by parathyroid hormone (PTH), vitamin D, and calcitonin levels. Primary hyperparathyroidism is often secondary to a parathyroid adenoma, whereas secondary disease is most commonly related to renal failure, vitamin D deficiency, and osteomalacia. Arthralgias are common in both primary and secondary disease, and can involve small joints of the hands, often sparing the proximal interphalangeal (PIP) joints. Radiographic changes include osteitis fibrosa cystica, erosions, phalangeal subperiosteal resorption along the radial edges, and even distal tuft resorption. Rheumatoid factor is typically negative and erythrocyte sedimentation rate normal. Calcium pyrophosphate deposition is associated with hyperparathyroidism, and acute gout attacks can also occur (Table 22.2). Either calcium pyrophosphate or uric acid crystals can be found in aspirated joint fluid from an acutely inflamed joint of a patient with hyperparathyroidism. Brown tumors (Fig. 22.4), which are lytic bone lesions, can be seen on radiographs and represent localized areas of fibrous tissue with increased osteoclastic activity.

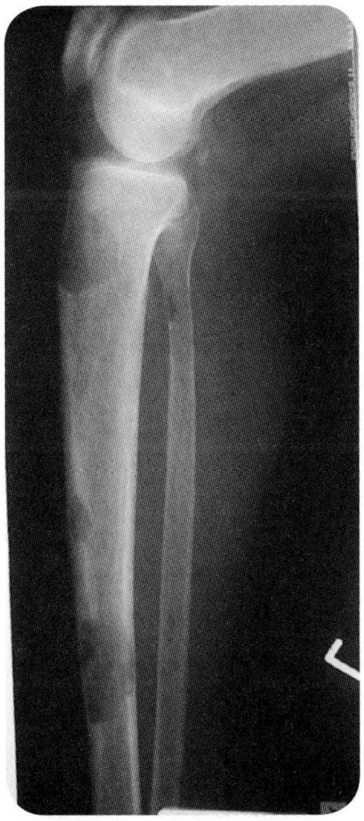

ACROMEGALY

Acromegaly is a rare condition with an estimated annual incidence of 4 cases per million persons and is typically due to hypersecretion of growth hormone secondary to a benign pituitary adenoma (6). While cardiovascular disease accounts for the majority of mortality in these patients, articular manifestations are the leading cause of morbidity. Acromegalic arthropathy affects both the axial and appendicular skeleton, with the knees being the most commonly involved peripheral joint. Noninflammatory arthritis with joint stiffness and swelling is common. Articular widening with soft-tissue hypertrophy and joint hypermobility predominates in early stages when control of growth hormone and insulin-like growth factor 1 (IGF-1) may reverse the arthropathy (6). Later stages manifest in cartilage ulcers, subchondral cyst formation, articular thickening, limited ROM, and ultimately severe degenerative arthritis. Radiographic abnormalities include distal tufting of the phalanges, osteophyte formation, especially at the base of distal phalanges, and subchondral cyst formation. Up to one half of patients have symptomatic carpal tunnel syndrome; however, this is likely related to median nerve edema rather than extrinsic compression in these patients.

Figure 22.4 Brown tumors hyperparathyroid. (Courtesy of Gerald F. Moore, MD.)

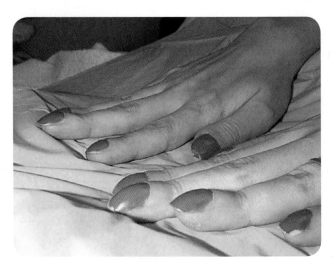

Figure 22.5 Digital Clubbing. (Courtesy of Gerald F. Moore, MD.)

Malignancies with Associated Arthropathies

HYPERTROPHIC OSTEOARTHROPATHY

Clinical Presentation

Hypertrophic osteoarthropathy (HOA) is a syndrome classically comprising digital clubbing and periostitis of tubular bones. It is diagnosed in the setting of comorbid malignancy over 80% of the time. Lung cancer, both primary and metastatic, is most commonly associated with the condition. The majority of cases involve non–small-cell malignancies, including squamous cell and adenocarcinoma (7). Intrathoracic lymphomas along with several other extrathoracic malignancies are also associated. Other pulmonary processes including infections, interstitial disease, and cystic fibrosis, as well as chronic liver disease, have also been associated with HOA. Symptoms of HOA include a deep sensation of pain within the long bones. Swelling of the extremities, particularly the lower limbs, and an associated symmetrical noninflammatory arthritis of large joints can be painful (7). However, some patients may be completely asymptomatic.

Examination

Digital clubbing is the most notable physical finding in patients with HOA (Fig. 22.5). Periungual skin may be thin and shiny. Dermal involvement of the face and extremities can also occur because of skin and bone proliferation. Relatively large joint effusions are possible.

Studies

Although no specific laboratory tests are used for diagnosis, radiographs can be helpful. Periostitis, or cortical thickening of long bones, remains the classic finding on radiographs (Fig. 22.6). Bone scans may reveal uptake in the cortex of long bones, reflecting proliferation because of periostitis. Acro-osteolysis of the fingers and toes can also be seen. Notably, joint spaces remain normal and erosions are not typical (7). Arthrocentesis reveals a viscous synovial fluid with minimal WBCs on fluid analysis. Importantly, the diagnosis of HOA warrants evaluation for and treatment of potential underlying causes.

Treatment

Asymptomatic patients do not require specific treatment for HOA. Nonsteroidal anti-inflammatory drugs (NSAIDs) may be useful for symptoms of pain. Case studies have reported improved pain control in refractory cases with administration of intravenous bisphosphonate therapy (7).

Clinical Course

In general, the clinical condition is most dependent on treatment of the underlying systemic disease. For example, clubbing can improve or even resolve with chemotherapy or resection of the associated malignancy.

CARCINOMATOUS POLYARTHRITIS

Generally a seronegative polyarthropathy, carcinomatous polyarthritis represents a condition that can mimic rheumatoid

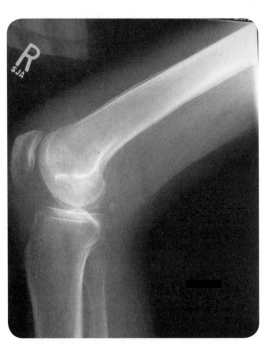

Figure 22.6 Periostitis in hypertrophic osteoarthropathy. (Courtesy of Gerald F. Moore, MD.)

arthritis with a volatile presentation. Typically found in older adults, symptoms often develop in close temporal relationship to the diagnosis of a malignancy. Asymmetrical involvement of lower extremity joints is most frequent with relative sparing of the hands. The most commonly reported co-occurring malignancies are colon, breast, ovarian, and lung. Arthropathy can improve with treatment of the malignancy.

COMPLEX REGIONAL PAIN SYNDROME

Complex regional pain syndrome (CRPS) is defined as pain, autonomic dysfunction, trophic changes, and functional impairment without identifiable nerve damage (8). History may reveal recent surgery or trauma. However, in the absence of such etiology, underlying malignancy must be considered. Pain is described as burning, throbbing, searing, or aching, and may be aggravated by heat, cold, or contact. Patients with CRPS experience significant skin tenderness, chronic mild swelling, limited relief with narcotics, and difficulty sleeping. Physical examination can reveal classic finger posturing with MCP extension and PIP flexion or extension. Conversely, flexion of both MCP and PIP joints, or clenched fist, may suggest malingering (8). Other signs and symptoms may include stiffness, local osteopenia, atrophy of nails and hair, skin hypertrophy, and fine motor difficulties. Magnetic resonance imaging and three-phase bone scan can be positive in late disease, showing increased periarticular uptake in involved joints. A multidisciplinary approach to management is important, with input from an internist, surgeon, pain specialist, physical therapist, psychologist or psychiatrist, and rheumatologist. Pharmacologic therapy includes antidepressants, anticonvulsants, calcium channel blockers, adrenergic compounds, and corticosteroids, as well as anti-inflammatory and analgesic agents. A combination of agents with concurrent hand therapy is most beneficial (8).

MULTICENTRIC RETICULOHISTIOCYTOSIS

A rare disorder with unknown pathogenesis, multicentric reticulohistiocytosis (MR) is characterized by progressive erosive polyarthritis and nodular skin and mucosal lesions (Fig. 22.7). Multicentric reticulohistiocytosis has been reported in association with several malignancies, most often breast and stomach carcinoma. Middle-aged women are most commonly affected, with arthralgias followed by skin manifestations months to years later. The long clinical course makes diagnosis difficult. Confirmation is by histologic presence of mononuclear histiocytes and multinucleated giant cells. Symmetrical arthropathy primarily affects the interphalangeal joints of the hands and causes moderate pain, stiffness, and swelling. Distal interphalangeal (DIP) joint involvement can help distinguish the process from other diseases, although any joint can be affected. Natural progression leads to severe destruction and disfiguration. Aggressive treatment with immunosuppressive medications is important in such cases (9).

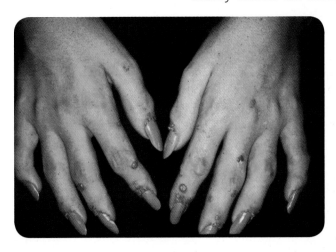

Figure 22.7 Multicentric reticulohistiocytosis. (Courtesy of Gerald F. Moore, MD.)

REMITTING SERONEGATIVE SYMMETRICAL SYNOVITIS WITH PITTING EDEMA

Described as a limited syndrome of synovitis to the bilateral hands and wrists, remitting seronegative symmetrical synovitis with pitting edema (RS3PE) has been reported almost exclusively in the elderly male population. Painful pitting edema of the dorsal surface of the hands is usually present. Very rapid onset is typical, with patients commonly able to pinpoint onset of symptoms to nearly the hour. Inflammatory markers including erythrocyte sedimentation rate and C-reactive protein levels are usually markedly elevated. Nonsteroidal anti-inflammatory drugs are often of little benefit. However, oral corticosteroids provide rapid clinical response, and subsequent remission persists after discontinuation of steroids (10). Malignancies including lymphoma, myelodysplastic disorder, and solid tumors are reported, and should be suspected in cases poorly responsive to glucocorticoids.

Hematologic Disorders with Associated Arthropathies

SICKLE CELL DISEASE

Clinical Presentation

Because of an abnormal β-globulin chain within hemoglobin, sickle cell disease is manifested as anemia. Additional important consequences include vaso-occlusion and infarction of bone with resultant osteonecrosis. Approximately 50% of patients with sickle cell disease develop avascular necrosis by 35 years of age (11). Hyposplenism also portends heightened risk of infection, including osteomyelitis and septic arthritis. Infarction can occur anywhere within the skeleton and is a direct result of sickled cells, causing stasis of blood and ischemia. Cold-induced vasoconstriction can also contribute. Infarcts typically occur in the medullary cavities and epiphyses, causing painful bone crises. However, asymptomatic silent infarcts do occur and are found incidentally on radiographs.

Examination

Signs and symptoms include joint or bone tenderness and swelling with limited ROM. Fever can also be seen. However, patients can be asymptomatic. Children may present with sickle cell dactylitis.

Studies

Acute infarcts cause osteolysis, with later development of intramedullary lucency and sclerosis in a patchy distribution. Epiphyseal ischemic necrosis in patients with sickle cell anemia is commonly seen in the humeral and femoral heads, with bilateral involvement more frequently seen than in other diseases with associated avascular necrosis. Initial radiographs can be normal, with the earliest signs of necrosis seen on MRI. (11). With progression, radiographic changes include lucency, sclerosis, and eventually depression of the articular surface with collapse and fragmentation (Fig. 22.8).

Treatment

Acute therapy for sickle cell crisis includes hydration and pain control. Conservative management versus surgical intervention for osteonecrosis is based on the patient and staging of severity. Core decompression, structural bone grafting, osteotomy, and arthroplasty are available options. Conservative measures include limitations in weight bearing and pain control with analgesic agents (11).

Clinical Course

Progression and prognosis of osteonecrosis is dependent on the size and location of the infarcted lesion. Range of motion typically declines slowly over time. Eventually, collapse can occur. Therefore monitoring is warranted.

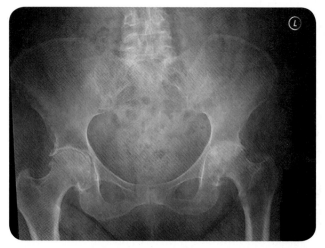

Figure 22.8 Osteonecrosis of left femoral head. (Courtesy of Gerald F. Moore, MD.)

HEMOPHILIA

Joint disease is one of the most important causes of morbidity in patients with severe hemophilia. Recurrent bleeding into the joint leads to cartilage damage, synovial hypertrophy, narrowed joint space, and even alterations in bone structure (12). Patients may present with pain, swelling, stiffness, or "locking" with instability of the knees or elbows. Magnetic resonance imaging is a sensitive tool showing low signal intensity on T_1- or T_2-weighted images where persistent hemosiderin deposition occurs from repeated intra-articular hemorrhage. Physical therapy and rehabilitation—including physiotherapy, hydrotherapy, splinting, and orthotics—are important in both the treatment and the prevention of hemophilic arthropathy (12). Synovectomy and joint replacement are additional options.

Hereditary Disorders with Associated Arthropathies

HEMOCHROMATOSIS

Clinical Presentation

Hereditary hemochromatosis is a relatively common autosomal-recessive disorder with approximately 1 in 200 persons affected. A substitution of tyrosine for cysteine at a specific location on each allele results in increased intestinal iron absorption and eventual iron overload. The arthropathy associated with hemochromatosis is well recognized and reported in up to 81% of patients (13). Fatigue and arthralgias are common nonspecific early symptoms, while classic bronze diabetes, CHF, and cirrhosis are a much less common presentation, and suggest end-stage disease (14).

Painful arthralgias are a major cause of morbidity, disability, and reduced quality of life for patients with hereditary hemochromatosis. It can affect nearly any joint, but most commonly involves the MCP and radiocarpal joints, ankles, hips, elbows, knees, and shoulders (13). Long-standing unexplained joint pain or osteoarthritis in a patient younger than 55 years of age should warrant suspicion of possible hemochromatosis (14).

Examination

Bony swelling can be significant and resemble osteoarthritis. Involvement of the second and third MCP joints in a symmetrical pattern is a hallmark (15).

Studies

Serum levels of iron, total iron-binding capacity (TIBC), and ferritin should be obtained. If iron saturation is greater than 50%, or an elevated ferritin level present, genetic testing should follow (14). Referral to a gastroenterologist is warranted. Radiographic changes include broadening of metacarpal heads with classic "hook-like" osteophytes and joint space narrowing (Fig. 22.9). Secondary CPPD disease from hemochromatosis can also reveal crystals on arthrocentesis of involved joints.

Treatment

Treatment options are limited, with only symptomatic therapies available for management of arthropathy. Unfortunately, regular phlebotomy with systemic iron depletion is seldom helpful for joint symptom relief, and has no effect on the progressive deterioration of joint structure (13).

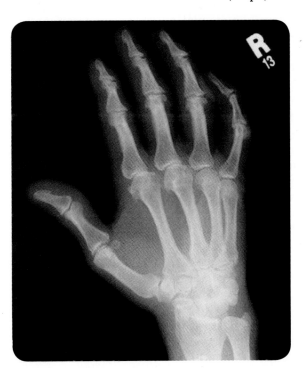

Figure 22.9 Joint space narrowing with "hook" osteophytes and hypertrophic changes seen in Hemochromatosis. (Courtesy of Gerald F. Moore, MD.)

Clinical Course

Although early diagnosis and treatment have little effect on the arthropathy, more serious complications secondary to systemic iron overload, notably cirrhosis, CHF, and diabetes mellitus, may be avoided.

WILSON'S DISEASE

Wilson's disease is a rare, but treatable, autosomal-recessive disorder caused by a mutation in copper-transporting ATPase. This results in an accumulation of free copper in organs including the liver, brain, and joints. Neurologic manifestations include dysarthria, dystonia, and tremor. Patients may complain of pain and stiffness, especially involving the knees, wrists, or other large joints. Musculoskeletal pain may be the only presenting symptom and is likely secondary to synovial inflammation and bone demineralization (16).

ALKAPTONURIA (OCHRONOSIS)

Alkaptonuria is a rare metabolic autosomal-recessive disease with estimated incidence of 1 in 250,000 to 1 million live births. A deficiency of homogentisate 1,2-dioxygenase enzyme results in excess homogentisic acid. Ochronotic pigment deposits in tissue, particularly joints, causing inflammation and articular degeneration (17). A child's first symptoms can include darkened or black urine. However, patients can be undiagnosed and present as an adult with long-standing back pain as their only complaint. Severe spondyloarthropathy is the most common presentation of ochronotic arthropathy. Clinical resemblance to ankylosing spondylitis exists; however, sacroiliac joints are typically spared.

Arthropathy begins in the third or fourth decade of life and results in ROM limitations, effusions, and eventually chronic pain. Knee, hip, or shoulder replacements are common. Spinal involvement leads to kyphosis, height loss, and decreased lumbar flexion. Densely calcified intervertebral discs are characteristic on imaging studies. Therapies include vitamin C because of antioxidant properties and protein restriction in an attempt to decrease homogentisic acid excretion. However, efficacy has not been proved. In general, surveillance for cardiac and renal complications and attention to pain control are most practical (17).

HEREDITARY DISORDERS OF CONNECTIVE TISSUES

Polyarticular hypermobility is present in up to 30% to 40% of young men and women, respectively. For most, however, hypermobility is of no medical consequence and termed *benign hypermobility syndrome*. Conditions including Ehlers–Danlos syndrome, osteogenesis imperfecta, and Marfan syndrome involve abnormalities of collagen, fibrillin, and matrix proteins with significant musculoskeletal manifestations. Patients with these diseases can present with localized or diffuse arthralgia, myalgias, tendinopathies, recurrent joint dislocation, subluxations, fragility fractures, ligament or capsular pathology, early onset osteoarthritis, and fatigue (18). Pain is the most common reason these patients seek medical attention. In most cases there is no evidence of significant damage to joints, muscles, or surrounding structures to account for the widespread pain. Physical and occupational therapy methods need to be modified to account for laxity of tissues, including splints to protect unstable joints, development of muscles responsible for core stability, restoration of proprioception, and orthotics to correct mechanical discrepancies (18).

For most heritable disorders, referral to a geneticist is warranted for appropriate reproductive risk stratification and counseling. Although musculoskeletal manifestations are discussed here, inherited diseases often have a wide array of systemic and multiorgan involvement necessitating interdisciplinary approach to management.

Miscellaneous Diseases with Associated Arthropathies

AMYLOIDOSIS

Amyloidosis is a heterogeneous group of diseases characterized by deposition of plasma proteins in an abnormal, insoluble, fibrillar form (19). Congo red stain makes the deposits appear apple green with birefringence under polarized microscopy. Amyloid deposition into the joint and periarticular tissues occurs in most forms of the disease. Diagnosis relies on histology and may be easily obtained by fine-needle aspiration of abdominal fat, confirming amyloid deposits in 80% to 88% of patients (19).

- *AL amyloidosis:* It is the most common form of systemic amyloid and is due to deposition of immunoglobulin light chains. Approximately 9% of patients, especially males, have musculoskeletal symptoms as a dominant clinical feature (19). Joint stiffness and swelling occur, occasionally with painful contractures because of amyloid infiltration of periarticular and synovial tissues. The "shoulder pad" sign is the most classic articular manifestation of AL amyloidosis and is due to infiltration of tendons and capsular structures of the shoulder, leading to swelling and motion limitation. When coupled with macroglossia and periorbital cutaneous ecchymosis ("raccoon eyes"), the shoulder pad sign is considered nearly pathognomonic. Patients with AL amyloidosis have the worst prognosis secondary to associations with heart failure. Treatment focuses on reduction of amyloidogenic protein concentration by chemotherapy.
- *AA amyloidosis:* Any chronic inflammatory process that causes persistent elevation of acute-phase reactants can lead to deposition of serum amyloid A (SAA) protein and result in AA amyloidosis. Rheumatic diseases including rheumatoid arthritis, ankylosing spondylitis, psoriatic arthritis, juvenile idiopathic arthritis, and familial Mediterranean fever (FMF) account for 70% of AA amyloidosis (19). Patients have a much better prognosis than those with AL amyloidosis, with a median survival of 4 to 10 years, depending on cardiac involvement. Therapy focuses on treating the underlying disorder to suppress chronic inflammation and thus reduce circulating levels of SAA protein. Colchicine is highly effective in preventing the AA amyloidosis of familial Mediterranean fever.
- *β_2-microglobulin (β2M) amyloidosis:* Patients on long-term hemodialysis are at risk of developing amyloidosis caused by deposition of fibrillar β2M protein. Pathogenesis is unknown but felt to be multifactorial and associated with age and duration of hemodialysis. Early manifestations include carpal tunnel syndrome and chronic arthralgia, commonly involving the shoulders. Unfortunately, an erosive and disabling arthropathy of large joints can develop. Radiographic signs of axial involvement include erosions of vertebral corners and severe intervertebral space narrowing. Magnetic resonance imaging can show amyloid deposits as well (Fig. 22.10). Approximately 50% to 60% of patients receiving hemodialysis for more than 10 years will have subchondral radiolucent bone cysts in the shoulder, hips, wrists, or vertebrae on imaging. Bony cysts can account for fractures of the femoral neck and vertebrae. Therapy aims at promoting clearance of β2M protein and preventing amyloid deposition; however, the use of high-flux dialysis membranes has not been proved to be effective (19).

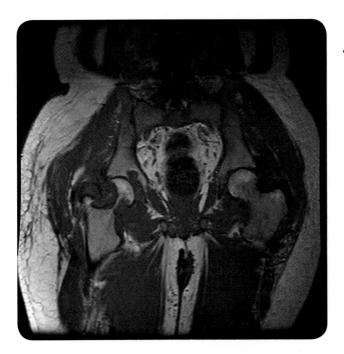

Figure 22.10 Magnetic resonance imaging of amyloid infiltrating right femoral head. (Courtesy of Gerald F. Moore, MD.)

WHEN TO REFER ⑦

- For assistance in difficult diagnoses
- When conservative measures are not helpful
- When the clinical picture no longer fits the diagnosis
- For management of immunosuppressant medications
- For therapeutic measures including special procedures

SARCOIDOSIS

Sarcoidosis is a poorly understood disease of noncaseating granuloma development, typically in the lungs and lymph nodes. It affects virtually any organ, although patients may be completely asymptomatic. Musculoskeletal manifestations include inflammatory arthritis, tenosynovitis, dactylitis, periarticular soft-tissue swelling, myopathy, and granulomatous bone infiltration (20). Löfgren's syndrome is bilateral hilar adenopathy with acute erythema nodosum, and may include fever, anterior uveitis, and arthritis, especially of the ankles. Two types of arthritis are recognized. Acute sarcoid arthritis is self-limited and resolves without permanent sequelae. Chronic arthritis is less common and can progress to joint deformity because of proliferative and inflammatory changes in the synovium. Nonsteroidal anti-inflammatory drugs, corticosteroids, colchicine, antimalarials, and/or immunosuppressive medications have all been used as drug therapy of sarcoid arthritis (20).

ICD9

726.90 **Capsulitis** *(joint)*
726.0 adhesive (shoulder)
250.0 **Diabetes, diabetic** *(brittle) (congenital) (familial) (mellitus) (severe) (slight) (without complication)*
244.9 **Hypothyroidism** *(acquired)*
715.9 **Osteoarthropathy**
757.39 chronic idiopathic hypertrophic
757.39 familial idiopathic
731.2 hypertrophic pulmonary
731.2 secondary
757.39 idiopathic hypertrophic
731.2 primary hypertrophic
731.2 pulmonary hypertrophic
731.2 secondary hypertrophic
716.59 **Polyarthritis, polyarthropathy** *NEC*
714.9 inflammatory

References

1. Caudill-Slosberg MA, Schwartz LM, Woloshin S. Office visits and analgesic prescriptions for musculoskeletal pain in US: 1980 vs. 2000. *Pain* 2004;109(3):514–519.
2. Prevention, C.f.D. C. a., *National Diabetes Fact Sheet: General Information and National Estimates on Diabetes in the United States, 2007.* US Department of Health and Human Services; 2008.
3. Burner TW, Rosenthal AK. Diabetes and rheumatic diseases. *Curr Opin Rheumatol* 2009;21(1):50–54.
4. Rajbhandari SM, Jenkins RC, Davies C, et al. Charcot neuroarthropathy in diabetes mellitus. *Diabetologia* 2002;45(8):1085–1096.
5. Kelley MJ, McClure PW, Leggin BG. Frozen shoulder: Evidence and a proposed model guiding rehabilitation. *J Orthop Sports Phys Ther* 2009;39(2):135–148.
6. Colao A, Ferone D, Marzullo P, et al. Systemic complications of acromegaly: Epidemiology, pathogenesis, and management. *Endocr Rev* 2004;25(1):102–152.
7. Yao Q, Altman RD, Brahn E. Periostitis and hypertrophic pulmonary osteoarthropathy: Report of 2 cases and review of the literature. *Semin Arthritis Rheum* 2009;38(6):458–466.
8. Li Z, Paterson Smith B, Smith TL, et al. Diagnosis and management of complex regional pain syndrome complicating upper extremity recovery. *J Hand Ther* 2005;18(2):270–276.
9. Trotta F, Castellino G, Lo Monaco A. Multicentric reticulohistiocytosis. *Best Pract Res Clin Rheumatol* 2004;18(5):759–772.
10. Keenan RT, Hamalian GM, Pillinger MH. RS3PE presenting in a unilateral pattern: Case report and review of the literature. *Semin Arthritis Rheum* 2009;38(6):428–433.
11. Ejindu VC, Hine AL, Mashayekhi M, et al. Musculoskeletal manifestations of sickle cell disease. *Radiographics* 2007;27(4):1005–1021.
12. Bossard D, Carrillon Y, Stieltjes N, et al. Management of haemophilic arthropathy. *Haemophilia* 2008;14(Suppl 4):11–19.
13. Carroll G, Breidahl WH, Bulsara MK, et al. Hereditary haemochromatosis (HH) is characterized by a clinically definable arthropathy that correlates with iron load. *Arthritis Rheum* 2011;63(1):286–94.

14. Carlsson A. Hereditary hemochromatosis: A neglected diagnosis in orthopedics: A series of 7 patients with ankle arthritis, and a review of the literature. *Acta Orthop* 2009;80(3):371–374.
15. von Kempis J. Arthropathy in hereditary hemochromatosis. *Curr Opin Rheumatol* 2001;13(1):80–83.
16. Soltanzadeh A, Soltanzadeh P, Nafissi S, et al. Wilson's disease: A great masquerader. *Eur Neurol* 2007;57(2):80–85.
17. Al-Mahfoudh R, Clark S, Buxton N. Alkaptonuria presenting with ochronotic spondyloarthropathy. *Br J Neurosurg* 2008;22(6):805–807.
18. Hakim AJ, Sahota A. Joint hypermobility and skin elasticity: The hereditary disorders of connective tissue. *Clin Dermatol* 2006;24(6):521–533.
19. Perfetto F, Moggi-Pignone A, Livi R, et al. Systemic amyloidosis: A challenge for the rheumatologist. *Nat Rev Rheumatol* 2010;6(7):417–429.
20. Torralba KD, Quismorio FP, Jr. Sarcoid arthritis: A review of clinical features, pathology and therapy. *Sarcoidosis Vasc Diffuse Lung Dis* 2003;20(2):95–103.

Infectious Arthritis

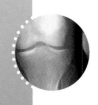

Chapter 23 **Bacterial Arthritis**

Arthur Kavanaugh and Maika Onishi

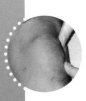

Chapter 24 **Lyme Disease**

William F. Iobst and Kristin M. Ingraham

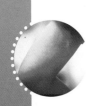

Chapter 25 **Viral Arthritis**

Katherine Holman and Martin Rodriguez

CHAPTER **23** # Bacterial Arthritis

Arthur Kavanaugh and Maika Onishi

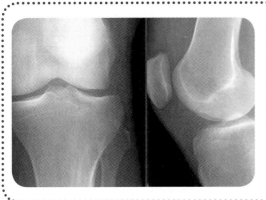

A 30-year-old male presenting with acute-onset left knee pain, warmth, and swelling (Fig. 23.1).

Introduction

Bacterial arthritis is a true rheumatologic emergency that can lead to irreversible joint destruction, increased morbidity, and accelerated mortality, without prompt diagnosis and treatment. Although many infectious agents may cause arthritis, bacterial arthritis is the most significant because of its rapidly progressive and highly destructive nature. Despite recent advances in antimicrobial therapy, diagnostic testing, and general medical care, the prognosis for patients with bacterial arthritis continues to be guarded with 25% to 50% of patients suffering permanent joint damage and an estimated 5% to 15% case fatality secondary to complications including sepsis. Perhaps the most important factor regarding the outcome of patients with bacterial arthritis is the speed with which appropriate therapy is instituted. Therefore, it remains true

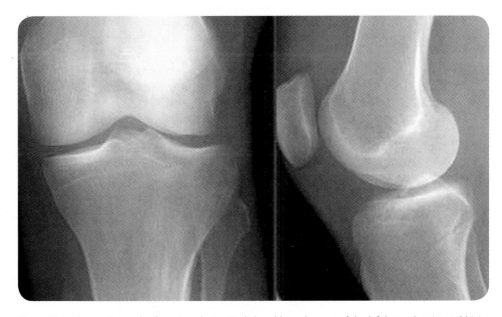

Figure 23.1 Plain radiograph of septic arthritis. Medial and lateral x-rays of the left knee showing mild joint effusion, but is otherwise normal.

at the start of the new millennium as it has for more than half a century; clinical suspicion of the diagnosis of bacterial arthritis is the most critical consideration for the clinician.

Bacterial arthritis ensues when foreign organisms invade the synovium or joint space. In the majority of cases, infection is introduced via hematogenous spread from a distant site. Less commonly, bacterial pathogens reach the joint space via direct inoculation through a penetrating trauma or procedure (e.g., arthrocentesis, surgery) or via contiguous spread from adjacent soft-tissue or bone infections, including cellulitis, osteomyelitis, and bursitis. Upon entry into the joint space, bacteria induce an acute inflammatory response, which rapidly progresses to synovial hyperplasia and infiltration by inflammatory cells. Without prompt treatment initiation, this can lead to enzymatic and cytokine-mediated cartilage and bone degradation within days. Additionally, in bacterial arthritis, the urgency of treatment is further heightened because of potential infection with bacterial strains with virulence factors (e.g., toxins, adhesins), which are associated with increased pathogenicity and disease severity (1).

The two major classes of bacterial arthritis are nongonococcal and gonococcal arthritis (discussed below), with nongonococcal arthritis accounting for the majority of cases across all age and risk groups. *Staphylococcus aureus* is the most common organism infecting naïve joints in 60% to 70% of cases. Because it is such a frequent cause of bacterial arthritis, the increasing prevalence of community- and hospital-acquired methicillin-resistant *Staph. aureus* (MRSA) is an important consideration when initially treating bacterial arthritis. Additionally, staphylococci infections are associated with higher rates of fulminant disease and residual joint damage, thus necessitating prompt diagnosis and aggressive treatment.

The main remaining causes of bacterial arthritis include streptoccci, gram-negative bacilli, and anaerobes. Host–pathogen associations may be helpful in guiding initial antimicrobial treatment. Streptococci (e.g., *Streptococcus viridans*, *Strep. pneumoniae*, group A and B streptococci) account for 15% to 20% of nongonococcal arthritis and may be preceded by primary skin or soft-tissue infections. Group A streptococci are the most common streptococcal species and are often isolated after dental procedures. Gram-negative bacilli infections (e.g., *Pseudomonas aeruginosa*, *Escherichia coli*, *Proteus mirabilis*) are responsible for 5% to 25% of cases, and are associated with chronic systemic illness, immunosuppression, intravenous drug use, and advancing age (e.g., in elderly patients). These infections may begin as urinary tract or skin infections with subsequent hematogenous spread to a joint. Lastly, anaerobic bacteria (e.g., *Bacteroides*, *Clostridium*, *Fusobacterium*) account for 1% to 5% of bacterial arthritis, although this may be an underestimate as anaerobes have historically been more difficult to isolate. While most bacterial arthritis infections are monomicrobial, anaerobic infections may be polymicrobial in nature. Predisposing factors include diabetes mellitus, immunocompromised states, and postoperative wound infections. Suspicion for an anaerobic agent should be raised in the case of foul-smelling synovial fluid or plain radiographs depicting gas in the joint space. Adequate drainage of the joint is a key adjunct to antimicrobial therapy in the case of anaerobic infection.

Less commonly, other organisms may also be associated with bacterial arthritis. One worth mentioning is the *Brucella* species (e.g., *B. melitensis*), which is becoming more prevalent worldwide (2). Risk factors include consumption of unpasteurized milk or cheese or direct contact with infected animals. Presentation is usually characterized by monoarthritis of the hip or knee, although oligoarthritis, sacroiliitis, or spondylitis may also be seen. Further work-up should be guided by the clinical setting if one of the common etiologic agents is not identified.

Gonococcal arthritis is the most common cause of bacterial arthritis in young, sexually active individuals without a history of joint disease. Women are at greatest risk for disseminated gonococcal infection, especially during pregnancy and menses, and are affected two to three times more often than men. While, overall, the prognosis for gonoccocal arthritis is better than that for nongonococcal arthritis, rapid diagnosis is equally important in this setting given the potential for joint destruction with delays in treatment.

Diagnosis of gonococcal arthritis can be difficult, as only 25% of patients may recall signs of mucosal involvement of the urethra, genitalia, or rectum. Clinical suspicion should be raised in the setting of purulent monoarticular arthritis, as well as in the setting of arthritis–dermatitis syndrome, the typical presentation of gonococcal arthritis in 60% of cases. It is characterized by a triad of migratory polyarthritis, tenosynovitis, and dermatitis. At disease onset, patients commonly experience migratory arthralgias in the upper extremities (e.g., wrist, elbows) and, less frequently, in the lower extremities. Later, patients may develop tenosynovitis, a finding not commonly seen in infectious arthritis related to other organisms. Gonococcal tenosynovitis most often occurs in the dorsum of the wrist, hand, or ankle. The skin lesions of disseminated gonococcal infection are typically painless, nonpruritic, maculopapular lesions distributed over the distal extremities, especially the palms and soles.

Diagnosis of gonococcal arthritis is further complicated by the difficulty in isolating gonococci in synovial fluid and blood. Even with attention to proper culture technique (e.g., chocolate agar, rapid plating), gram stains and cultures of synovial fluid are positive in fewer than 40% of cases, and blood cultures are almost always negative (3). Mucosal cultures of the urethra, pharynx, cervix, and rectum should be performed in all patients, since they have a higher yield and may be positive even in the absence of symptoms. More sensitive techniques for identification of gonococci, such as polymerase chain reaction, are currently not routinely used, but may provide additional diagnostic value in the future.

Although most patients respond dramatically to antibiotics within 24 to 48 hours and nearly all make a complete recovery, when gonoccocal arthritis is suspected, patients should be considered for hospital admission to confirm diagnosis, exclude complications such as meningitis and endocarditis, and receive parenteral therapy.

Clinical Presentation

Clinical suspicion for bacterial arthritis should be raised in patients with underlying joint disease, compromised immune function, and increased infection risk, all of which are key risk factors for joint infection. Joints that have been damaged by arthritis (e.g., rheumatoid arthritis, osteoarthritis, crystalline arthritis) or trauma are more susceptible to infection than normal joints. This may be secondary to structural damage, neovascularization, or local factors. As the synovium serves an important protective role in joint defense, patients with rheumatoid arthritis are particularly susceptible. Patients with impaired host defenses because of extremes of age, systemic illness (e.g., diabetes mellitus, malignancy, liver or kidney disease), immunosuppressive medications, or immunocompromised conditions (e.g., HIV/AIDs) are also at increased risk. Likewise, it follows that risk factors for infection such as prosthetic joints in which foreign bodies serve as a nidus for infection, intra-articular joint injections, skin infections, and intravenous drug abuse may predispose patients to bacterial arthritis. As a clinician, obtaining a thorough history regarding these risk factors plays an important role in diagnosis and treatment.

Examination

The classic presentation for bacterial arthritis is acute monoarticular joint pain with swelling, warmth, and erythema. On examination, patients typically exhibit

- The classic presentation is acute monoarticular joint pain with swelling, warmth, and erythema.

- Patients with gonococcal arthritis may exhibit migratory polyarthralgias, tenosynovitis, and characteristic skin lesions.

- Joint aspiration should be performed in all patients with suspected bacterial arthritis prior to starting empiric antibiotic therapy.

- Synovial fluid will be inflammatory with white blood cell (WBC) count >2,500/mm^3 and >75% neutrophils; infectious arthritis may be associated with very high WBC counts in the synovial fluid, for example, WBC count >50,000/mm^3.

- A negative gram stain and culture does not exclude a diagnosis of bacterial arthritis.

Table 23.1 **Differential Diagnosis of Bacterial Arthritis**

Other infectious arthritides
   Viral arthritis
   Mycobacterium arthritis
   Fungal arthritis
   Lyme disease

Crystalline arthritis
   Gout
   Pseudogout

Spondyloarthropathies
   Reiter's syndrome
   Ankylosing spondylitis

Reactive arthritis (e.g., poststreptococcal)

Nonarthritic conditions
   Cellulitis
   Bursitis
   Trauma/fracture
   Foreign body reaction

obvious joint effusion, tenderness to palpation, and restricted range of motion. Large joints are more commonly affected than small joints, and in up to 70% of cases, the knee or hip is involved. Intravenous drug users may present with sternoclavicular or sacroiliac joint involvement. Fever is the most commonly associated symptom on presentation and is found in >50% of patients, while sweats and chills are less common (4).

Clinical acuity for the diagnosis of bacterial arthritis is particularly important in atypical presentations, given the rapid pace of joint destruction over a matter of days. Clinical suspicion should remain high with polyarticular presentations, which may account for a quarter of septic arthritis cases (5). Polyarticular infection is more likely in the setting of *Staph. aureus* infection, gonococcal disease, and in patients with rheumatoid arthritis and other systemic connective tissue diseases. On the other hand, preexisting polyarticular joint disease may confound the diagnosis of a monoarticular infection. In these patients, bacterial arthritis should be suspected in those who present with new symptoms in one joint that are out of proportion to the other joints. Additionally, it is important not to exclude a diagnosis of bacterial arthritis in patients with a gradual onset of symptoms, which may be found in patients with prosthetic joints, rheumatic disease, or immunocompromised states.

Given the risks associated with a delay in diagnosis, it is not unreasonable to suggest that absent a clearly established other cause, acute monoarticular arthritis is infectious until proven otherwise. Likewise, a high degree of clinical suspicion for bacterial arthritis should be held in patients with predisposing risk factors for septic arthritis. The differential diagnosis for bacterial arthritis is reviewed in Table 23.1. A thorough history and physical examination may help distinguish between an infectious and inflammatory process. To distinguish periarticular conditions, diagnosis will be facilitated if the clinician is confident in his or her physical examination skills regarding differentiation of arthritis from involvement of structures surrounding the joint (e.g., skin, bursas, tendons).

Studies

The cornerstone of the diagnosis of bacterial arthritis is prompt arthrocentesis and synovial fluid analysis (Table 23.2). Samples should be sent for WBC count

> ## Table 23.2 Suspected Bacterial Arthritis: Key Points in Joint Aspiration
>
> Never aspirate a joint through infected skin or soft tissues
>
> Obtain WBC count with differential, gram stain and culture, and possibly crystal analysis from the aspirated synovial fluid
>
> When there is clinical suspicion of infection, initiate antimicrobial therapy immediately after aspiration
>
> Joint aspiration may be performed serially to remove infected fluid and assess WBC counts over time to monitor response to therapy
>
> Consider orthopedic consultation for prosthetic joints, hip joints (particularly in children), or open drainage if clinical response is suboptimal
>
> Use extreme care in aspirating a prosthetic joint
>
> WBC, white blood cell.

NOT TO BE MISSED

- A thorough history and physical examination are critical, although it may still be difficult to distinguish between an infectious cause and an inflammatory arthritis of other etiology (e.g., crystalline, autoimmune).

- Septic arthritis may be superimposed on other joint diseases and may be mistaken for exacerbation of the preexisting condition.

- Keep a high index of suspicion in patients who are elderly, young, immunocompromised, or have preexisting joint disease.

- Pediatric patients may present with subtle and nonspecific findings; heightened clinical suspicion is especially critical given the potential for catastrophic outcomes.

and differential, gram stain, culture, and crystal analysis; these are the only tests of proven diagnostic value in this clinical setting (6). Infected fluid is characteristically inflammatory (i.e., with WBC count $>2,500/mm^3$ and $>75\%$ neutrophils) in the differential ($>75\%$); not uncommonly, it is purulent with synovial WBC counts of 30 to $50,000/mm^3$ or higher. The likelihood of infection increases with rising WBC count (4). The predominant differential diagnosis for highly inflammatory synovial fluid is crystalline arthritis (e.g., gout). Synovial fluid gram stains give a positive result in 50% to 70% of cases of nongonoccocal arthritis and should be used to guide initial therapy. Positive cultures increase the yield to 70% to 90% of cases of nongonococcal arthritis, but a negative gram stain or culture does not rule out an infected joint (7). For example, false negatives may occur in patients previously treated with antibiotic therapy or in patients with gonococcal infections.

Additional tests that should be performed include blood cultures, which are positive in up to 50% of cases, and should be obtained to exclude a bacteremic origin of the infected joint. When clinically appropriate, urethral, nasal, throat, rectal, or cervical swabs may be performed to evaluate for gonococcal infection. Other laboratory studies such as peripheral WBC count, erythrocyte sedimentation rate, and C-reactive protein are usually elevated and may help in monitoring treatment.

Imaging studies are of limited diagnostic value early in the disease course of bacterial arthritis. Plain radiographs may only reveal soft-tissue swelling or joint effusion (Fig. 23.1). Despite this, they should be obtained as a baseline and to exclude osteomyelitis. In later stages of bacterial arthritis (>10 days after infection onset), cartilage and bone destruction may be visualized on plain radiographs, highlighting its rapid course. Of note, untreated septic arthritis tends to be characterized by erosions with relatively indistinct margins as opposed to other joint pathology (e.g., gout, rheumatoid arthritis [RA]), which is characterized by erosions with clearly defined edges. Other methods of imaging such as computed tomography (CT) and magnetic resonance imaging (MRI) are more sensitive for distinguishing osteomyelitis, joint effusions, and periarticular abscesses, but are not commonly used for the evaluation of joint infections. Usually they are reserved for evaluating the sternoclavicular or sacroiliac joints, which are difficult to visualize using plain radiography. Lastly, radionuclide scans may help localize areas of inflammation, but are unable to definitively establish infection. Given their low specificity, they are rarely used in the diagnosis of bacterial arthritis.

Treatment

All patients with suspected bacterial arthritis should be considered for hospital admission. Bacterial arthritis is not frequently treated as an outpatient as it typically requires intravenous antibiotics and possibly repeated drainage of the affected joint depending on the clinical course. Consideration should be given to rheumatology or orthopedic surgery consultation, and in more complicated cases, an infectious disease consult may be helpful in guiding work-up and treatment.

Early initiation of antibiotic treatment is critical for improving prognosis and outcomes. If there is a high suspicion for bacterial arthritis, empiric therapy should be started immediately after cultures have been drawn. Currently, there are no randomized controlled trials evaluating antibiotic regimens for bacterial arthritis (8). Thus, choice of initial therapy should be guided by gram stain, risk factors, and clinical setting. Furthermore, resistance patterns of potential organisms should also be taken into account during selection of initial therapy. In general, treatment duration is 3 to 6 weeks, intravenous, and oral combined.

Joint drainage and lavage is the other mainstay of treatment and is important in removing the inflammatory cells and mediators that cause permanent joint destruction. While there is controversy regarding whether closed needle aspirations, arthroscopy, or open arthrotomy is better, in most circumstances, repeated needle aspiration is usually sufficient. Serial synovial fluid analyses should demonstrate a downward trend in WBC numbers and decrease in effusion volume with response to treatment.

Clinical Course

Long-term prognosis for joint preservation correlates with the organism involved, promptness of diagnosis, and institution of appropriate antimicrobial therapy, as well as host-related characteristics. In general, patients with gonococcal arthritis have the best prognosis with prompt resolution of symptoms and rare long-term joint morbidity from this infection. Patients with significant comorbidities, especially those who are immunosuppressed, are most vulnerable to joint damage because of their inability to effectively clear infections in spite of appropriate antimicrobial therapy. Infections with particularly virulent organisms such as *Staph. aureus* can produce long-term articular damage in spite of appropriate timing and selection of antibiotic therapy.

Patients with prosthetic devise pose a difficult challenge as successful joint recovery requires surgical debridement in conjunction with antibiotic therapy; on occasions, this combined fails to clear the infection necessitating removal of the prosthetic device followed by prolonged antibiotic therapy and eventual joint replacement.

Special Circumstances

BACTERIAL ARTHRITIS IN CHILDREN

There are several characteristics of bacterial arthritis in children who are distinct from those in adults. Because of the immature vascular anatomy of their joints, neonates and young children often have coexisting septic arthritis and osteomyelitis. The spectrum of common pathogens also varies because of their less developed immune system. While *Staph. aureus* remains the most common organism, group B streptococci and gram-negative bacilli (*Kingella kingae*, *N. gonorrhoeae*) may also be found. *Haemophilus influenzae* was a dominant pathogen in the past although less so nowadays, given widespread use of vaccines. Additionally, one of the main concerns in children is hip involvement, which can lead to potentially catastrophic consequences. Physical examination should include careful assessment of the hip, buttocks, and groin, and work-up should include ultrasound, which has a high negative predictive value for bacterial arthritis in the hip.

BACTERIAL ARTHRITIS IN IMMUNOCOMPROMISED PATIENTS

Impairments in immune defense are important factors in the development of bacterial arthritis in most affected patients. In addition, patients with defects in specific components of the immune response tend to develop particular infections reflective of their immunodeficiency. For example, patients with defects in antibody-mediated responses (e.g., common variable immunodeficiency, X-linked agammaglobulinemia) are more susceptible to infection by encapsulated coated organisms (e.g., *Streptococcus pneumococci*, *H. influenzae*). Patients with defects in cellular immunity (e.g., AIDS) are particularly susceptible to infection with intracellular organisms, including viruses, mycobacteria, and *Listeria* among others. Patients with impaired neutrophil function (e.g., chronic granulomatous disease) are more susceptible to infection with catalase-positive organisms, such as *Staph. aureus*. Thus, patients with known immunodeficiencies should be considered to be at particular risk for certain organisms.

PROSTHETIC JOINT INFECTIONS

As joint replacement procedures become increasingly common, it is important to keep in mind the unique characteristics associated with prosthetic joint infections. The etiology, microbiology, and treatment of an infection can vary depending on the timing of infection. Early postoperative infections (within the first 3 months) are usually secondary to contamination acquired during implantation and are associated with virulent organisms such as *Staph. aureus* and gram-negative bacilli. As time passes, the likelihood of hematogenous seeding and infection with low-virulence organisms (e.g., *Staph. epidermidis*, *Diptheroides*) introduced during surgery increases. It is these organisms that produce biofilms and account for the more indolent presentation in prosthetic joint infections. While management for prosthetic joint infections depends on the clinical setting, in general, treatment for early onset infections involves surgical debridement, an extended course of antibiotics, and implant retention, whereas for late-onset infections, it requires prosthesis removal with either immediate or delayed reimplantation (9). In cases of suspected infection of joint prostheses, consultation with an orthopedist should be strongly considered.

Conclusions

Bacterial arthritis continues to be an important health problem. Clinical suspicion, rapid diagnosis, and prompt therapy are key to improving outcomes.

WHEN TO REFER

- All patients should be considered for hospital admission.

- Consider consulting rheumatology or orthopedics if a septic joint is suspected or confirmed.

- Consider consultation with an infectious disease specialist in the immunocompromised host or when unusual organisms are implicated in the process.

- All patients with prosthetic joint infections should be considered for referral to an orthopedic surgeon for further evaluation and possible removal of prosthesis.

SECTION 5 Infectious Arthritis

ICD9

716.9 **Arthritis, arthritic** *(acute) (chronic) (subacute)*
040.89 [711.4] due to or associated with bacterial disease NEC
098.50 gonococcal
727.3 **Bursitis** *NEC*
726.79 ankle
726.33 elbow
726.8 finger

(Continued)

ICD9 (Continued)

726.79 foot

726.4 hand

726.5 hip

726.60 knee

726.33 olecranon

726.61 pes anserinus

726.65 prepatellar

726.10 shoulder

726.5 trochanteric area

726.4 wrist

730.2 **Osteomyelitis** *(general) (infective) (localized) (neonatal) (purulent) (pyogenic) (septic) (staphylococcal) (streptococcal) (suppurative) (with periostitis)*

730.1 sicca

References

1. Shirtliff ME, Mader JT. Acute septic arthritis. *Clin Microbiol Rev*2002;15(2):527–544.
2. Franco MP, Mulder M, Gilman RH, et al. Human brucellosis. *Lancet Infect Dis* 2007;7(12):775–786.
3. Ross JJ. Septic arthritis. *Infect Dis Clin North Am* 2005;19(4):853–861.
4. Margaretten ME, Kohlwes J, Moore D, et al. Does this adult patient have septic arthritis? JAMA 2007; 297(13):1478–1488.
5. Dubost JJ, Fis I, Denis P, et al. Polyarticular septic arthritis. *Medicine (Baltimore)* 1993;72(5):296–310.
6. Schmerling RH, Delbanco ML, Tosteson AN, et al. Synovial fluid tests: What should be ordered? JAMA 1990;264:1009–1014.
7. Ryan MJ, Kavanagh R, Wall PG, et al. Bacterial joint infections in England and Wales: Analysis of bacterial isolates over a four-year period. *Br J Rheumatol* 1997;36(3):370–373.
8. Stengal D, Bauwens K, Sehouli J, et al. Systematic review and meta-anaylsis of antibiotic therapy for bone and joint infections. *Lancet Infect Dis* 2001;1(3):175–188.
9. Zimmerli W, Trampuz A, Ochsner PE. Prosthetic-joint infections. *N Engl J Med* 2004;351(16):1645–1654.

24 Lyme Disease

William F. Iobst and Kristin M. Ingraham

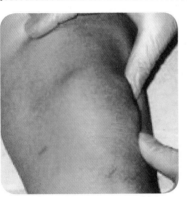

A 39-year-old white male presents to your office with a 3-month history of a painful, swollen left knee. He currently denies other significant joint pain, but describes what he thought was a flu-type illness, characterized by fatigue, headache, malaise, and arthralgias 3 to 4 months prior to the onset of his knee pain. He also notes altered sensation in his hands and feet. He has no history of knee injury, and believes that use of over-the-counter ibuprofen has helped take the edge off the pain. This medication has not reduced the swelling or sensation of warmth when he touches the knee.

The patient lives in rural southeastern Pennsylvania, and is an active hunter. He denies family history of arthritis or arthritis-related diseases. He is aware that Lyme disease is a common illness in this area and wonders if he in fact has this illness.

Introduction

The clinical presentation described above is that of late-stage Lyme disease. While Lyme disease is the most common tick-borne illness in the United States, accurate diagnosis requires an appreciation of regional variation in disease prevalence (Fig. 24.1). Lyme disease is endemic in the northeastern, midwestern, and western regions of the United States. In 2009, approximately 30,000 cases of confirmed and suspected disease were reported by the Centers for Disease Control and Prevention (CDC). The states with the highest total number of reported cases are New York, Pennsylvania, and Massachusetts. The highest incidence of disease occurred in Delaware and was reported at 111.2 per 100,000 individuals (Fig. 24.2).

Reported Cases of Lyme Disease – United States, 2009

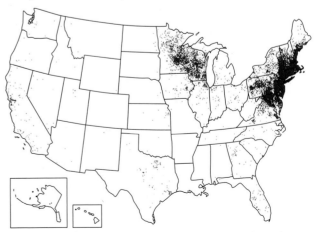

Figure 24.1 2009 representation of distribution of Lyme disease cases. Courtesy of Yehia Mishriki, MD. Centers for Disease Control and Prevention, available at http://www.cdc.gov/ncidod/dvbid/lyme/ld_Incidence.htm. Accessed January 21, 2011.

1 dot placed randomly within county of residence for each confirmed case

Reported Lyme disease cases by state, 1995-2009

State	1995	1996	1997	1998	1999	2000	2001	2002	2003	2004	2005	2006	2007	2008[†]	2009		
															Confirmed	Probable	Incidence*
Alabama	12	9	11	24	20	6	10	11	8	6	3	11	13	6	3	0	0.1
Alaska	0	0	2	1	0	2	2	3	3	3	4	3	10	6	7	0	1.0
Arizona	1	0	4	1	3	2	3	4	4	13	10	10	2	2	3	4	0.0
Arkansas	11	27	27	8	7	7	4	3	0	0	0	0	1	0	0	0	0.0
California	84	64	154	135	139	96	95	97	86	48	95	85	75	74	117	0	0.3
Colorado	0	0	0	0	3	0	0	1	0	0	0	0	0	2	0	1	0.0
Connecticut	1548	3104	2297	3434	3215	3773	3597	4631	1403	1348	1810	1788	3058	2738	2751	1405	78.2
Delaware	56	173	109	77	167	167	152	194	212	339	646	482	715	772	984	0	111.2
DC	3	3	10	8	6	11	17	25	14	16	10	62	116	71	53	8	8.8
Florida	17	55	56	71	59	54	43	79	43	46	47	34	30	72	77	33	0.4
Georgia	14	1	9	5	0	0	0	2	10	12	6	8	11	35	40	0	0.4
Hawaii	0	1	0	0	0	0	0	0	0	0	0	0	0	0	0	0	0.0
Idaho	0	2	4	7	3	4	5	4	3	6	2	7	9	5	4	12	0.3
Illinois	18	10	13	14	17	35	32	47	71	87	127	110	149	108	136	0	1.1
Indiana	19	32	33	39	21	23	26	21	25	32	33	26	55	42	61	22	0.9
Iowa	16	19	8	27	24	34	36	42	58	49	89	97	123	85	77	31	2.6
Kansas	23	36	4	13	16	17	2	7	4	3	3	4	8	16	18	0	0.6
Kentucky	16	26	20	27	19	13	23	25	17	15	5	7	6	5	1	0	0.0
Louisiana	9	9	13	15	9	8	8	5	7	2	3	1	2	3	0	0	0.0
Maine	45	63	34	78	41	71	108	219	175	225	247	338	529	780	791	179	60.0
Maryland	454	447	494	659	899	688	608	738	691	891	1235	1248	2576	1746	1466	558	25.7
Massachusetts	189	321	291	699	787	1158	1164	1807	1532	1532	2336	1432	2988	3960	4019	1237	61.0
Michigan	5	28	27	17	11	23	21	26	12	27	62	55	51	76	81	22	0.8
Minnesota	208	251	256	261	283	465	461	867	474	1023	917	914	1238	1046	1063	480	20.2
Mississippi	17	24	27	17	4	3	8	12	21	0	0	3	1	1	0	0	0.0
Missouri	53	52	28	12	72	47	37	41	70	25	15	5	10	6	3	0	0.1
Montana	0	0	0	0	0	0	0	0	0	0	0	1	4	6	3	0	0.3
Nebraska	6	5	2	4	11	5	4	6	2	2	2	11	7	8	4	1	0.2
Nevada	6	2	2	6	2	4	4	2	3	1	3	4	15	9	10	3	0.4
New Hampshire	28	47	39	45	27	84	129	261	190	226	265	617	896	1211	996	419	75.2
New Jersey	1703	2190	2041	1911	1719	2459	2020	2349	2887	2698	3363	2432	3134	3214	4598	375	52.8
New Mexico	1	1	1	4	1	0	1	1	1	1	3	3	5	4	1	4	0.0
New York	4438	5301	3327	4640	4402	4329	4083	5535	5399	5100	5565	4460	4165	5741	4134	1517	21.2
North Carolina	84	66	34	63	74	47	41	137	156	122	49	31	53	16	21	75	0.2
North Dakota	0	2	0	0	1	2	0	1	0	0	3	7	12	8	10	5	1.5
Ohio	30	32	40	47	47	61	44	82	66	50	58	43	33	40	51	7	0.4
Oklahoma	63	42	45	13	8	1	0	0	0	3	0	0	1	1	2	0	0.1
Oregon	20	19	20	21	15	13	15	12	16	11	3	7	6	18	12	26	0.3
Pennsylvania	1562	2814	2188	2760	2781	2343	2806	3989	5730	3985	4287	3242	3994	3818	4950	772	39.3
Rhode Island	345	534	442	789	546	675	510	852	736	249	39	308	177	186	150	85	14.2
South Carolina	17	9	3	8	6	25	6	26	18	22	15	20	31	14	25	17	0.5
South Dakota	0	0	1	0	0	0	0	2	1	1	2	1	0	3	1	0	0.1
Tennessee	28	24	45	47	59	28	31	28	20	20	8	15	31	7	10	27	0.2
Texas	77	97	60	32	72	77	75	139	85	98	69	29	87	105	88	188	0.4
Utah	1	1	1	0	2	3	1	5	2	1	2	5	7	3	6	3	0.2
Vermont	9	26	8	11	26	40	18	37	43	50	54	105	138	330	323	85	51.9
Virginia	55	57	67	73	122	149	156	259	195	216	274	357	959	886	698	210	8.9
Washington	10	18	11	7	14	9	9	11	7	14	13	8	12	22	15	1	0.2
West Virginia	26	12	10	13	20	35	16	26	31	38	61	28	84	120	143	58	7.9
Wisconsin	369	396	480	657	490	631	597	1090	740	1144	1459	1466	1814	1493	1952	637	34.5
Wyoming	4	3	3	1	3	3	1	2	2	4	3	1	3	1	1	2	0.2
U.S. TOTAL	11,700	16,455	12,801	16,801	16,273	17,730	17,029	23,763	21,273	19,804	23,305	19,931	27,444	28,921	29,959	8,509	13.4

[†] confirmed cases presented for all years except most recent
* confirmed cases per 100,000 population

Figure 24.2 2009 reported Lyme disease cases by state, 1995 to 2009. Courtesy of Yehia Mishriki, MD. Centers for Disease Control and Prevention, available at http://www.cdc.gov/ncidod/dvbid/lyme/ld_rptdLymeCasesbyState.htm. Accessed January 21, 2011.

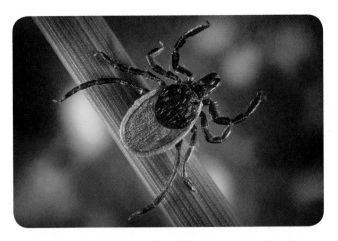

Figure 24.3 Black-legged tick or deer tick. Courtesy of James Gathany. Centers for Disease Control and Prevention, available at http://www.cdc.gov/ncidod/dvbid/lyme/ld_transmission.htm. Accessed January 21, 2011.

Effective prevention, diagnosis, and treatment of this disease also require an understanding of the prevalence, transmission vector, and natural history of Lyme disease. The disease is caused by the spirochete *Borrelia burgdorferi* and is transmitted through the bite of the black-legged tick or deer tick *Ixodes scapularis* (Fig. 24.3). The spirochete is most frequently transmitted by the bite of the nymphal stage of the tick in the spring of the year. The nymphal-stage tick is very small, not being larger than a poppy seed (Fig. 24.4). Less frequently, adult ticks transmit the disease in the fall of the year. Cases typically cluster in children younger than 15 years and in middle-aged adults, and are associated with histories of outdoor activities that expose individuals to the tick. Lyme disease is a reportable illness and both confirmed and probable cases have been tracked by the CDC since 1995. From 1995 to 2009, more than 400,000 cases of confirmed and probable Lyme disease have been reported with the number of cases increasing on a yearly basis (Fig. 24.5). While infection with B. *burgdorferi* is a worldwide occurrence, this chapter discusses only the manifestations, diagnosis, and treatment of this illness in North America.

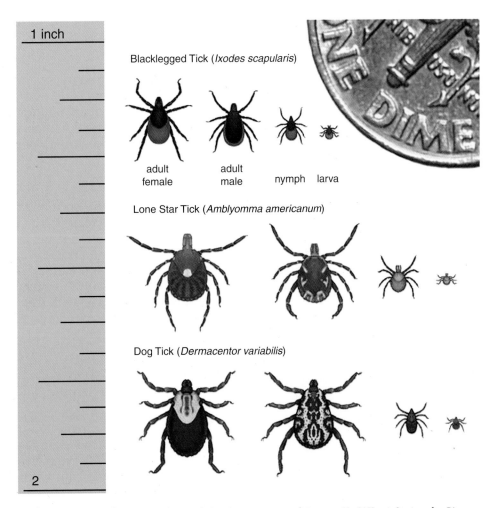

Figure 24.4 Dime ticks transmission and size. Image accessed January 11, 2011, at Centers for Disease Control and Prevention Web site http://www.cdc.gov/ncidod/dvbid/lyme/ld_transmission.htm.

SECTION 5 Infectious Arthritis

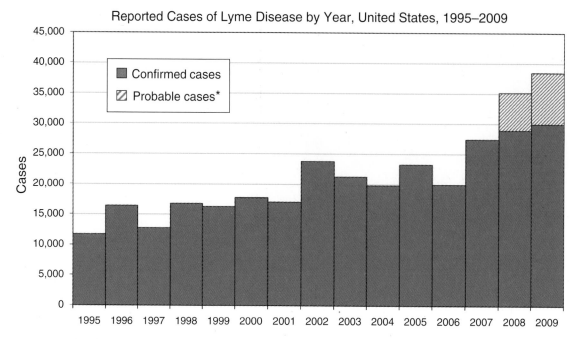

Reported Cases of Lyme Disease by Year, United States, 1995–2009

*National Surveillance case definition revised in 2008 to include probable cases; details at http://www.cdc.gov/ncphi/disss/nndss/casedef/lyme_disease_2008.htm

Figure 24.5 Lyme disease incidence by year. Courtesy of James Gathany. Centers for Disease Control and Prevention, available at http://www.cdc.gov/ncidod/dvbid/lyme/ld_UpClimbLymeDis.htm. Accessed January 21, 2011.

Clinical Presentation

The clinical presentation of Lyme disease is generally divided into three stages: early localized, early disseminated, and late-stage disease. Two additional stages have also been described, but are not universally accepted as part of the natural history of the disease. An understanding of these stages is critical for effective diagnosis and treatment of Lyme disease.

EARLY LOCALIZED DISEASE

Early localized Lyme disease occurs within days to up to 1 month of initial tick bite and is characterized by a skin rash and constitutional symptoms including malaise, fatigue, headache, mild stiff neck, myalgias, and arthralgias. Examination can reveal regional lymphadenopathy. Erythema migrans (EM) occurs in only 80% of patients diagnosed, and only 25% of patients with this rash ever recall a tick bite. Furthermore, not all patients present with the classically described skin rash. The classical rash has an expanding and slightly raised erythematous border with an area of central clearing and is frequently referred to as a "target lesion" (Fig. 24.6).

EARLY DISSEMINATED DISEASE

Early disseminated disease typically occurs within a few weeks to months after tick bite, and can present in the absence of a clear history of early localized disease. In addition to constitutional symptoms similar to those described in early Lyme disease, patients can present with musculoskeletal, neurologic, and cardiac symptoms. Approximately 60% of patients report migratory arthralgias; 15% experience neurologic symptoms, which can range from meningitis (lymphocytic), encephalitis, cranial neuropathy (facial nerve), peripheral neuropathy, myelitis,

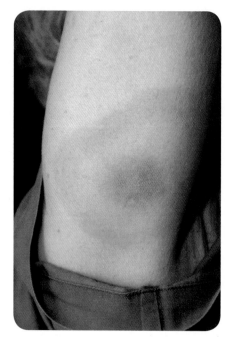

Figure 24.6 Target lesion. Courtesy of James Gathany. Centers for Disease Control and Prevention, available at http://www. cdc.gov/ncidod/dvbid/lyme/ld_LymeDiseaseRashPhotos.htm. Accessed January 21, 2011.

and cerebellar ataxia. Up to 8% of patients develop cardiac abnormalities. Cardiac abnormalities frequently present with symptoms of light-headedness, palpitations, and syncope. Heart block is the most frequent abnormality and can occur in up to 8% of patients. Heart block can range from first degree to complete heart block. Myocarditis has also been reported but is rare.

LATE-STAGE DISEASE

Late-stage disease occurs months to years following tick bite. Musculoskeletal symptoms are the most common finding in late-stage disease, with slightly more than half of patients developing intermittent mono- or oligoarticular arthritis. Approximately 10% of patients develop persistent monoarthritis of the knee. Even with appropriate treatment, a small number of late-stage patients persist with objective finding such as mono- or oligoarthritis. Persistence of these findings is not an indication to extend antibiotic therapy. Currently there is no conclusive evidence to suggest that such findings are due to ongoing active infection unless there is reason to suspect treatment noncompliance. One potential explanation for ongoing joint manifestations following appropriate antibiotic therapy is the development of a secondary autoimmune response in the joint. Posttreatment joint symptoms typically subside within months to a few years and do not necessarily require additional treatment. Ongoing symptomatic joint pain can be treated with anti-inflammatory medications.

Late-stage patients can also present with chronic low-grade encephalopathy, encephalomyelitis, and/or peripheral neuropathy. Peripheral neuropathy typically presents with paresthesias in the setting of unremarkable sensory and motor examinations. These symptoms are similar to those of early disseminated disease, and differentiating between early disseminated and late-stage disease can be difficult unless there is a clear history of tick bite or early stage symptoms. Encephalopathy and encephalomyelitis can present years after infection and can be subtle and difficult to diagnose.

In addition to the three classical phases of Lyme disease, clinicians should be aware of two additional, but controversial, stages called "post–Lyme disease syndrome" and "chronic Lyme disease" (1).

Chronic Lyme disease describes a condition some physicians and patients believe to be persistent B. burgdorferi infection. Frequently, these patients have no reproducible or convincing scientific evidence linking symptoms to B. burgdorferi infection.

Chronic Lyme disease can be approached as having four categories. In category one, patients present with nonspecific symptoms with no objective clinical or laboratory evidence of infection.

In category two, patients present with a history of potential Lyme disease, by have evidence of illness other than Lyme disease.

Category three patients have antibodies against B. burgdorferi, but have no objective clinical findings.

Finally, category four patients have symptoms of what has been termed "post-Lyme disease syndrome".

Post–Lyme disease syndrome is characterized by subjective symptoms, including fatigue, malaise, headache, and cognitive dysfunction. The Infectious Disease Society of America (IDSA) has proposed the following criteria for this syndrome (2):

- Symptoms must occur within 6 months of the diagnosis of Lyme disease and must persist for 6 months after recommended treatment.
- Prior diagnosis of Lyme disease with resolution of objective symptoms following appropriate antibiotic therapy.
- Exclusion of other comorbid disease states including fibromyalgia, abnormal thyroid function, long-standing history of unexplained neurologic or musculoskeletal symptoms clearly preceding the diagnosis of Lyme disease, sleep

CLINICAL POINTS

- Lyme disease is the most common tick-borne illness in the United States.

- Cases are most commonly seen in children younger than 15 years and in middle-aged adults.

- Effective treatment requires an understanding of the three stages of Lyme disease and an understanding that not all patients report progressing through each of these stages.

- Persistent symptoms following appropriate treatment of Lyme disease should prompt reinvestigation for other potential comorbid disease states.

SECTION 5 Infectious Arthritis

apnea, established autoimmune disease, liver disease, psychiatric illness, or documented history of drug or alcohol abuse.

The care of patients presenting with possible chronic Lyme disease or post-Lyme disease syndrome is challenging. The primary care clinician should consider referring such patients to a recognized specialist for second opinion before initiating treatment.

UNIQUE SITUATIONS

Reinfection

Reinfection with B. burgdorferi has been reported in patients following effective treatment. Patients who receive antibiotics for early localized or early disseminated Lyme disease are at greater risk for reinfection than patients who are treated for late-stage Lyme disease. In late-stage disease, host antibody response to B. burgdorferi is robust and usually provides protection against reinfection. Antibody production in early and early disseminated stages of disease is less robust and unlikely to provide the same level of immunity to reexposure (3).

Pregnancy

Current evidence does not support the occurrence of congenital Lyme disease. With adequate treatment, future parents should be reassured that there is not significant risk of transmission to the fetus and no increased risk of adverse outcomes or fetal demise. There is also no evidence that Lyme disease can be transmitted through breast-feeding. In pregnancy, use of tetracycline and doxycycline are contraindicated (4).

Coinfection

In addition to B. burgdorferi, the black-legged tick or deer tick can also transmit the parasites Theileria microti and Anaplasma phagocytophilum. These parasites cause babesiosis and human granulocytic anaplasmosis (HGA), respectively, and should be suspected in the setting of incomplete or atypical response to appropriate antibiotic treatment for Lyme disease. Up to 40% of early Lyme disease cases can be coinfected with T. microti (babesiosis) and 12% with A. phagocytophilum (HGA).

The finding of a hemolytic anemia suggests the possibility of babesiosis coinfection.

The findings of thrombocytopenia, leucopenia, and elevated serum transaminase levels should prompt an evaluation for HGA. Coinfection has also been reported with Bartonella, Ehrlichia, and Rickettsia (5).

Physical Examination

Physical examination of potential patients with Lyme disease is required to confirm the diagnosis, identify the stage of the disease, and prescribe appropriate treatment. Given the overlap of physical findings across multiple disease stages, the following discussion of physical findings is presented by organ system.

SKIN

Occasionally, patients present for examination with a tick firmly attached to the skin. If engorged, the tick is feeding and the likelihood of disease transmission increases. Unengorged (flat) and unattached ticks are unlikely to transmit disease. The likelihood of disease transmission can be estimated on the basis of the duration of feeding. Given the mechanism of spirochete transmission, feeding periods of less than 48 to 72 hours reduce the likelihood of disease transmission.

In early localized and early disseminated disease, the finding of an EM rash can provide an important clue to the diagnosis of this disease. Erythema migrans develops days to weeks after the initial tick bite, and is typically located in the axilla, inguinal region, popliteal fossa, or belt line. At the time of the tick bite,

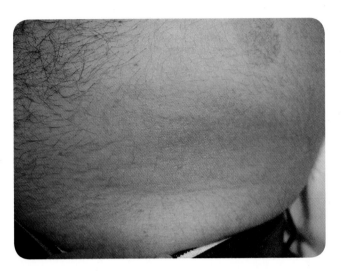

Figure 24.7 Solid erythema migrans skin rash. Courtesy of Alison Young, MD. Centers for Disease Control and Prevention, available at http://dermatlas. med.jhmi.edu/derm/indexdisplay.cfm?ImageID=-323138275. Accessed January 21, 2011.

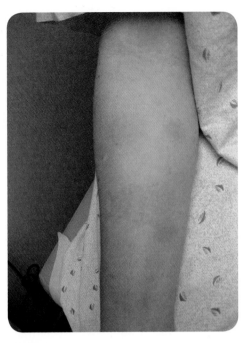

Figure 24.8 Multiple erythema migrans skin lesions indicating early disseminated disease. Courtesy of Yehia Mishriki.

the spirochete is inoculated into the skin. After a period of time ranging from 3 to 30 days, the spirochete begins to migrate outwards from the inoculation site causing the rash. The rash is minimally painful, but is frequently hot to touch. It expands slowly over days to weeks and is ultimately characterized by a region of central clearing. A fully mature rash has a characteristic appearance described as a "target lesion" (Fig. 24.6). Early lesions can be atypical and appear uniformly red (Fig. 24.7). The average time from discovery of a rash to medical evaluation has been demonstrated to be about 3 days (6). Presenting rashes in these patients were uniformly red in almost 60% of cases, with only 9% of rashes demonstrating central clearing. Clinicians should therefore be willing to diagnose EM even when the classic target lesion is absent. Clinicians should also remember that only 80% of patients develop ECM following a tick bite.

When multiple ECM (EM?) lesions are identified (Fig. 24.8), the disease has progressed from early localized to early disseminated disease. This finding does not represent multiple tick-bite exposures.

Patients presenting for evaluation immediately following tick removal can also demonstrate a nonspecific local irritation at the bite site. These patients should be reassured that this local irritation is not EM and does not require specific treatment for Lyme disease.

CARDIAC

Cardiac symptoms are typically seen in early disseminated (stage 2) disease. On physical examination, cardiac arrhythmias can indicate the presence of heart block, which can range from first-degree atrioventricular (AV) block to complete heart block. In addition, carditis can occur and present with findings of ventricular ectopy or congestive heart failure.

NEUROLOGIC

Neurologic abnormalities develop in both early disseminated (stage 2) and late-stage (stage 3) Lyme disease. Abnormal neurologic findings include peripheral neuropathy, cranial neuropathy, meningitis, and radiculoneuritis.

Peripheral neuropathies without objective sensory or motor abnormalities occur in both early disseminated and late-stage disease. Cranial neuropathies develop in up to 10% to 20% of early disseminated presentations and frequently include either unilateral or bilateral facial nerve palsies. When facial nerve palsy presents with headache and/or signs of ménage irritability (nuchal rigidity), evaluation for possible meningitis is warranted. Lymphocytic meningitis presenting with typical signs of meningeal irritation can also occur without cranial nerve palsy during early disseminated disease. Radiculoneuritis typically presents with acute onset of severe pain or motor weakness. Even without treatment, these symptoms typically resolve within months of onset.

Chronic encephalopathy and encephalomyelitis can also present with memory change and fatigue, and may present years after the onset of disease. These findings do not typically remit spontaneously and require antibiotic treatment for treatment.

MUSCULOSKELETAL

Intermittent, migratory arthralgia syndromes are frequently seen in the first two stages of Lyme disease. On examination, painful joints can be identified in the absence of erythema, swelling, or warmth.

Weeks to years after initial infection (stage 3), patients can present with oligo- or monarticular arthritis. Up to 60% of patients with late-stage disease report an asymmetric relatively painless arthritis. While multiple large joint can be involved, the most typical site of involvement is the knee. While relatively painless, knee arthritis can be associated with joint effusions and Baker's cysts (6).

Studies

The diagnosis of Lyme disease requires knowledge of the incidence of the disease, the patient's clinical presentation, and when appropriate, serologic confirmation of immune response to the spirochete. Serologic testing is not recommended as a screening test for disease in the setting of possible tick-bite exposure in the absence of supporting clinical presentation and is useful for confirmation of diagnosis in only certain instances. Guidelines for the assessment and treatment of suspected Lyme disease have been issued by the IDSA (7).

NONSPECIFIC EVALUATION

Evaluation of patients presenting with signs of meningitis or arthritis frequently require further evaluation. While joint and spinal fluid analysis may not confirm the diagnosis of Lyme disease, evaluation of these fluids can serve the important purpose of excluding other causes of joint or meningeal irritation.

The meningitis of Lyme disease is typically a lymphocytic meningitis characterized by spinal fluid cell counts ranging from occasional to a few hundred lymphocytes. Mild spinal fluid protein elevations can also occur, but glucose levels are usually normal. Spinal fluid analysis for Lyme antibodies can be performed, but interpretation of test results can be challenging given the lack of assay standardization. Because neurologic symptoms develop in the early disseminated stage of disease, the absence of serum antibodies makes the diagnosis of Lyme disease highly unlikely and should call into question attributing neurologic findings to *B. burgdorferi* infection.

Joint fluid can also be analyzed when joint effusions are identified on physical examination. Knee effusions can range from minimally to highly inflammatory effusions with synovial fluid white blood cell counts of predominantly neutrophils ranging from 500 to 100,000 cells. Synovial fluid can also be analyzed of *B. burgdorferi* DNA using polymerase chain reaction (PCR) testing. This

---

NOT TO BE MISSED

- Coinfection with other tick-borne illness. Incomplete or atypical response to standard antibiotic therapy or abnormalities on peripheral blood analysis should raise the possibility of either babesiosis or HGA coinfection.

- Patients presenting with multiple ECM lesions do not have multiple initial exposures. Multiple ECM lesions indicate early disseminated disease.

- The diagnosis of Lyme disease does not require a positive Lyme serology in early disease presentations.

test is positive in most untreated patients and becomes negative with treatment. However, while synovial fluid PCR testing may be commercially available, it has not been standardized or validated for routine clinical use (8).

Skin biopsy of EM lesions can demonstrate the presence of B. burgdorferi, but is generally not required for diagnosis in patients presenting with lesions consistent with early or more classical EM presentations.

SEROLOGIC EVALUATION

Serologic studies should be ordered when the history and physical examination strongly suggest Lyme disease. Most laboratories begin with the sensitive enzyme-linked immunosorbent assay (ELISA). If this is positive, a reflex Western blot should be performed as other infections and conditions may cause a positive ELISA. The criteria for a positive Western blot test include two of the following IgM bands early in the disease: 24, 39, 41, or five of the following IgG bands later in the disease: 18, 23, 28, 30, 39, 41, 45, 58, 66, 93 (9). Patients with early localized disease presenting with EM are often seronegative and should be treated immediately on the basis of clinical grounds. This two-step approach has been endorsed by the CDC and should guide the serologic evaluation of potential cases of Lyme disease. While additional testing is offered for the diagnosis of Lyme disease, the accuracy of these tests has not been established. Such testing includes urine antigen testing, immunofluorescent staining for cell-wall–deficient forms of B. burgdorferi, and lymphocyte transformation testing.

Antibodies to Lyme disease may persist even after appropriate treatment; therefore, repeated courses of antibiotics are not necessary if the clinical symptoms have resolved. Patients who have received the vaccine (LYMErix) may exhibit positive ELISA and Western blot bands. The Lyme vaccine is no longer available.

Treatment

The treatment of Lyme disease depends on age of the patient as well as clinical stage of the disease at the time of presentation. Doxycycline is not recommended in children younger than 8 years or patients who are pregnant or lactating. Relapse after treatment is possible; however, only patients with objective clinical signs of disease should be considered for a second course of antibiotics.

The following reflect the clinical practice guidelines from the IDSA (7).

Prophylaxis with doxycycline 200 mg one-time dose is indicated if the tick is identified as a deer tick, the length of exposure (feeding) was at least 36 hours, prophylaxis is begun within 72 hours of tick removal, local rate of infection of ticks with B. burgdorferi is at least 20%, and the patient is able to take doxycycline. While prophylaxis can be given to children 8 years and older (doxycycline 4 mg/kg up to a maximum dose of 200 mg), this recommendation has not been formally evaluated for efficacy or safety. When doxycycline cannot be prescribed, the IDSA does not recommend prophylaxis.

EARLY LOCALIZED DISEASE (ERYTHEMA MIGRANS)

Doxycycline 100 mg PO BID for 10 to 21 days
Amoxicillin 500 mg PO TID for 14 to 21 days

Early Disseminated Disease

Isolated facial nerve palsy is treated the same as early localized; however, it may require 14 to 28 days of therapy.
Meningitis or encephalitis is treated with ceftriaxone 2 g intravenously (IV) daily for 28 days.

WHEN TO REFER ?

- Patients who request ongoing IV antibiotic therapy for nonspecific symptoms including chronic fatigue or fibromyalgia.

- Patients who believe they have post–Lyme disease syndrome or chronic Lyme disease.

- Persistent mono- or oligoarticular arthritis after appropriate antibiotic therapy that has not responded to recommended anti-inflammatory treatment.

Carditis with first-, second-, or third-degree AV block is treated with ceftriaxone 2 g IV daily for 21 days. Oral regimens may be considered for first-degree AV block with PR interval <300 ms.

Late-stage Disease

Lyme arthritis is treated with the same oral regimens as earlier disease; however, therapy should be continued for 28 days. If synovial inflammation persists, treatment with nonsteroidal anti-inflammatory drugs (NSAIDs) or hydroxychloroquine 200 mg BID should be considered (10).

A Jarisch–Herxheimer reaction has been observed in up to 10% of patients during the first 24 hours of treatment (11). The reaction can include fever, rash with or without pruritus, nonspecific gastrointestinal complaints, myalgias, and arthralgias.

Clinical Course

Treated Lyme disease should not result in chronic symptoms. Patients complaining of diffuse body pain without objective findings of inflammation or infection should be evaluated for fibromyalgia. Coexisting migraine headaches, endometriosis, irritable bowel syndrome, interstitial cystitis, and underlying psychiatric disease should also prompt the physician to consider fibromyalgia or other possible diagnosis.

Lyme disease can present a diagnostic and therapeutic challenge unless careful attention is given to completing an accurate history and thorough physical examination. With appropriate data collection, clinicians can utilize evidence-based approaches to treatment and prevention that will ensure safe and effective care for all patients diagnosed with this illness.

ICD9

088.81 **Lyme**

References

1. Feder H, Johnson BJ, O'Connell S, et al. Current concepts: A critical appraisal of "chronic Lyme disease." N Engl J Med 2007;357:1422.
2. Centers for Disease Control and Prevention. Case definitions for infectious conditions under public health surveillance. MMWR Morb Mortal Recomm Rep 1997;46(RR-10):1.
3. Nadelman RB, Wormser GP. Reinfection in patients with Lyme disease, Clin Infect Dis 2007;45:1032.
4. Silver HM. Lyme disease during pregnancy. Infect Dis Clin North Am 1997;11:93.
5. Wormser GP. Clinical practice. Early Lyme disease. N Eng J Med 2006;354(26):2794–801.
6. Smith RP, Schoen RT, Rahn DW, et al. Clinical characteristics and treatment outcome of early Lyme disease in patients with microbiologically confirmed erythema migrans. Ann Intern Med 2002;136:421.
7. Wormser GP, Dattwyler RJ, Shapiro ED, et al. The clinical assessment, treatment, and prevention of Lyme disease, human granulocytic anaplasmosis, and babesiosis: Clinical Practice Guidelines by the Infectious Disease Society of America. Clin Infect Dis 2006;43:1089.
8. Nocton JJ, Dressler F, Rutledge BJ, et al. Detection of Borrelia burgdorferi DNA by polymerase chain reaction in synovial fluid from patients with Lyme arthritis. N Engl J Med 1994;330(4):229–234.
9. Dressler F, Whalen JA, Reinhardt BN, et al. Western blotting in the serodiagnosis of Lyme disease. J Infect Dis 1993;167(2):392–400.
10. Steere AC, Angelis SM. Therapy for Lyme arthritis: Strategies for the treatment of antibiotic-refractory arthritis. Arthritis Rheum 2006;54(10):3079–3086.
11. Steere AC, Hutchinson GJ, Rahn DW, et al. Treatment of the early manifestations of Lyme disease. Ann Intern Med 1983;99:22–26.

CHAPTER 25 Viral Arthritis

Katherine Holman and Martin Rodriguez

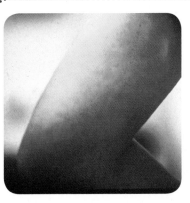

A 21-year-old Caucasian woman with no significant past medical history presents with a 3-day history of joint pain and swelling. She states that the symptoms started with fever up to 102°F and diffuse myalgias. The joint pain began abruptly in her knees and spread to involve multiple joints over the next few days. She notes that her pain and stiffness are worse in the mornings. Her social history is significant for working at an establishment that held parties for children. Physical examination is notable for a temperature of 102.7°F, and tenderness to palpation with limited range of motion over knees, wrists, elbows, and proximal interphalangeal (PIP) joints symmetrically. Rash is noted as shown in Figure 25.1. Laboratory data were significant for white blood cell (WBC) 11.3 with a normal differential, erythrocyte sedimentation rate (ESR) 25 mm/hour, and C-reactive protein (CRP) 12.2 mg/L; human immunodeficiency virus (HIV) and hepatitis B and C serologies were negative. Antinuclear antibodies (ANA), anticyclic citrullinated peptide antibodies (anti-CCP), and rheumatoid factor (RF) were negative. Parvovirus IgM and IgG were positive at 3.4 and 5.3 respectively.

Introduction

Viruses affecting humans are ubiquitous, and their clinical syndromes are diverse. Their ability to either cause an acute illness with full recovery or establish a latent course—progressing to a relapsing syndrome or chronic progressive illness—can make their diagnoses difficult (1). Among the wide manifestations of viral illnesses, arthritis is an uncommon symptom; however, in the case of specific viruses, arthritis can be one of the most common symptoms (i.e., alphaviruses). Therefore, various viral illnesses should be considered in the differential diagnosis of a patient presenting with undifferentiated arthritis.

Parvovirus B19

CLINICAL PRESENTATION

Parvovirus B19 was identified in human serum in the mid-1970s (2). However, its disease manifestations have been recognized since the 1800s, with the initial description of "fifth disease" or erythema infectiosum in children (3). The classic forms of parvovirus B19 infection occur at either the viremic stage (transient aplastic crisis and pure red cell aplasia) or the postviremic stage (erythema infectiosum and arthropathy; 2). While children commonly present with the classic "slapped cheek" and reticular rash of erythema infectiosum, rash is usually absent or subtle in adults (1). Conversely, arthralgias or arthritis is far more common in adults with acute infections (4). The classic arthritis begins precipitously in a few joints, spreads rapidly in 24 to 48 hours, and is characterized by severe, prolonged morning stiffness.

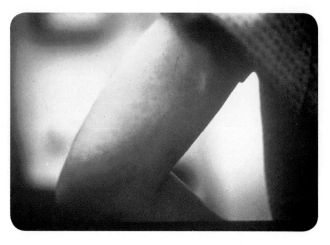

Figure 25.1 Parvovirus infection. Photograph demonstrates the lacelike reticulated rash on the arm of a youngster with fifth disease. From Sweet RL, Gibbs RS. *Atlas of Infectious Diseases of the Female Genital Tract.* Philadelphia: Lippincott Williams & Wilkins; 2005.

EXAMINATION

Patients tend to present with a low temperature. A lacy rash, most commonly present in the extremities, can be found. Tender, swollen joints are commonly seen, but no deformities are present. Both small- and medium-size joints are predominantly affected usually in a symmetrical fashion (1). Axial joints are spared.

DIAGNOSIS

Viremia is evident by 5 to 6 days postexposure, with a peak at 8 to 9 days. The virus clears quickly, and IgM is present by days 10 to 12 and may persist for 2 to 3 months (2). Serum of infected patients can show transient autoantibodies, including, but not limited to, ANA, RF, and anti-DNAs (4). Diagnosis therefore relies on serum IgM antibodies to parvovirus B19, with or without IgG and demonstrable parvovirus DNA.

TREATMENT

Treatment is supportive, with nonsteroidal anti-inflammatory drugs (NSAIDs) as needed for pain and inflammation. Intravenous immunoglobulin has been used in cases of pure red cell aplasia in immunocompromised patients, but it is not recommended in arthritis (4).

CLINICAL COURSE

Acute arthritis resolves within weeks although, uncommonly, cases have persisted for months. Whether parvovirus B19 infection causes a chronic arthritis remains controversial (4), as does its possible association with RA and other inflammatory arthropathies. Some studies have found ongoing B19 DNA in serum, bone marrow, and synovium of patients with chronic arthritis and/or RA, but they have been found in healthy controls as well, making a determination of the cause difficult (1, 2, 4–6).

Hepatitis C

CLINICAL PRESENTATION

Hepatitis C (HCV) is a single-stranded RNA *Flavivirus*. It is estimated that greater than 170 million people worldwide are infected with the virus (7). Parenteral infection occurs most commonly, often in the setting of intravenous drug use. Transmission in health care settings has become rare in developed countries since routine testing of blood products began in the early 1990s; however, occasional cases continue to be reported (7). Following acute infection with HCV, 74% to 86% of patients develop persistent viremia and 15% to 20% of these patients with chronic infection develop cirrhosis (7), which can progress to hepatocellular carcinoma and end-stage liver disease.

Extrahepatic manifestations of HCV infection are varied, with joint pain being a common one. Studies estimate that 9% to 29% of all patients with HCV complain of arthralgias, while 2% to 4% of patients have arthritis (1, 8). True inflammatory arthritis appears to manifest in four distinct ways: (1) relating directly to HCV infection (2) as a sign of mixed cryoglobulinemia (3) coexisting, but separate rheumatic disease (4) occurring rarely secondary to therapy for HCV (4). As therapy-related arthritis is exceedingly rare, further discussion of 1 to 3 follows.

CLINICAL POINTS

- There is no "classic" presentation that is typical of virally associated arthritis.

- Many virally associated arthritides can be mistaken for early rheumatoid arthritis (RA).

- Arthritis may occur before the onset of a typical clinical viral syndrome (i.e., HBV, HIV).

PATIENT ASSESSMENT

- Thorough history, including immunizations, exposures, occupation, travel, sexual, and social.

- Close examination for signs of other rheumatologic conditions.

- Specific laboratories on the basis of risk assessment above.

HCV-RELATED ARTHRITIS

Patients can develop an inflammatory arthritis directly related to HCV, which occurs in fewer than 5% of patients (4). Physical examination reveals evidence of synovitis of small joints in a symmetrical pattern.

Diagnosis

Demonstration of HCV antibody or RNA in serum and ruling out other causes of both HCV-related, such as mixed cryoglobulinemia, and nonrelated inflammatory arthritis.

Treatment/Clinical Course

Most commonly used treatments are analgesics and low-dose corticosteroids. Disease-modifying antirheumatic drugs (DMARDs) and biologic agents, such as antitumor necrosis factor (anti-TNF), have also been used, albeit uncommonly (4). Studies of antiviral therapy show mixed results, with evidence of benefit and occasionally exacerbation of symptoms; however, most of these studies did not clearly define if these patients had cryoglobulinemia-related versus HCV-related arthritis (9).

MIXED CRYOGLOBULINEMIA

Essential mixed cryoglobulinemia is associated with HCV infection, and symptoms include purpura, glomerulonephritis, lymphadenopathy, skin ulcers, and peripheral neuropathy. Many patients complain of arthralgias; however, less than 10% develop frank arthritis (4). The classic triad is described as that of purpura, glomerulonephritis, and arthralgias. Physical examination seldom reveals evidence of synovitis or deformity; skin examination shows palpable purpura most frequently in the lower extremities.

Diagnosis

Diagnosis requires demonstration of the clinical syndrome in addition to serologic, including serum cryoglobulins, low C4 level, and positive RF (serologic), with histologic findings such as evidence of leukocytoclastic vasculitis (4). Notably, tests for HCV antibodies can be falsely negative in this condition, requiring tests directed toward HCV RNA for diagnosis (7).

Treatment/Clinical Course

Treatment generally involves antiviral therapy directed toward HCV, but corticosteroids, rituximab, cyclophosphamide, and plasmapheresis are sometimes required for the more severe cases (4).

COEXISTING INFLAMMATORY ARTHRITIS

Given the prevalence of chronic HCV, a number of these patients also have a coexisting rheumatic disease, including, but not limited to, rheumatoid arthritis (RA), systemic lupus erythematosus (SLE), and Sjogren syndrome (4).

Diagnosis

Clinical findings combined with overlapping laboratory findings—positive RF, cytopenias, ANA, low C4 level—make a firm diagnosis difficult. To address this, anti-CCP antibody, a fairly specific test for RA, has been evaluated in patients with HCV. In patients with RA, 76.6% had positive anti-CCP antibodies, but no HCV patients with or without joint involvement were positive. Notably, in 10 patients initially thought to have HCV-associated arthritis but who were ultimately found to have RA, 60% of their initial blood samples showed anti-CCP antibodies (10).

Treatment/Clinical Course

Inflammatory arthritis, such as RA, requires early immune-modifying approaches that can worsen the underlying liver dysfunction, making accurate diagnosis crucial. More data are needed regarding the use of immunomodulatory therapies in the setting of HCV-associated liver disease. Methotrexate is known to have hepatic complications associated with its use; anti-TNF agents are just beginning to be evaluated in these patients (6). Therapy requires a multidisciplinary approach.

Hepatitis B

CLINICAL PRESENTATION

Hepatitis B virus (HBV) is a small DNA virus of the family Hepadnaviridae. Transmission occurs most commonly in three ways: perinatally, sexually, or parenterally (11). Persistence of viral infection is largely determined by age at infection. Perinatal infection often results in chronic HBV infection, whereas clearance of HBV is more common when contracted in adulthood, with only 5% to 10% of people infected developing chronic HBV (1). Arthritis occurs in two forms. The first form appears during the presymptomatic phase of acute infection, mostly a few days and unusually weeks prior to the onset of jaundice or evidence of hepatitis. Chronic arthritis, the second form, occurs in the setting of HBV-associated polyarteritis nodosa (PAN; 1).

EXAMINATION

Acute HBV-associated arthritis presents as a symmetric polyarthritis involving the PIP joints, knees, and ankles (1, 4), which is similar to RA; however, distinguishing features are an abrupt onset, accompanied by a concomitant rash. In HBV-associated PAN, arthralgias are commonly reported. Frank arthritis affects the mid-size joints (wrist, ankles, and knees) and is much less common.

DIAGNOSIS

In the acute form, the diagnosis of arthritis is made retrospectively after the appearance of jaundice and/or transaminitis. Hepatitis B surface antigen (HBsAg) is detectable in serum approximately 4 to 10 weeks after infection, accompanied by a significant viremia, and hence is helpful to diagnose only the chronic form of this disease. Antibodies to core antigen (anti-Hbc) develop shortly after (12; Fig. 25.2). Similar to HCV, erosive arthritis and anti-CCP antibodies are not usually seen and should prompt work-up for additional causes (4, 6).

TREATMENT/CLINICAL COURSE

Presymptomatic arthritis is self-limited, requires no specific therapy, and usually resolves around the time that jaundice develops. Treatment for arthritis related to HBV-associated PAN involves immunomodulatory plus antiviral agents, with initial remission indicative of good overall prognosis (4).

Alphaviruses

EPIDEMIOLOGY AND CLINICAL PRESENTATION

The alphaviruses, a genus of the family Togaviridae, are arthropod borne and divided into "Old World" and "New World" species. The former cause a syndrome of fever, rash, and arthralgias, whereas their "New World" counterparts commonly cause encephalitis (13). The arthritis-inducing alphaviruses have a wide geographic distribution and can cause vast outbreaks. O'Nyong-nyong and Igbo-Ora occur mainly in Africa, Barmah Forest and Ross River mainly in

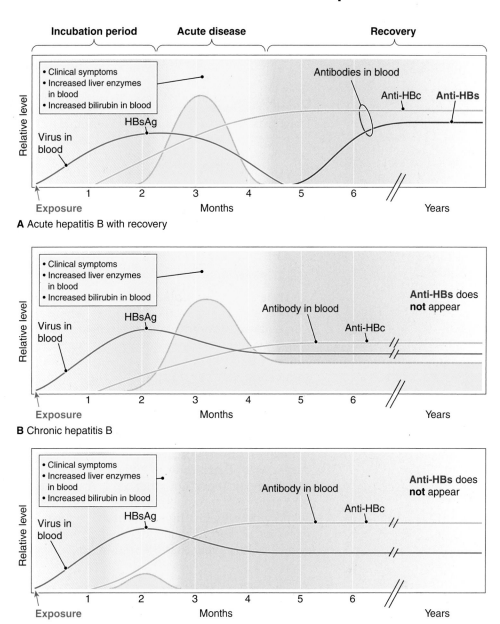

Figure 25.2 Hepatitis B clinical phases and blood markers of infection. **A:** Acute infection is characterized by rapid appearance of the virus in blood before symptoms appear, disappearance of the virus from blood, and appearance in blood of antibodies to hepatitis B surface antigen (HBsAg). **B:** Chronic hepatitis is signaled by continuing jaundice or clinical symptoms, or the continued presence of virus in blood (as is indicated by the detection in blood of HBsAg). **C:** The carrier state is indicated by disappearance of clinical symptoms and the persistence of virus in blood (as is indicated by the detection in blood of HBsAg).

Australia, and Mayaro in South America, whereas chikungunya and Sindbis have wider geographic range (14). Symptoms from these viruses occur abruptly, with fever, malaise, myalgias, retro-orbital pain, and headache occurring early. Arthralgias, often incapacitating, are nearly ubiquitous in those who present with symptomatic infection.

EXAMINATION

The arthropathy typically affects multiple small joints, especially those previously injured; patients often try to limit movement (13). Rash frequently occurs, and in certain infections, notably chikungunya, o'nyong-nyong, and Mayaro, petechiae, purpura, as well as bleeding from gastrointestinal tract, gums, and nasopharynx can occur (14).

DIAGNOSIS

Diagnosis of a specific alphavirus remains a challenge, as they clinically resemble each other and many other viral illnesses. In endemic areas, differentiating between the major alternate diagnoses is key: dengue for chikungunya or Mayaro; malaria for o'nyong-nyong (15). The Centers for Disease Control and Prevention (CDC) has testing capability for chikungunya, o'nyong-nyong, Ross River, Barmah Forest, and limited testing for Sindbis (16). Detailed travel history and knowledge of recent and ongoing outbreaks are essential in the evaluation of returning travelers.

TREATMENT

Treatment for the alphaviruses is largely supportive, with NSAIDs for pain. Aspirin should be avoided in cases where dengue or other hemorrhagic illnesses are in the differential as this can exacerbate bleeding manifestations (15). Prevention remains the mainstay of therapy. The CDC specifically recommends that a person diagnosed with chikungunya fever should limit exposure to mosquitoes to avoid spread of the infection (17).

CLINICAL COURSE

As study of the alphaviruses is limited in most cases, clinical course can only be estimated. Chikungunya and Ross River are the most studied of these alphaviruses. With regard to Ross River, symptoms generally resolve within 6 months (15). However, reports of other alphaviruses have described chronic and/or recurrent arthritis (14). Reports from the recent chikungunya outbreaks have described joint symptoms lasting frequently for longer than 6 months (18) and in some cases for 18 months following severe clinical infection (19). As more data become available, it is likely that the natural progression will be further elucidated.

Rubella and Rubella Vaccine

RUBELLA

Epidemiology and Clinical Presentation

Rubella, another member of the family Togaviridae, is an RNA virus spread by airborne droplets. While the clinical manifestations of the disease are generally mild in children—usually fever, rash, and coryza (1)—exposure to rubella during pregnancy, particularly during the first trimester, can have devastating consequences for the fetus. Thus, a major focus has been vaccination, resulting in a marked decrease in its incidence.

In adults, symptoms are both more common and severe, including fever, malaise, coryza, and posterior cervical lymphadenopathy, which present approximately 1 week postexposure (1). Rash, which may be subtle, generally occurs 2 to 3 weeks after exposure (1), with arthralgias or frank arthritis usually developing within 1 week of the rash (20). Nearly one third of patients may experience joint symptoms (21). With increasing numbers of individuals refusing vaccines we may see a resurgence of this viral illness in the future.

Examination

Hands and knees are most frequently affected, usually symmetrically; however a migratory pattern can also occur (1). Frank arthritis occurs more commonly in adult women compared to men and children (21).

Diagnosis

Diagnosis rests on isolation of virus from throat culture or demonstration of serum antibodies to rubella. Presence of IgM to rubella indicates infection likely in the past 1 to 2 months; IgG can be used for diagnosis only if paired acute and convalescent sera are used (1).

Treatment

SUPPORTIVE AND SYMPTOMATIC

Clinical Course

Symptoms generally resolve within a few weeks; however, cases have been reported in which joint symptoms were persistent for months to years (1, 20).

RUBELLA VACCINE

While vaccination prevents rubella infection, it carries a risk of arthritis as well, with highest incidences in adult women. Generally, postvaccination arthritis occurs 10 to 28 days after rubella vaccination (22). Although it is postulated that the initial HPV77/DK12 strain carried the greatest risk of postimmunization arthritis, reports postvaccination with the presently used RA 27/3 have emerged (1, 23). The Institute of Medicine released a report reviewing the evidence and concluded, it "... is consistent with a causal relation between the RA 27/3 rubella vaccine strain and chronic arthritis in adult women, although the evidence is limited in scope" (23). Thus, despite widespread vaccination in the United States, both wild rubella and its vaccine should be considered in the differential certainly for acute, and possibly chronic, arthritis, particularly in adult women.

Human Immunodeficiency Virus

Joint complaints are described at all stages of HIV infection, even during acute infection, where arthralgias can be seen in 28% to 54% of cases (24). A painful articular syndrome was described early in the HIV epidemic, most commonly as severe pain involving the knees (less frequently, shoulders and elbows). Typically, it lasts 2 to 24 hours and resolves, but may require NSAIDs or opiates (24, 25). It is not commonly seen nowadays. Frank arthritis also occurs, either directly related to HIV or in the setting of a secondary inflammatory arthropathy. HIV-associated arthritis, defined as a disabling arthritis commonly affecting the knees and ankles, has a self-limited course. Definition of this disorder involves a nonerosive oligoarthritis, with negative studies for RF, ANA, and HLA-B27 (24–26).

Highly active antiretroviral therapy (HAART) has changed the spectrum of joint diseases in HIV. Human immunodeficiency virus–associated arthritis and psoriatic arthritis occur more commonly with advanced stages of disease; the severity of these articular manifestations decreases with effective antiretroviral therapy. Conversely, coexisting inflammatory disorders such as RA and SLE tend to improve with advancing stages of HIV disease (24, 27). This observation provided both an eloquent proof of the effectiveness of antiretroviral therapy and a clue toward the pathogenesis of these rheumatic conditions. While treatment of HIV-associated arthritides generally involves treating the HIV infection, most importantly, patients presenting with a similar arthritis have an indication for HIV testing. It is important to remember that the CDC recommends universal HIV testing in adults aged 13 to 64 in the United States at least once and more frequently in those at risk (28).

Others

Other viruses have been implicated in the setting of arthritis. Human T-cell lymphotrophic virus-1 (HTLV-1) can cause inflammatory arthropathies, mostly

SECTION 5 Infectious Arthritis

NOT TO BE MISSED

- Rash.
  - May indicate parvovirus, acute HIV, acute HBV, rubella, arbovirus.
- Joint deformity.
  - More likely to be nonviral.

WHEN TO REFER ?

- Arthritis needs specific treatment of causal virus for recovery (i.e., HIV, HCV, HBV).
- Inflammatory arthritis (i.e., RA) diagnosed in setting of HCV.

in endemic areas (4). Epstein–Barr virus and coxsackievirus have been implicated in a few cases of polyarthritis; however, a causal relationship remains difficult to prove (4, 21).

Conclusion

Although virally associated arthritis remains a rare etiology of the common complaint of arthritis, it is important for clinicians to be aware of the possibility. Diagnosing a viral etiology of arthritis can spare a patient an invasive workup, as well as prevent potentially harmful therapy (4). Diagnosing HIV, hepatitis, or an alphavirus has both individual and public health benefits. Given their ubiquity, viruses should always be included in the differential of a patient presenting with arthritis.

> *ICD9*
>
> *716.9* **Arthritis, arthritic** *(acute) (chronic) (subacute)*
> *079.99 [711.5] viral disease NEC*

References

1. Calabrese LH, Naides SJ. Viral arthritis. *Infect Dis Clin N Am* 2005;19:963–980.
2. Young NS, Brown KE. Parvovirus B19. *N Engl J Med* 2004;350:586–597.
3. Brown KE. Human parvoviruses, including parvovirus B19 and human bocavirus. In: Mandell GL, Bennett JE, Dolin R, eds. *Mandell, Douglas, and Bennett's: Principles and Practice of Infectious Diseases*. Vol. II. 7th ed. Philadelphia, PA: Elsevier; 2010:2087–2095.
4. Vassilopoulos D, Calabrese LH. Virally Associated Arthritis 2008: Clinical, epidemiologic, and pathophysiologic considerations. *Arthritis Res Ther* 2008;10:215.
5. Lundqvist A, Isa A, Tolfvenstam T. High frequency of parvovirus B19 DNA in bone marrow samples from rheumatic patients. *J Clin Virol* 2005;33:71–74.
6. Becker J, Winthrop KL. Update on rheumatic manifestations of infectious diseases. *Curr Opin Rheumatol* 2010;22:72–77.
7. Lauer GM, Walker BD. Hepatitis C virus infection. *N Engl J Med* 2001;345:41–52.
8. Vassilopoulos D, Calabrese LH. Rheumatic manifestations of hepatitis C infection. *Curr Rheumatol Rep* 2003;5:200–204.
9. Zuckerman E, Yeshurun D, Rosner I. Management of hepatitis C virus-related arthritis. *BioDrugs* 2001;15:573–584.
10. Bombardieri M, Alessandri C, Labbadia G, et al. Role of anti-cyclic citrullinated peptide antibodies in discriminating patients with rheumatoid arthritis from patients with chronic hepatitis C infection-associated polyarticular involvement. *Arthritis Res Ther* 2004;6:R137-R141.
11. Koziel MJ, Thio CL. Hepatitis B virus and hepatitis delta virus. In: Mandell GL, Bennett JE, Dolin R, eds. *Mandell, Douglas, and Bennett's: Principles and Practice of Infectious Diseases*. Vol II. 7th ed. Philadelphia, PA: Elsevier; 2010:2059–2086.
12. Ganem D, Prince AM. Hepatitis B virus infection—natural history and clinical consequences. *N Engl J Med* 2004;350:1118–1129.
13. Markoff L. Alphaviruses. In: Mandell GL, Bennett JE, Dolin R, eds. *Mandell, Douglas, and Bennett's: Principles and Practice of Infectious Diseases*. Vol II. 7th ed. Philadelphia, PA: Elsevier; 2010:2117–2125.
14. Toivanen A. Alphaviruses: An emerging cause of arthritis? *Curr Opin Rheumatol* 2008;20:486–490.
15. Suhrbier A, Linn ML. Clinical and pathologic aspects of arthritis due to Ross River virus and other alphaviruses. *Curr Opin Rheumatol* 2004;16:374–379.
16. Diagnostic Testing/CDC Chikungunya. Centers for Disease Control and Prevention Web site. http://www.cdc.gov/ncidod/dvbid/Chikungunya/CH_Diagnostic.html. Accessed October 29, 2010.
17. Fact Sheet/CDC Chikungunya. Centers for Disease Control and Prevention Web site. http://www.cdc.gov/ncidod/dvbid/Chikungunya/CH_FactSheet.html. Accessed October 5, 2010.
18. Taubitz W, Cramer JP, Kapaun A, et al. Chikungunya fever in travelers: Clinical presentation and course. *Clin Infect Dis* 2007;45:e1–4.
19. Borgherini G, Poubeau P, Jossaume A, et al. Persistant arthralgia associated with chikungunya virus: A study of 88 adult patients on reunion island. *Clin Infect Dis* 2008;47:469–475.
20. Tingle AJ, Allen M, Petty RE. Rubella-associated arthritis. I. Comparative study of joint manifestations associated with natural rubella infection and RA 27/3 rubella immunisation. *Ann Rheumatic Dis* 1986;45:110–114.
21. Ytterberg SR. Viral arthritis. *Curr Opin Rheumatol* 1999;11:275–280.
22. Geier DA, Geier MR. Rubella vaccine and arthritic adverse reactions: An analysis of the vaccine adverse events reporting system (VAERS) database from 1991 through 1998. *Clin Exp Rheumatol* 2001;19:724–726.
23. Howson CP, Katz M, Johnston RB, Jr. Chronic arthritis after rubella vaccination. *Clin Infect Dis* 1992;15:307–312.
24. Walker UA, Tyndall A, Daikeler T. Rheumatic conditions in human immunodeficiency virus infection. *Rheumatology* 2008;47:952–959.

25. Tehranzadeh J, Ter-Oganesyan RR, Steinbach LS. Musculoskeletal disorders associated with HIV infection and AIDS. Part II: Non-infectious musculoskeletal conditions. *Skeletal Radiol* 2004;33:311–320.

26. Allroggen A, Frese A, Rahmann A. HIV associated arthritis: Case report and review of the literature. *Eur J Med Res* 2005;10:305–308.

27. Nguyen BY, Reveille JD. Rheumatic manifestations associated with HIV in the highly active antiretroviral therapy era. *Curr Opin Rheumatol* 2009;21:404–410.

28. Centers for Disease Control and Prevention. Revised recommendations for HIV testing of adults, adolescents and pregnant women in health-care settings. *MMWR* 2006;55(No. RR-14):1–17. http://www.cdc.gov/mmwr/preview/mmwrhtml/rr5514a1.htm. Accessed October 27, 2010.

Special Diagnostic and Therapeutic Conditions

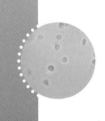

Chapter 26   **Use of the Laboratory in Diagnosing Rheumatic Disorders**

Terry Shaneyfelt and Gustavo R. Heudebert

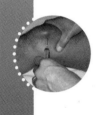

Chapter 27   **Techniques of Arthrocentesis**

Dennis W. Boulware

Chapter 28   **Monitoring of Patients on Antirheumatic Therapy**

W. Winn Chatham

26 Use of the Laboratory in Diagnosing Rheumatic Disorders

Terry Shaneyfelt and Gustavo R. Heudebert

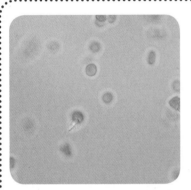

Patient 1: An 80-year-old retired carpenter presents for evaluation of diffuse joint pain. He reports gradual onset and progression of pain in the right first metacarpophalangeal (MCP) joint and bilateral proximal interphalangeal (PIP) and distal interphalangeal (DIP) joints over the past 5 years.

He also has pain in both knees. He has some stiffness in all the affected joints, which lasts approximately 15 to 30 minutes each morning. Pain is worse with activity. He denies any swelling, rashes, fevers, or other joint involvement. Physical examination of the hands reveals hard enlargement of the second through fourth DIP and PIP joints, and painful range of motion of the right first MCP joint. No synovitis is detected. Knee examination reveals crepitance with preserved range of motion and no joint effusion.

Patient 2: A 25-year-old female presents for evaluation of fatigue, myalgias, and intermittent hand pain. She reports that the pain tends to "move around" both the hands and is moderate in severity and can resolve within 24 hours. On further questioning, she reports an erythematous rash on her cheeks after working out in the sun a few weeks earlier, but it resolved and has not recurred. She also reports a short-lived episode of pleuritic chest pain a month earlier. Physical examination reveals mild pain with range of motion in several PIP joints and her left wrist. No effusions or deformities are seen. No pleural or cardiac rubs are heard on auscultation and no rashes are noted on skin examination.

As clinicians, we combine clinical skills with information from diagnostic tests to establish accurate diagnoses so that we may initiate appropriate treatment for our patients. In this chapter, we focus on probabilistic diagnostic reasoning in which pretest probability is informed by diagnostic testing resulting in posttest probabilities. We do not focus on the commonly used diagnostic method of pattern recognition. We recognize that both diagnostic methods are appropriate and complementary. Probabilistic diagnostic reasoning is useful especially for more challenging or less familiar clinical situations where pattern recognition fails.

The generation of a differential diagnosis relies on us, having both general medical knowledge and disease prevalence knowledge. Key features derived from the history, in conjunction with physical examination findings, serve to either increase or decrease the likelihood of each diagnosis under consideration in a process of hypothesis testing. In establishing hypotheses, it is important that we accurately assess the *pretest probability* of the diagnoses we are considering so that subsequent testing can help us to rule in or rule out those possibilities. Pretest probability is the chance or probability that the patient under consideration has the target disorder before any testing is carried

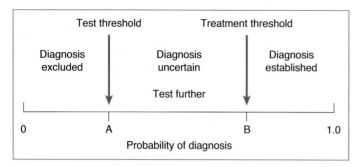

	Disease Present	**Disease Absent**
Test Positive	*True Positive* (a)	False Positive (b)
Test Negative	False Negative (c)	*True Negative* (d)

Figure 26.1 Test and treatment thresholds.

out. It can be determined in several ways. Validated clinical prediction rules are decision aids that combine elements of history, physical examination, and basic diagnostic or laboratory testing to accurately estimate pretest probability. Disease probability studies, in which representative samples of patients with certain symptoms (e.g., syncope) undergo extensive diagnostic work-ups and report the frequency of the underlying disorders that caused the patients' illnesses, can provide very accurate estimates of pretest probability but are available for few disorders. Most commonly, and least accurate, clinicians use clinical intuition and experience to guess at the pretest probability. However, there are few well-validated clinical prediction rules in general as well as specifically in the area of rheumatologic disorders; as such it is of crucial importance to understand the interplay between results of diagnostic tests and the clinician intuition of the likelihood of the diagnosis for which the test is being ordered. Since pretest probability informs posttest probability, clinicians must begin with an accurate pretest probability. The consequences of inaccurate pretest probability assessment include poor selection of tests, poor interpretation of results, and ultimately diagnostic error.

Once pretest probability is determined, clinicians must decide whether to initiate treatment or to perform further diagnostic testing. The treatment threshold is the threshold above which the probability of disease is so high that further testing is unnecessary and treatment can be initiated. The testing threshold is the threshold below which the probability of disease is so low that further testing is unnecessary and the diagnosis is considered excluded (Fig. 26.1). Diagnostic testing is only useful to inform intermediate probabilities between the testing and treatment thresholds. These thresholds vary on the basis of the disease prognosis under consideration, the properties of the diagnostic tests, and the nature of the treatment. The safer the testing strategy, the more serious the condition if left undiagnosed, and the more effective and safe the available treatment, the lower the test threshold. For the treatment threshold, the more benign the prognosis of the illness and the higher the morbidity associated with therapy, the higher we would place the threshold. For example, our testing threshold would be low if a clinician suspects deep venous thrombosis as the duplex ultrasonography is a test that is both safe and easily available; on the other hand, our treatment threshold would be relatively high as anticoagulation, especially when considering short- and long-term courses of therapy, is potentially dangerous for a patient.

The first patient likely has osteoarthritis. No validated clinical prediction rules for the diagnosis of osteoarthritis of the knee or hand exist, nor any disease probability study has been conducted. Clinical intuition would place the pretest probability of osteoarthritis at around 85% to 90%. For most clinicians, the treatment threshold to initiate acetaminophen in this patient is fairly low and could be initiated without further testing (as we are fairly confident he has osteoarthritis and the consequences of moderate doses of acetaminophen are low). The alternative would be to order hand films, which we suspect would be done to rule out other conditions (i.e., rheumatoid arthritis), although the clinical scenario would make this diagnosis highly unlikely (<5%). Of interest, a relatively nondiagnostic radiologic study likely would not stop most clinicians

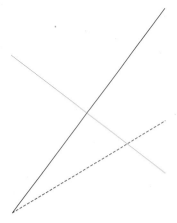

$Sensitivity = TP / TP + FN = a / a+c$
$Specificity = TN / TN + FP = d / d+b$
$PPV = TP / TP + FP = a / a+b$
$NPV = TN / TN + FN = d / d+c$

Figure 26.2 2 × 2 table.

to initiate acetaminophen therapy; in other words, ordering a hand film had no bearing on our treatment decision but perhaps made us feel better regarding other diagnostic possibilities. The difficult question then becomes if the cost or inconvenience of the hand film is worth excluding highly unlikely diagnoses.

Patient 2, on the other hand, likely has systemic lupus erythematosus (SLE). No validated clinical prediction rules to determine the pretest probability of SLE have been published. One population-based screening study (1) of SLE reported a prevalence of 200 cases per 100,000 women (18 to 65 years of age) in England, whereas another review estimated the overall U.S. prevalence of definite SLE plus incomplete SLE (disease meeting only some diagnostic requirements for SLE) to be 40 to 50 cases per 100,000 persons (2). Population prevalence studies such as these two can give misleading estimates of pretest probability because they have the wrong denominator, namely both healthy and diseased persons, both men and women. What we want to know is what is the proportion of all young women presenting with arthritis, malar rash, and possible pleuritis, similar to our second patient, who are ultimately diagnosed with SLE. Again we have to rely on clinical intuition and estimate this patient's pretest probability to be >50%. The treatment threshold to initiate immunosuppressive therapy in this case would be fairly high (i.e., the clinician would want to be certain of or rule in the diagnosis of SLE). The consequences of undiagnosed SLE are great, making the testing threshold fairly low. Thus further testing for SLE is indicated in patient 2 prior to initiating disease-specific therapy.

Choosing a Diagnostic Test

The main determinant of diagnostic test choice (assuming more than one test is available) is the intended role of the test—whether the clinician wants to rule in or rule out a particular disease. Pretest probability informs this decision. When pretest probability is low, the goal of diagnostic testing should be to rule out disease. With high pretest probabilities the goal is to rule in disease. Once the decision to rule in or rule out disease is made, clinicians then choose among diagnostic tests on the basis of their test properties (i.e., sensitivity, specificity, and likelihood ratios).

Sensitivity of a diagnostic test is the proportion of people with disease who test positive. ("PID," positive in disease, is a mnemonic to help remember this association.) It reflects the *true positive rate* of a test (Fig. 26.2). Tests with 100% sensitivity detect every single person with disease. Tests with 80% sensitivity miss 20% of persons with disease, resulting in a 20% false negative rate. Sensitivity is calculated by dividing the true positive rate by the true positive plus false negative rates. Sensitive tests are most useful to rule out disease when pretest probability is low (i.e., using fecal occult testing to screen for colorectal cancer in average-risk individuals).

Specificity of a diagnostic test is the proportion of people without disease who test negative. ("NIH," negative in health, is a mnemonic to help remember this association.) It reflects the *true negative rate* of a test (Fig. 26.2). Tests with 100% specificity have no false positives and are negative when disease is absent. Tests with 80% specificity are falsely positive 20% of the time. Specificity is calculated by dividing the true negative rate by the true negative plus false positive rates. Specific tests are used to rule in disease. For example, colonoscopy has a higher specificity than fecal occult testing and would be used to follow up positive fecal occult testing.

Patient 1 has such a low pretest probability of SLE that further testing for SLE is not useful (i.e., pretest probability is below the test threshold). Patient 2, on the other hand, has a fairly high pretest probability of having SLE. In this case we want to rule in SLE and would choose the test with the highest specificity. Table 26.1 shows the test properties and associations of different

KEY POINT 1

- Sensitive tests, when negative, rule out disease (SnNout) when the pretest probability is low.

- Specific tests, when positive, rule in disease (SpPin) when the pretest probability is high.

SECTION 6 Diagnosis and Therapy

Table 26.1 Sensitivity and Specificity of Different Antinuclear Antibodies in Systemic Lupus Erythematosus

| | ANTIBODY | | | | | | |
	ds-DNA (%)	ss-DNA (%)	HISTONE (%)	SMITH (%)	RIBONUCLEAR PROTEIN (%)	RO (%)	LA (%)
Sensitivity	70	80	30–80	30	27	25–35	15
Specificity	95		50	96	82	87–94	

antinuclear antibodies with SLE. Clinicians should choose either anti-ds DNA or anti-SM antibody tests as they have the highest specificity, and if positive, will increase the posttest probability of SLE in this patient. Of interest, most clinicians would also appropriately order an antinuclear antibody (ANA) test for this patient, with the thought of "ruling out" the possibility of SLE. Unfortunately, if the test returned negative, this does not decrease the probability of disease enough to exclude the diagnosis in the setting of high clinical suspicion.

Many tests have multiple cutoff points that can be used to determine positivity (i.e., they are not just positive or negative). For example, ANA tests are positive at a variety of titers (>1:40, >1:320, etc.). Different positive cutoff points affect sensitivity and specificity of diagnostic tests. In general, lowering the positivity criterion increases sensitivity (tests finds more disease) while lowering specificity (more false positives). Conversely, raising the positivity criterion lowers sensitivity (test detects less disease) but raises specificity (less false positives). For example, requiring a treadmill stress test to be positive with only 0.5-mm ST elevation would detect most every body with coronary artery disease (CAD) at a significant risk if erroneously labeling many patients without CAD with this diagnosis; the opposite effect would be achieved by requiring 4-mm ST elevation as the diagnostic criterion for positivity as in this scenario we would miss many patients with CAD but not label as diseased those without CAD. This interesting paradox is known as the trade-off phenomenon when changing the criterion to interpret a test as positive or negative.

Interpreting Diagnostic Test Results

The role of diagnostic testing is to lower or increase intermediate pretest probabilities. It is important to remember that not every positive test indicates the presence of disease, nor does every negative test indicate disease is absent. Most tests yield at least some false positive and false negative results (unless the test is both 100% sensitive and specific). A positive test result is more likely to be falsely positive when the pretest probability was low. Likewise, a negative test result is more likely to be false negative when the pretest probability was high (see examples below).

There are two methods to determine posttest probability predictive value method and likelihood ratio method; in the interest of brevity and clarity, we discuss only the former here. Most diagnostic test study manuscripts report the predictive value of the diagnostic test under study. *Positive predictive value* is the probability that a person with a positive test result has disease. *Negative predictive value* is the probability that a person with a negative test result does not have disease. These can be calculated from a 2 × 2 table (see Fig. 26.2) or using online EBM calculators (http://ktclearinghouse.ca/cebm/toolbox/statscalc). Clinicians must be cautious in using predictive values reported in diagnostic test study manuscripts because predictive values are affected by prevalence or pretest probability of disease. Unless your patient has the same pretest probability of disease as those in the study, you cannot use the predictive value reported

ADVANCED TOPIC 2

- Readers wanting more information on adjusting predictive values reported in diagnostic test studies are referred to Altman and Bland (6).

- Alternatively, likelihood ratios can be used to calculate posttest probability (3,4,5).

- Several diagnostic test calculators are available on the Internet to aid clinicians in these calculations. Epocrates (www.epocrates.com) is a popular online drug reference that contains several clinical and EBM calculators. The Centre for Evidence-Based Medicine also has several EBM calculators (http://ktclearinghouse.ca/cebm/practise/ca/calculators).

in the manuscript. It must be recalculated adjusting for your patient's pretest probability (which is beyond the scope of this chapter; 4,5)

Summary

The first step in making an accurate diagnosis is to integrate evidence from our knowledge of disease and disease prevalence with a patient's history and physical examination to formulate a differential diagnosis and estimate pretest probability. Several resources can be used to help guide our estimation of pretest probability, such as clinical prediction rules. Clinicians should be wary of ordering tests when the pretest probability of disease is high or low. Tests are unlikely to alter disease probability and only confuse the situation as unexpected results are usually false positives or false negatives.

ICD9

796.4 **Findings,** *(abnormal), without diagnosis (examination) (laboratory tests)*
795.79 antibody titers, elevated
795.79 antigen-antibody reaction
790.95 C-reactive protein (CRP)
791.9 crystals, urine
790.1 sedimentation rate, elevated
795.79 skin test, positive

References

1. Johnson AE, Gordon C, Hobbs FD, et al. Undiagnosed systemic lupus erythematosus in the community. *Lancet* 1996;347:367–369.
2. Lawrence RC, Helmick CG, Arnett FC, et al. Estimates of the prevalence of arthritis and selected musculoskeletal disorders in the United States. *Arthritis Rheum* 1998;41:778–799.
3. McGee S. Simplifying likelihood ratios. *J Gen Intern Med* 2002;17:646–649.
4. Fagan TJ. Letter: Nomogram for Bayes theorem. *N Engl J Med* 1975;293:257
5. Grimes DA, Schulz KF. Refining clinical diagnosis with likelihood ratios. *Lancet* 2005;365:1500–1505.
6. Altman DG, Bland JM. Statistics notes: Diagnostic tests 2: Predictive values. *BMJ* 1994;309:102.

SECTION 6 Diagnosis and Therapy

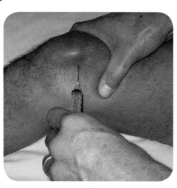

A 52-year-old man with rheumatoid arthritis presents with a 36-hour history of acute knee pain with fever after a week of moderate fever and a productive cough. His oral temperature is 39.6°C, and his knee has a large, warm, tense effusion with limited range of motion secondary to pain. His white blood cell count is 24,100 with many immature polymorphonuclear white blood cells. There is concern of septic arthritis, and he requires arthrocentesis for culture and relief.

Arthrocentesis is a frequent part of the evaluation and/or treatment of a patient with a musculoskeletal condition. This chapter focuses on the technique for accessing certain joints with a sterile needle with specific indications for arthrocentesis and treatment recommendations located in the specific chapters regarding that musculoskeletal condition.

CLINICAL POINTS

- Knowledge of local anatomy is essential.
- Weigh benefits and risks of arthrocentesis in bacteremia and bleeding diathesis.
- Have all needed equipment (syringe, needle, gauge, Band-Aid, etc.) readily accessible to the operator.

Contraindications to arthrocentesis are relative and typically related to the potential for bleeding and/or infection. Caution in performing arthrocentesis should be exercised in the following clinical settings:

1. *Infection of the overlying skin:* Passing a sterile needle through an area of skin that is infected or cannot be prepped to retain the needle's reasonable sterility creates risk of introducing an infection into a joint. Areas of obvious or potential infection must be avoided to preserve the sterility of the joint.

2. *Bacteremia:* Performing arthrocentesis in the clinical setting of known bacteremia similarly increases the risk of introducing an infection into the joint. Clinical judgment must be exercised on the relative benefit and risk of performing the arthrocentesis for diagnostic purposes in documenting a polymicrobial infection or therapeutic benefit of the removal of synovial fluid.

3. *Bleeding diathesis:* Patients on anticoagulation, with thrombocytopenia, hemophilia, or other causes leading to a bleeding diathesis, are at risk of hemarthrosis from the arthrocentesis. Complications can be avoided by using the smallest needle gauge feasible and providing adequate hemostasis after the procedure. In reality, we are not hesitant to perform venipuncture in these settings with adequate attention to hemostasis postprocedure, so we should have a similar attitude toward arthrocentesis in these settings.

4. *Prosthetic joints:* Arthrocentesis of a prosthetic joint can be more challenging because of scarring from the surgical procedure and the risk of infection since the prosthesis can act as a foreign body. Aspiration of the prosthetic joint is possible, but better deferred to the orthopedic surgeon or interventional radiologist under imaging.

5. *Uncooperative patient:* Arthrocentesis requires significant cooperation from the patient in positioning and should be performed only on patients who can be fully cooperative.

- Presence of systemic or local infection.
- Evidence of local rash overlying injection site.
- Consider bleeding diathesis.

Table 27.1 Necessary Equipment

- Disposable gloves
- Povidone–iodine antiseptic solution
- Alcohol wipes
- Syringe or multiple syringes if draining large effusions
- Appropriate needle
- Ethyl chloride spray (optional)
- Hemostat to assist in changing syringes during the procedure
- Gauze for postprocedure hemostasis
- Bandage

Equipment

Appropriate equipment (see Table 27.1) should be assembled at the bedside prior to the procedure and easily accessible to the operator during the procedure, without the operator changing position. An assistant is optional and dependent on the operator, but he or she will be helpful if there is concern of patient cooperation or a larger effusion is to be drained requiring changing syringes.

Technique

After selecting an appropriate entry site, the entry site can be marked using a ball-point pen with the pen tip retracted. The pen's aperture can be pressured to the site to leave an impression of the selected entry site before cleansing the area. The selected entry point is cleansed appropriately with an antiseptic solution followed by removal of the antiseptic solution using the alcohol wipes. After cleansing the area, caution should be exercised to avoid contaminating the site by further palpation with an unsterile gloved finger. If further palpation is desired, then a sterile glove can be used or a sterile 4 × 4 gauze can be placed over the area and palpation done over the sterile gauze to preserve the site's antiseptic condition. Some topical anesthesia is obtained by spraying the site with ethyl chloride until the area "frosts." Alternatively, a small amount of lidocaine can be injected subcutaneously into the proposed injection area.

When advancing the needle into the joint cavity, the patient experiences discomfort when the needle passes through the skin and again when it crosses the synovium. Less discomfort is experienced when the skin and synovium is crossed quicker as opposed to slowly and deliberately. Once the needle is introduced into the joint cavity, fluid should flow easily into the syringe if using a needle gauge of 20 or larger. If no fluid can be aspirated, or fluid stops flowing, the most common cause is that synovial tissue or solid material (clot, fibrin, cartilage fragments, etc.) within the fluid is obstructing the needle. Rotating the needle or injecting back a small amount of the aspirated fluid into the joint cavity may remove the obstruction. At that point. gentle negative pressure can be placed and the fluid may aspirate. As the total effusion approaches complete drainage, the synovial lining becomes closer to the needle tip and further difficulty is typically experienced or fresh blood now appears in the aspirated fluid. Discomfort by the patient is common at this point, and a decision to continue aspirating at the patient's discomfort should be weighed by the benefit of removing more fluid at this time. Once sufficient fluid is removed, the needle can be withdrawn and appropriate hemostasis applied to the injection site. Alternatively, if steroids or medication are planned to be injected after aspiration, the syringe can be separated from the needle that remains in the joint and a syringe with the medication attached to the needle and the medication injected. This situation where an injection follows an aspiration is where a hemostat can be helpful to grasp the hub of the needle while changing syringes. Injecting medication into a joint cavity should not require much pressure on the plunger, although the larger the discrepancy between a large syringe bore and a small-gauge needle, the greater the pressure required. If significant pressure is required, the needle has left the joint space and should be positioned again properly.

When aspiration is not planned and only injection of medication is planned, aspiration of fluid is not always possible when using small-gauge needles of less than 20 and the operator must be confident of the needle position. Again, injecting medication into a joint cavity should not require much pressure on the plunger except when there is a greater discrepancy between a large-bore syringe and a small-gauge needle, when greater pressure required. If significant pressure is required, the needle is not positioned in the joint space and should be positioned properly.

When injecting medication only without aspiration, using a 27-gauge needle is more comfortable to the patient, although it requires greater plunger pressure from the operator. If limiting the syringe to a 3-cc volume, the pressure should not be too difficult. If injecting viscous solutions such as in viscosupplementation or certain depot steroid products, the operator requires a larger bore needle than a 27-gauge needle and should consider a 25-gauge needle for depot steroids and a 22-gauge needle for viscosupplementation.

Complications

Procedure-related complications such as infection or bleeding are rare if antiseptic techniques are practiced, selection of injection site is prudent, and appropriate hemostasis is implemented. Complications from the steroid injected are more common and the patient should be informed prior to the procedure. When injected into soft tissues, corticosteroids can cause fat atrophy, cutaneous hypopigmentation along the needle track, and atrophy of ligament and tendon structures, making rupture a risk. Fat atrophy and hypopigmentation usually resolve, although they may take years. A crystal-induced arthritis (postinjection flare) is not common, but it can occur within hours of injection and last for several. The flare occurs likely because of the inflammatory effect of the steroid crystals, causing a transient crystal-induced synovitis. If injecting a combination of steroids and a local anesthetic such as lidocaine, the patient should be warned of the therapeutic window of effect when using this combination, as the anesthetic may wear off before the steroid starts to work. Finally, patients with diabetes should be cautioned to observe the effect of the steroids on their glucose control over the next several days following injection.

Technique for Specific Joints

KNEE

- *Patient position:* Supine with the knee to be aspirated fully extended or extended as much as is tolerable to the patient. Support placed under a knee unable to fully extend provides greater comfort to the patient and allows for greater relaxation.
- *Entry site:* Medial or lateral.
- *Technique:* With the patient relaxed, the patella should be movable and the landmarks of the patella identified, particularly the superior medial or lateral corner, as the entry point will be inferior to that landmark (Fig. 27.1). Position the needle perpendicular to the leg and angled to be parallel to the inferior

NOT TO BE MISSED

- Systemic or local infection.
- Rash overlying injection site.
- Bleeding diathesis, as it requires more attention to hemostasis postprocedure.

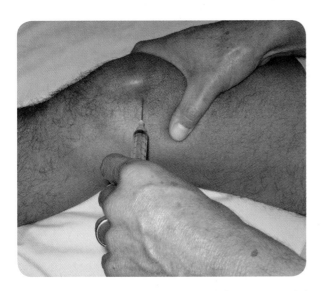

Figure 27.1 Medial entry point of knee beneath the superior medial pole of the patella. Needle is positioned parallel to the inferior surface of the patella.

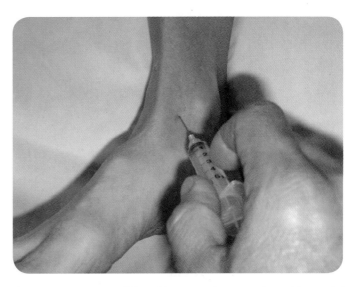

Figure 27.2 Entry point of the ankle joint, at the same plane of the medial malleolus and medial to the anterior tibialis tendon.

surface of the patella, typically about 30 to 45 degrees from horizontal. Advance the needle quickly through the skin and then advance further until the synovium is crossed.

ANKLE (TIBIOTALAR) JOINT

- *Patient position:* Patient supine and ankle relaxed.
- *Entry site:* Anteromedial.
- *Technique:* Identify the patient's medial malleolus and anterior tibialis tendon. The entry point will be in the sagittal, or horizontal, plane of the medial malleolus and immediately medial to the anterior tibialis tendon (Fig. 27.2). The needle should be directed toward the center of the concave distal end of the tibia. This trajectory will position the needle between the talus and the distal tibia.

METATARSOPHALANGEAL, METACARPOPHALANGEAL, AND INTERPHALANGEAL JOINTS

- *Patient position:* Patient supine and joint relaxed.
- *Entry site:* Dorsal, medial, or lateral to the extensor tendon.
- *Technique:* Identify the base of the distal phalanx and the extensor tendon as it crosses the joint space. Select the area medial or lateral to the extensor tendon that avoids any visible subcutaneous veins. Use this as your entry point and direct the needle toward the center of the concave proximal end of the distal phalanx (Figs. 27.3 and 27.4). This trajectory will position the needle between the convex head of the proximal bone and the distal phalanx.

SHOULDER

- *Patient position:* Patient seated, elbow flexed to 90 degrees, forearm resting on the lap, and joint relaxed.
- *Entry site:* Posterior.

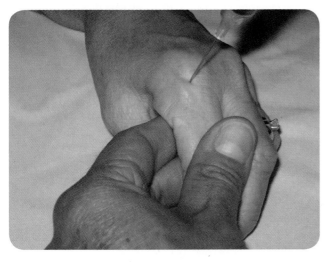

Figure 27.3 Entry point of the hand—metacarpophalangeal joint.

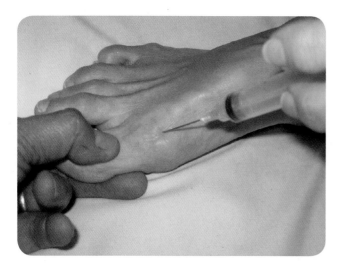

Figure 27.4 Entry point of the foot—metatarsophalangeal joint.

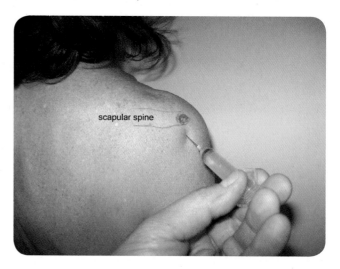

Figure 27.5 Posterior entry point into the shoulder beneath the scapular spine's acromian with the needle directed toward the coracoid process.

- *Technique:* Standing behind the patient, identify the scapular spine and distal acromian on the back of the patient, and the coracoid process on the anterior chest of the patient. Place the hand not holding the needle on the shoulder and identify or palpate the coracoid process. The entry point will be immediately inferior to the distal acromian and the needle tip directed toward the palpable coracoids process (Fig. 27.5).

SUBACROMIAL BURSA

- *Patient position:* Patient seated, elbow flexed to 90 degrees, forearm resting on the lap, and joint relaxed.
- *Entry site:* Lateral.
- *Technique:* Standing on the side of the patient, identify the acromian process. The entry point will be inferior to the lateral most point of the acromian process and the needle directed superiorly roughly 30 degrees below the horizontal level. This will place the needle above the humeral head and below the acromian process (Fig. 27.6).

ELBOW

- *Patient position:* Patient lying, elbow flexed to 90 degrees, forearm resting on the abdomen, and joint relaxed.
- *Entry site:* Lateral.
- *Technique:* Identify the lateral epicondyle, radial head, and olecranon process, and establish the center of this triangle (Fig. 27.7). The needle will enter in the center of the triangle, directed perpendicular to the skin's entry point, and end up in the elbow's lateral paraolecranon groove.

WRIST

- *Patient position:* Patient seated or lying, wrist in mild passive flexion of 10 degrees with a support beneath the wrist for comfort, and relaxed.
- *Entry site:* Dorsal.

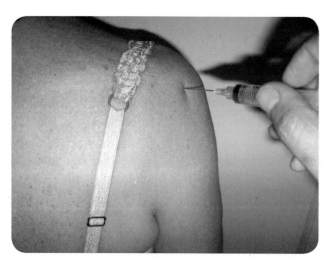

Figure 27.6 Entry point of the subacromial bursa.

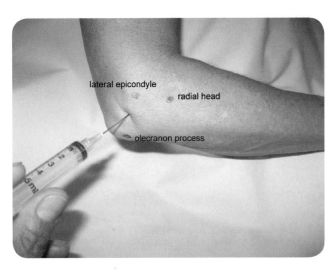

Figure 27.7 Entry point of the elbow between lateral epicondyle, radial head, and olecranon process.

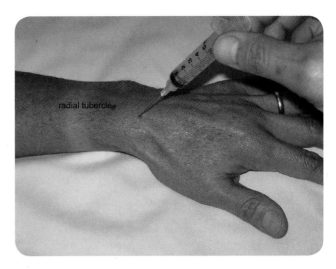

Figure 27.8 Entry point between the distal radius and scaphoid bone in the wrist distal to the radial tubercle.

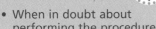

WHEN TO REFER

- When in doubt about performing the procedure.
- Joints inaccessible without imaging guidance.

- *Technique:* Identify the radial tubercle on the distal radius and an indentation between the distal radius and the scaphoid bone in the wrist. Entry point will be distal to the radial tubercle in the indentation and directing the needle perpendicular to the skin (Fig. 27.8).

ICD9

81.91 **Arthrocentesis**
Joint aspiration

Additional Reading

1. Moore GF. Techniques of arthrocentesis and injection therapy. In: Koopman WJ, Boulware DW, Heudebert GR, eds. *Clinical Primer of Rheumatology*. Philadelphia: Lippincott Williams and Wilkins; 2003:354–367.
2. Lotke PA. Injection techniques for joints and bursa. In: Lotke PA, Abboud JA, Ende J, eds. *Lippincott's Primary Care Orthopaedics*. Philadelphia: Lippincott Williams and Wilkins; 2008:389–394.
3. Moore GF. Arthrocentesis technique and intra-articular therapy. In: Koopman WJ, Moreland LW, eds. *Arthritis and Allied Conditions*. 15th ed. Philadelphia: Lippincott Williams and Wilkins; 2005:755–774.

SECTION 6 Diagnosis and Therapy

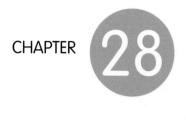

28 Monitoring of Patients on Antirheumatic Therapy

W. Winn Chatham

The chronicity of the majority of rheumatic diseases often involves the long-term use of antirheumatic therapies. Multiple inflammatory mediators and mechanisms of tissue injury operative in both acute and chronic inflammation frequently require the concurrent use of several reagents to adequately suppress disease activity. Moreover, the increased prevalence of rheumatic disease with age dictates that use of antirheumatic and immunomodulating therapies must often be prescribed in the context of comorbidities. As such, it is important for clinicians involved in the care of patients with rheumatic disease to be mindful of the short-term as well as long-term consequences of antirheumatic therapies, not only on organ systems affected by therapy, but also on the course or treatment of coexisting disease.

Corticosteroids

Glucocorticoids have broad inhibitory effects on specific immune responses mediated by T- and B-cell lymphocytes as well as potent suppressive effects on the effector functions of monocytes and neutrophils. Although these attributes coupled with their rapid onset of action render steroids extremely valuable in suppressing undesired inflammatory processes, corticosteroids have similar broad effects on the function of cells comprising other organ systems. The immunocompromised status and catabolic consequences associated with use of corticosteroids limit their long-term use in high doses and dictate the need for careful surveillance and preventive interventions to avoid undesired complications.

Use of high doses of corticosteroids first and foremost requires vigilance for the development of intercurrent infections. Patients with either rheumatoid arthritis or systemic lupus erythematosus (SLE) have an intrinsic susceptibility to infection, and the administration of glucocorticoids enhances the risk of infection. In addition to typical bacterial organisms, infections with mycobacteria, cryptococci, listeria, and nocardia have been associated with corticosteroid therapy. The combination of steroid use with cytotoxic agents, such as cyclophosphamide, has been associated with higher risk of infection with *Pneumocystis jirovecii* pneumonia, most notably among patients with lymphopenia. Unless life- or organ-threatening disease complications dictate otherwise, in the setting of serious intercurrent infection, doses of corticosteroids should be attenuated to that required to avoid adrenal crisis.

Given the significant catabolic effects of glucocorticoids on muscle, skin, and bone, patients taking moderate or high doses of steroids for prolonged intervals require periodic assessment for the evolution of steroid myopathy or

COMMON PITFALLS TO AVOID WHEN USING GLUCOCORTICOSTEROIDS

1. Infection with mycobacteria, listeria, cryptococci, and nocardia

2. Salt and water retention

3. Glucose intolerance

4. Muscle and skin wasting

5. Osteoporosis

6. Osteonecrosis

development of steroid-induced osteoporosis. Since steroid myopathy most commonly affects the proximal hip-girdle musculature, assessment of hip-girdle strength by having the patient squat or arise from a chair unassisted are simple maneuvers that can be employed during clinic visits. Corticosteroid-induced muscle wasting and weakness may be difficult to distinguish from inflammatory muscle diseases for which they are prescribed. Muscle tenderness and elevation in creatine kinase favor the presence of active myositis. On muscle biopsy, loss of type I and type II fibers as well as vacuolar changes may be observed in steroid-induced myopathy or myositis.

Periodic assessment for osteoporosis is now a standard of care for patients on chronic corticosteroids. The employment of alternate-day dosing regimens does not appear to confer protection from steroid-induced osteopenia. Exogenous administration of calcium and vitamin D may suffice to protect patients from steroid-induced osteopenia. Glucocorticoid-induced suppression of adrenal dehyrdoepiandrosterone (DHEA) production may render women at increased risk for the catabolic effect of steroids on bone, but a role for DHEA administration in the prevention of bone complications has not yet been confirmed. Bisphosphonates (alendronate, risedronate, ibandronate, and zoledronic acid) and have emerged as proven therapies for the prevention and treatment of glucocorticoid-induced osteoporosis (1). Periodic assessment of bone density at 1- to 2-year intervals is recommended to assess the efficacy of these interventions in patients on chronic steroid therapy.

The predictable metabolic consequences of steroids include salt and water retention as well as variable degrees of insulin resistance with hyperglycemia. The mineralocorticoid effects of steroids warrant expectant observation for the development of hypertension or heart failure exacerbations in patients who have or are at risk for these cardiovascular disorders. Long-term metabolic consequences of corticosteroid use in patients with rheumatic disease may include accelerated atherogenesis. Attention to other cardiovascular risk factors including assessment for and treatment of hypercholesterolemia may slow the progression of atherogenesis and lower the risk for vascular events in patients who require long-term steroid use for management of rheumatic disease manifestations.

Other complications of corticosteroid therapy are less predictable but nonetheless require vigilance for their occurrence so as to avoid unfavorable outcomes. Corticosteroids may have untoward effects on the central nervous system, including emotional irritability, difficulty in concentration, depression, confusion, or psychosis. High-dose corticosteroids therapy has been implicated as a possible inducer of pancreatitis. Since pancreatitis may be a manifestation of lupus, the occurrence of pancreatitis in patients with lupus receiving glucocorticoid therapy may result in a therapeutic dilemma. Osteonecrosis is a recognized complication of high-dose steroid use. In patients with lupus, other disease-related factors may account for the development of osteonecrosis, but the incidence appears to correlate with the cumulative steroid dose. Since routine radiographs typically fail to reveal the presence of osteonecrosis during its early stages, patients on high doses of steroids who develop otherwise unexplained pain in the shoulders, hips, knees, or ankles should be evaluated with magnetic resonance imaging to rule out the presence of osteonecrosis.

COMMON PITFALLS TO AVOID WHEN USING NSAIDs

1. Decline in glomerular filtration rate
2. Gastropathy including ulceration and bleeding
3. Platelet dysfunction and bleeding
4. Salt and water retention

NSAIDs, nonsteroidal anti-inflammatory drugs.

Nonsteroidal Anti-inflammatory Drugs

Nonsteroidal anti-inflammatory drugs constitute the most frequently prescribed class of medication used in the treatment of patients with rheumatic disorders. A rapid onset of action and their combined analgesic or anti-inflammatory attributes render NSAIDs very useful in the management of rheumatic disease. Although a number of cellular effects distinct from those related to prostaglandin production have been described for various NSAIDs, the major therapeutic effect of NSAIDs relates to their ability to inhibit cyclooxygenase-mediated synthesis of prostaglandins, affecting vascular permeability and hyperalgesia. However, prostaglandins generated by cyclooxygenase also play an important role in hemostasis, in maintaining the integrity of the intestinal mucosa, and in regulating renal blood flow. These physiologic effects of prostaglandins account for the majority of NSAID side effects and toxicity, most notably bleeding, intestinal ulceration, azotemia, and retention of salt and water.

Certain toxic effects of a given NSAID may be governed by its specificity for the respective isoforms of cyclooxygenase, COX-1 and COX-2. COX-1 is expressed constitutively in most organ systems and is the isoform primarily responsible for synthesis of prostaglandins maintaining the integrity of the gastrointestinal (GI) mucosa and the hemostatic function of platelets. COX-2 is primarily induced and expressed in response to cytokines at sites of tissue injury and inflammation and is not expressed in platelets. Traditional nonselective NSAIDs inhibit both COX-1 and COX-2, whereas celecoxib selectively inhibits COX-2, substantially sparing activity of COX-1.

Monitoring of patients taking NSAIDs, particularly those not selective for COX-2, entails careful attention to symptoms referable to the GI tract and the possibility of bleeding complications. As the majority of NSAID-induced ulcerations are silent, periodic assessment of the hematocrit and red cell indices are prudent in patients taking NSAIDs for extended durations. Although there are no published studies to provide guidelines for how frequently such monitoring should occur, risk factors for NSAID-induced GI bleeding and perforation are now well recognized (Table 28.1) (2,3), and the presence of these risk factors in a given patient should guide the frequency of blood count or hemoccult monitoring.

Both COX-1 and COX-2 are constitutively expressed in the kidney and generate prostaglandins (PGE_2 and PGI_2) that regulate renal blood flow under conditions of volume contraction and/or decreased effective arterial blood volume. PGE_2 and PGI_2 furthermore stimulate secretion of renin with attendant release of aldosterone and potassium secretion. Accordingly, diminution in GFR with salt

---

Table 28.1 Risk Factors for NSAID-Induced Gastrointestinal Bleeding and Perforation

Previous peptic ulcer disease

Previous gastrointestinal bleed

Previous hospitalization for gastrointestinal disease

History of NSAID-induced gastritis or dyspepsia

Use of H_2-blocker or antacid for dyspepsia

Concurrent corticosteroid use

Older age

Higher dose of NSAID

History of cardiovascular disease

Higher arthritis-related disability score

Concurrent anticoagulant use

Smoking

Alcoholism

NSAID, nonsteroidal anti-inflammatory drugs.
Risk factors compiled from the ARAMIS database and outcomes in the MUCOSA trial (2,3).

and water retention and/or hyperkalemia may occur as a consequence of treatment with either nonselective or COX-2 selective NSAIDs. Patients with preexisting renal disease or diminished effective arterial blood volume (congestive heart failure, cirrhosis, and renal vascular disease) are at particular risk for effects of NSAIDs on glomerular perfusion. Effects of NSAIDs on GFR may cause significant complications in patients with diabetes with type IV renal tubular acidosis (hyporeninemic hypoaldosteronism), as the attendant inhibition of renin release accompanied by diminution of salt load to distal nephrons may precipitate significant hyperkalemia. Careful monitoring for fluid retention and elevations of creatinine or potassium should be undertaken in these at-risk patient populations within several days of instituting treatment with an NSAID.

In addition to their potential effects on glomerular perfusion and renin secretion, NSAIDs may induce idiosyncratic, drug-specific complications of interstitial nephritis. While this complication may occur with any NSAID, interstitial nephritis has been reported most commonly in patients receiving fenoprofen. Although an appropriate frequency of monitoring renal function in patients taking NSAIDs has not been established by relevant outcome studies, at least semiannual assessment of creatinine and urinalysis is prudent for patients on long-term NSAID therapy to minimize the risk of permanent kidney damage from drug-induced interstitial nephritis.

> **COMMON PITFALLS TO AVOID WHEN USING COLCHICINE**
>
> 1. Dose-related diarrhea
> 2. Myopathy with chronic use

COLCHICINE

Colchicine is most commonly used in the treatment of acute gout or pseudogout; the drug may be used for extended periods of time to prevent repeated flares of acute crystalline-induced arthritis. The anti-inflammatory effects of colchicine are attributed to the drug's interference with the function of tubular microfilaments required for chemotaxis, migration, and release of granule constituents by neutrophils. The toxicity of colchicine when used acutely is primarily related to effects on the intestinal mucosa when administered excessively. When used in the appropriate setting of an acute attack of crystalline-induced arthritis of shorter than 24 hours' duration, it is seldom necessary to administer oral dosing of colchicine that induces diarrhea. Two oral doses of 0.6 mg administered 1 hour apart followed by a third dose 6 hours later is usually sufficient to manage an acute attack of gout or pseudogout. Attacks of crystalline-induced arthritis of longer than 24 hours' duration are less likely to resolve with administration of colchicine and alternative therapies, such as NSAIDs, or corticosteroids should be considered in this setting.

A vacuolar myopathy may evolve in the setting of chronic colchicine use, particularly among patients with renal sufficiency. For patients treated with colchicine over extended periods, monitoring for the development of myopathy with periodic assessment for serum elevations in creatine kinase is prudent. Patients with renal insufficiency may also be at greater risk for marrow toxicity and should also be monitored periodically for evidence of cytopenias when taking colchicine over extended periods.

Disease-modifying Antirheumatic Drugs

Use of one or more disease-modifying antirheumatic drugs (DMARDs) is now the standard of care for patients with active rheumatoid arthritis. Many DMARDs, including methotrexate, hydroxychloroquine, azathioprine, cyclosporine, and mycophenolate are used to manage manifestations of diseases other than rheumatoid arthritis, including lupus and polymyositis. Use of DMARDs entails titration of the dose to achieve the desired clinical benefit without inducing toxicity. Selection and successful use of a DMARD or DMARD combination for a given patient rests upon multiple clinical considerations, including stage and activity of the disease, patient comorbidities, concurrent medication use, and the known side-effect profiles of the respective DMARDs. Monitoring for DMARD toxicity and side effects is therefore critical to the appropriate use of these drugs.

METHOTREXATE

An analogue of folic acid, methotrexate inhibits folic acid–dependent pathways through numerous mechanisms. At high doses, methotrexate is an effective chemotherapeutic agent for the treatment of lymphoid neoplasms and some solid tumors. At lower doses, methotrexate has immunosuppressive and significant anti-inflammatory effects, most likely mediated by effects of its polyglutamated metabolites on AICAR transformylase. Inhibition of AICAR transformylase by polyglutamated methotrexate results in impaired synthesis of purines and pyrimidines, as well as accumulation of AICAR, a potent inducer of adenosine release. The latter may account for methotrexate's anti-inflammatory effects, as engagement of adenosine receptors on leukocytes attenuates their adherence to endothelial cells.

Although uncommon in the doses usually employed for management of rheumatoid arthritis, mucositis, bone marrow suppression, and hepatocellular injury constitute the primary toxicities associated with the use of methotrexate. Less common complications include acute interstitial pneumonitis, interstitial nephritis, and transient postdose syndromes that may include fever, neurocognitive impairment, arthralgia, and/or myalgia. The occurrence of mucositis or cytopenias may depend in part on folate stores, as these complications can be prevented or significantly reduced with folic acid supplementation (4). Folic acid does not impair the formation of polyglutamated methotrexate metabolites, and use of folic acid supplements has been shown not to alter the antirheumatic efficacy of methotrexate.

Effects of methotrexate on hematopoiesis are typically dose dependent, but there is considerable individual variability in the dose threshold for development of methotrexate-induced cytopenias. Rare, severe idiosyncratic cytopenias may develop even in the setting of low weekly doses and adequate folate stores. Renal insufficiency greatly enhances the likelihood of marrow toxicity, due in large part to the prominent role of renal excretion in elimination of the drug. Use of methotrexate in patients with end-stage renal disease, even while on regular hemodialysis, may have deleterious and irreversible consequences. Although serum levels of methotrexate can be efficiently lowered by hemodialysis using high-flux dialyzers, peritoneal dialysis is ineffective at lowering serum levels of methotrexate, and dialysis of any type likely has little effect on removal of the active polyglutamated metabolites within cells.

Guidelines for monitoring of patients with rheumatoid arthritis receiving methotrexate have been established (Table 28.2) (5,6). Prior to starting methotrexate, a complete blood count (CBC) with serum levels of liver transaminases (ALT, AST), albumin, and creatinine should be checked. Screening for hepatitis B and C infection is also advocated. Transaminase levels and CBC should be checked within 4 weeks of instituting therapy and within 4 weeks of any dose increment. More frequent assessment of blood counts may be indicated for patients with renal insufficiency. Alternatively, the interval between assessment of blood counts and liver function tests may be extended to 3 months for patients who have been on a stable dose of methotrexate in excess of 6 months. Creatinine levels should be checked at least every 6 months.

For patients who develop cytopenias (WBC <3,000; hematocrit <30; platelets <130,000), methotrexate should be withheld until the cause of the cytopenia is elucidated or the level of the depressed blood element recovers. A similar strategy should be employed for patients who develop elevation in liver transaminases in excess of twice the upper limit of normal. In either case, if it is deemed the abnormality was due to methotrexate, treatment with

Table 28.2 Guidelines for Monitoring Patients Receiving Methotrexate

Baseline evaluation:
  Complete blood count
  Liver function tests—AST, ALT, bilirubin, alkaline phosphatase, albumin
  Hepatitis B surface antigen, hepatitis C antibody

Pretreatment liver biopsy for patients with:
  Prior history of excessive alcohol consumption
  Persistent abnormal elevations in transaminases (AST, ALT) levels
  Evidence of persistent infection with hepatitis B or C

Monitor CBC, AST, ALT, and albumin at 4- to 12-week intervals

Monitor creatinine at 3- to 6-month intervals

In setting of cytopenia or elevation in AST, ALT twice upper range of normal:
  Hold methotrexate and resume at lower dose once laboratory
    abnormality resolves

Perform liver biopsy before continuing treatment if:
  Five of nine or six of twelve AST determinations in a 1-year time frame are
    abnormal, *or*
  Albumin decreases below normal range despite adequate control of synovitis

methotrexate at a lower dose can often be employed with success. Elevations of creatinine while on methotrexate warrant exclusion of interstitial nephritis and attention to the need for dose adjustment to avoid marrow toxicity. The occurrence of cough, dyspnea, and fever should prompt withholding of methotrexate until it can be established that the syndrome is not likely attributable to methotrexate pneumonitis.

The reported occurrence of cirrhosis among patients with psoriasis treated with long-term weekly methotrexate initially prompted recommendations for routine liver biopsy in patients with rheumatoid arthritis treated with methotrexate once the cumulative dose approached 2 g. However, given the infrequent occurrence of serious liver disease observed among patients with rheumatoid arthritis treated with methotrexate (estimated risk at 5 years <1 in 1,000), current guidelines do not advocate routine liver biopsy for patients treated with long-term methotrexate who have normal liver function. Liver biopsy is advocated pretreatment for patients with known history of previous heavy alcohol use, active hepatitis B, or hepatitis C infection, and for patients on methotrexate who develop persistent elevation in liver transaminases or a fall in serum albumin despite well-controlled rheumatoid arthritis.

ANTIMALARIALS—HYDROXYCHLOROQUINE, CHLOROQUINE, AND QUINACRINE

Most commonly employed in the management of lupus or rheumatoid arthritis, antimalarials have multiple effects on immunologic function and have a very favorable toxicity/benefit profile. Hydroxychloroquine and chloroquine do not suppress bone marrow function and liver toxicity is uncommon. Side effects consist primarily of cutaneous reactions, GI intolerance, and mild CNS symptoms. With the exception of severe skin eruptions, many of the GI and neurologic side effects may abate with reduction in the dose of antimalarials. Although rare, cardiac conduction abnormalities, cardiomyopathy, and neuromyopathy have been reported as more serious complications. As is recommended following initiation of therapy with most antirheumatic drugs, assessment of liver transaminases should be performed within the first 2 or 3 months of treatment to ensure the absence of idiosyncratic liver toxicity.

Although uncommon in the doses employed (200 to 400 mg daily), ocular toxicity may occur with use of antimalarials. Corneal deposits associated with perception of halos around lights may occur, but often remit spontaneously even with continued antimalarial use. Central nervous system (CNS) effects of hydroxychloroquine or chloroquine following initiation of either drug may result in transient defects in accommodation or convergence. Retinopathy is a more serious complication that may result in permanent visual impairment. Although opinion remains varied with regard to the appropriate frequency of monitoring, patients on hydroxychloroquine should undergo at least yearly ocular evaluation for evidence of hydroxychloroquine retinopathy (7,8). Antimalarial-induced retina toxicity is often, although not uniformly, identifiable before any perceived alterations in visual acuity. With regular ocular assessment for pigmentary abnormalities in the retina, alterations in visual field, and changes in acuity or color perception, permanent visual impairment from antimalarial use can usually be avoided.

SULFASALAZINE

Sulfasalazine consists of a salicylate (5-aminosalicylic acid) and a sulfapyridine molecule adjoined by an azo bond that is cleaved by bacterial organisms in the gut. In addition to the anti-inflammatory effects afforded by the liberated salicylate, sulfapyridine and/or its metabolites appear to have immunomodulatory effects that are of benefit in the management of patients with rheumatoid arthritis, ankylosing spondylitis, or one of the other spondyloarthropathies. Gastrointestinal symptoms are usually the most common side effects reported with use of sulfasalazine, but these often resolve with dose attenuation. The less common, but potentially more serious, hematologic consequences of sulfasalazine use include aplastic anemia, agranulocytosis, or hemolytic anemia, with the latter occurring predominantly in patients with glucose-6-phosphate dehydrogenase deficiency. Leukopenia most often occurs during the first several months of treatment, but may occur at any time. In decreasing order of frequency, cutaneous, hepatic, pulmonary, and renal hypersensitivity reactions may also occur.

When initiating therapy with sulfasalazine, it is advisable to check baseline blood counts and liver function tests, and screen for glucose-6-phosphate dehydrogenase deficiency. The drug is best introduced incrementally, starting with a 500 mg daily dose and then increasing by 500 mg weekly until the therapeutic target dose of 1 to 2 g twice daily is reached. Blood counts and liver function test should be assessed at 2-week intervals until the patient has been on the target maintenance dose for at least 1 month. Blood counts and liver transaminase levels can then be monitored less frequently, but should be assessed at least every 3 months. As leukopenia may occur precipitously, patients should be instructed to promptly report the occurrence of fever, malaise, mouth ulcers, or sore throat.

LEFLUNOMIDE

Leflunomide is an inhibitor of dihydro-orotate dehydrogenase, an enzyme mediating synthesis of pyrimidines. Leflunomide has significant inhibitory effects on proliferation of lymphocytes and has demonstrated efficacy in the management of rheumatoid arthritis. Adverse effects of leflunomide are relatively mild and infrequent, and include reversible alopecia, skin rash, diarrhea, and elevation in liver enzymes. Leflunomide is teratogenic in animals and contraindicated in women who are or wish to become pregnant.

Liver function tests should be assessed at baseline and at monthly intervals following initiation of therapy. Frequency of testing can be extended to every 3 months for patients who have been on therapy in excess of 6 months without signs of liver toxicity. Leflunomide should be promptly discontinued if significant elevations in liver transaminases occur. The serum half-life of the major active metabolite of leflunomide (referred to as M1) exceeds 2 weeks, but because of significant enterohepatic circulation, the serum levels of M1 can be rapidly decreased with administration of cholestyramine. In the setting of significant liver or the occurrence of pregnancy, a 10- to 14-day course of 8 g cholestyramine taken three times daily should be administered to enhance rapid elimination of drug and bring the serum levels of M1 below 0.02 µg/mL. It is recommended that sequential determinations of M1 be performed at 2-week intervals until it is established that elimination is complete.

GOLD SALTS—AUROTHIOGLUCOSE AND AURANOFIN

Gold salts have a variety of effects on cells and enzymes that regulate immune responses and inflammatory reactions relevant to the pathogenesis and expression of rheumatoid arthritis. Although parenteral gold salts, such as aurothioglucose, are very effective disease-modifying drugs, because of the frequency of side effects patients experience over time and newer therapies that are much better tolerated, the use of gold salts has diminished considerably. The preparations still currently in use in selected patients are aurothioglucose, administered parenterally, and auranofin, administered orally.

The most common adverse events limiting use of gold compounds are mucocutaneous reactions including stomatitis, pruritis, and any number of various forms of dermatitis. Although rarely reported with use of auranofin, proteinuria may be a complication of parenteral gold salt therapy that may require either dose attenuation or cessation of therapy. Leukopenia, thrombocytopenia, and aplastic anemia are rare, but potentially, fatal consequences that may occur at any time during the course of gold therapy.

For patients on parenteral gold therapy, blood counts and a urinalysis should be checked prior to each injection during the first year of treatment. Once a patient is on a stable regimen beyond the initial year, the monitoring interval for proteinuria and cytopenias can be extended to every other injection. The development of significant leukopenia ($<3,500/mm^3$), thrombocytopenia ($<100,000/mm^3$), or a persistent downward trend in the platelet count or hematocrit should prompt cessation of chrysotherapy. In the absence of other identifiable causes for observed cytopenia(s), treatment with gold compounds should not be reinstituted. Proteinuria during treatment with gold compounds is often transient, responding to temporary withholding of gold; most patients can resume treatment at lower doses without recurrence of the proteinuria. Gold should not be reinstituted in patients who develop nephrotic-range proteinuria (>1 g protein excreted/24 hours).

Monitoring of patients on gold therapy also requires attention to the occurrence of skin rash, pruritis, or mouth ulcers. Prior to each injection of parenteral gold, patients should be questioned as to the occurrence of mucocutaneous symptoms; patients on oral gold should be advised to report the occurrence of skin rash or symptoms of stomatitis that may arise between monthly blood checks. The majority of mucocutaneous side effects are best managed by interruption of therapy and then resuming treatment at a lower dose once the dermatitis or stomatitis has resolved.

Nitritoid reactions are vasomotor responses to injection of gold manifest by symptoms of flushing, nausea, vomiting, sweating, or dizziness. Such reactions are rarely seen following administration of aurothioglucose, but have been reported with use of auranofin. The peripheral vasodilatation associated with nitritoid reactions is usually well tolerated, but in elderly patients with arteriosclerotic vascular disease may, it result in stroke or myocardial infarction.

TETRACYCLINES—MINOCYCLINE AND DOXYCYCLINE

In addition to their well-established antimicrobial effects, tetracyclines have a variety of effects on leukocytes and enzymes involved in immune responses that likely account for their moderate efficacy in the management of rheumatoid arthritis. Tetracyclines inhibit the activity of matrix metalloproteases and have demonstrated efficacy in preventing bone resorption in patients with periodontal disease.

In controlled trials examining the efficacy of minocycline in the treatment of rheumatoid arthritis, very few side effects were experienced that required discontinuation of the drug. Side effects most commonly experienced among patients using tetracyclines over extended time periods include nausea and anorexia. Photosensitivity is not uncommon, particularly associated with use of doxycycline. Vertigo and the development of slate-gray skin pigmentation are most often associated with use of minocycline. Rare complications other than hypersensitivity reactions include hepatitis, interstitial nephritis, pronounced eosinophilia, leukemoid reactions, and drug-induced lupus syndromes.

Given the adverse effects of tetracyclines on skeletal development in the fetus as well as pigmentation of unerupted teeth, tetracyclines should not be given to pregnant women or young children. Although there are no published guidelines for adult patients taking tetracyclines over extended time periods, surveillance at 3-month intervals for possible hematologic, liver, or renal abnormalities with routine blood counts, serum creatinine, and liver transaminases is advisable. Flare of joint symptoms while on minocycline requires consideration of the possibility of an evolving drug-induced lupus syndrome; the syndrome is often associated with hepatitis, usually associated with a positive antinuclear antibody test and prompt resolution of joint symptoms upon withdrawal of the drug.

Cytotoxic and Antiproliferative Drugs

CYCLOPHOSPHAMIDE

The effects of cyclophosphamide are mediated through its active metabolites, hydroxycyclophosphamide and phosphoramide mustard, which alkylate DNA, resulting in breaks in DNA, decreased DNA synthesis, and cell apoptosis. Although the relationship between the drug's cytotoxic effects and its immunoregulatory effects remain unclear, T-cell proliferation and the proliferation and function of B-cell lymphocytes are significantly affected by cyclophosphamide. Daily oral cyclophosphamide is frequently the drug of choice for the management of patients with systemic necrotizing vasculitis and for patients with active lung inflammation associated with autoimmune disease. Intermittent intravenous "pulse" cyclophosphamide is commonly employed in patients with certain manifestations of lupus. The toxicities of cyclophosphamide include reversible myelosuppression, bladder toxicity, ovarian failure, and irreversible oligospermia.

The adverse effects of cyclophosphamide are dependent in part on the administered dose and whether the drug is given as a daily oral dose or as a periodic intravenous pulse. Effects of intravenous pulse dosing on peripheral leukocyte counts are fairly predictable, with a nadir in the leukocyte count occurring within 8 to 14 days following a single intravenous dose and full recovery 21 days postdose. To achieve the desired clinical effects in lupus patients without inducing severe leukopenia and the attendant risk of infection, subsequent doses of intravenous cyclophosphamide are usually adjusted on the basis of the WBC nadir 10 to 14 days postdose, attenuating the dose if the WBC nadir is $<1,500/mm^3$. It is also prudent to assess the WBC immediately prior to each intravenous dose. In the doses employed for management of rheumatologic disorders, pulse intravenous doses of cyclophosphamide generally have minimal, if any, impact on platelet counts.

The hematologic effects of daily oral cyclophosphamide are much less predictable. Drug-induced leukopenia as well as thrombocytopenia may occur at any time during the course of treatment. Blood counts should be monitored a minimum of every 2 weeks following initiation of therapy. For management of vasculitides such as microscopic polyangiitis or granulomatosis with angiitis (Wegener's granulomatosis), clinical efficacy does not require induction of cytopenia. Once a stable target dose (usually 2 mg/kg/day) has been established and blood counts have been stable for a minimum of 6 to 8 weeks, the interval between blood count determinations can be extended to every 4 weeks; longer intervals between blood count determinations are not recommended.

Toxic effects of cyclophosphamide on the bladder are also related to the route of administration as well as the duration of therapy. With attention to hydration at the time of administration, pulse intravenous cyclophosphamide in doses employed for management of lupus generally does not result in bladder toxicity. Bladder toxicity primarily occurs in the setting of long-term daily oral cyclophosphamide and is due to exposure of vesicular epithelium to acrolein, a cyclophosphamide metabolite. Microscopic or gross hematuria is the common presenting feature of acrolein toxicity. In the setting of either oral or intravenous cyclophosphamide therapy, urinalysis should be performed monthly with prompt urologic evaluation of nonglomerular hematuria. The risk of bladder cancer is significantly increased in patients who receive cyclophosphamide; major risk factors are daily oral dosing, a history of cyclophosphamide-induced cystitis, smoking, duration of therapy of more than 2 years, and a cumulative dose in excess of 100 g (9). For patients who have experienced an episode of cyclophosphamide-induced cystitis, life-long surveillance for bladder cancer is recommended with yearly urinalysis and urine cytologic evaluation.

Regardless of the route of administration, there is a 45% to 71% percent risk of ovarian failure following treatment with cyclophosphamide, with highest rates observed among women who are older and who have received higher cumulative doses. Similar rates of azoospermia are reported for males receiving alkylating agents, such as cyclophosphamide. To preserve future fertility, sperm or ova can be banked before treatment with cyclophosphamide is initiated. There is no evidence that prior treatment of either parent with cyclophosphamide is associated with genetic abnormalities in subsequent offspring.

Treatment with oral cyclophosphamide is associated with a two- to fourfold increased risk of malignancy. Bladder, skin, myeloproliferative, and oropharyngeal cancers have been reported more commonly among patients with RA treated with daily cyclophosphamide than patients with RA not treated with cyclophosphamide. Although there are insufficient data to render a quantifiable risk for malignancy following treatment with pulse intravenous cyclophosphamide, few malignancies have been reported in this setting.

CHLORAMBUCIL

Chlorambucil and its primary metabolite, phenylacetic acid mustard, are potent alkylating agents. The clinical effects are comparable to cyclophosphamide, although slower in onset. Chlorambucil does not induce bladder toxicity and is most often used as an alternative to cyclophosphamide when cytotoxic therapy is indicated. It is often the drug of choice to suppress clones of immunoglobulin light chain secreting cells in patients with primary (AL) amyloidosis. The primary toxicity of chlorambucil is that of myelosuppression, which may occur abruptly at anytime during the course of treatment. Although reversible, chlorambucil-induced leukopenia may persist for months following discontinuation of the drug.

Because of the occurrence of precipitous leukopenia in patients taking chlorambucil, frequent surveillance for cytopenia is imperative. Following the initiation of treatment, CBCs should be assessed a minimum of every 2 weeks. Once the dose and leukocyte count are stable, the monitoring interval can be extended to every 4 weeks. The risk of myeloid leukemias as well as lymphomas is increased among patients who have been treated with chlorambucil;

this association should be considered when patients treated with chlorambucil develop persistent cytopenia, adenopathy, or otherwise unexplained constitutional symptoms.

AZATHIOPRINE AND 6-MERCAPTOPURINE

Azathioprine is a purine analogue antimetabolite that is converted following ingestion by glutathione S-transferase and sulfhydryl groups to 6-mercaptopurine (6-MP). Thiopurine metabolites of 6-MP decrease the synthesis of purine nucleotides resulting in antiproliferative effects, while incorporation of thiopurine nucleotides into DNA and RNA results in cytotoxicity. The net immunosuppressive effects of azathioprine and 6-MP are comparable, but azathioprine is better tolerated, favoring its use. Although efficacious as a disease-modifying drug in the treatment of rheumatoid arthritis, azathioprine is used most commonly as a steroid-sparing agent in the management of lupus and inflammatory myositis.

The myelosuppressive effects of azathioprine are dose related and vary considerably among individuals. Severe myelosuppression is most often associated with a genetic polymorphism in the activity of thiopurine methyltransferase (TPMT), one of the two enzymes (xanthine oxidase being the other) that convert 6-MP to inactive metabolites. Thiopurine methyltransferase activity has a trimodal distribution, with 90% of the population having normal activity, just fewer than 10% having intermediate activity, and about 1 in 300 individuals homozygous for poorly functioning TPMT; median TPMT activity is reported to be lower among African Americans relative to Caucasians (10). Myelosuppression associated with impaired TPMT appears anywhere from 1 to 3 months following initiation of treatment with azathioprine. Assays for TPMT activity are commercially available; prudent approaches at present to avoid severe myelosuppression are either to assess TPMT activity upon initiation of therapy or to carefully follow blood counts in patients at 2-week intervals following initiation of treatment with azathioprine as the dose is sequentially increased by 25 to 50 mg to the target amount (usually 2 to 3 mg/kg/day). Once the target dose has been achieved with stable blood counts, the interval for blood count surveillance can be extended to every 1 to 3 months.

Azathioprine and 6-MP are metabolized by xanthine oxidase, and use of either drug is best avoided in patients taking a xanthine oxidase inhibitor, such as allopurinol or febuxostat. For patients requiring a xanthine oxidase inhibitor to manage gout, employing an alternative immunosuppressant such as mycophenolate is recommended. If no effective alternative options exist, the dose of azathioprine should be attenuated 75% to 80% and blood counts monitored weekly.

Gastrointestinal symptoms are the most common side effects associated with use of azathioprine. Nausea, vomiting, or diarrhea often responds to dose attenuation followed by more gradual dose increases (25 mg/week) as clinically indicated. It is important to recognize that relative leukopenia is not required to achieve therapeutic immunosuppression with azathioprine. Although severe hepatitis and cholestasis are rare complications of azathioprine use, mild increases in liver enzymes occur in up to 10% of patients. Liver function tests should be checked within the first month of initiating treatment and every 3 to 4 months thereafter. A reasonable approach to patients who develop serum levels of liver transaminases in excess of twice the upper limit of normal is to withhold therapy and reinitiate treatment at a lower dose.

Other rare complications of azathioprine use include acute hypersensitivity syndromes, eosinophilia, drug fever, and drug-induced pancreatitis. There is conflicting data with regard to any increased risk of malignancy associated with azathioprine use. Although not approved for use during pregnancy, favorable outcomes have been reported when azathioprine has been used to manage and suppress the emergence of severe lupus complications through the course of pregnancy.

MYCOPHENOLATE MOFETIL

Mycophenolate mofetil is an established therapy for the suppression of graft rejection in organ transplant recipients that is acquiring an expanded role as an immunosuppressant in the management of patients with autoimmune disease. Following ingestion the drug is hydrolyzed to its active metabolite, mycophenolic acid, an inhibitor of inosine monophosphate dehydrogenase. As lymphocytes are particularly dependent on this enzyme for de novo synthesis of purines, mycophenolate selectively targets proliferation of T- and B-cell lymphocytes without a significant impact on granulopoiesis, erythropoiesis, or thrombopoiesis.

Mycophenolate has been studied as an alternative to cyclophosphamide in the management of lupus nephritis and is generally well tolerated. Most adverse events relate to GI intolerance including nausea, vomiting, diarrhea, and abdominal pain. For patients experiencing significant GI intolerance, use of mycophenolic acid preparations may be better tolerated. Liver enzyme abnormalities may occur, and patients taking mycophenolate should have liver function test performed at baseline, 1 month following initiation of therapy and every 3 to 4 months thereafter.

Other Immunomodulating Drugs

CYCLOSPORINE A AND TACROLIMUS

Originally developed and employed to suppress graft rejection in recipients of organ transplants, cyclosporine and tacrolimus are used as a disease-modifying drugs in the management of rheumatoid arthritis and other autoimmune disorders, including chronic recurrent anterior uveitis, psoriatic arthritis, and Behcet's syndrome. These drugs inhibit the activation of T cells and secretion of IL-2 (a major T-cell growth factor) by forming a cytoplasmic complex with cyclophilin. The resulting complex inactivates a phosphatase (calcineurin) required for the translocation of a factor to the nucleus that activates transcription of IL-2 and other genes associated with activation of T cells.

Although cyclosporine and tacrolimus are generally well tolerated, measurable but reversible decreases in renal function occur in the majority of patients treated. A small rise in serum creatinine within the first 3 months of treatment is fairly predictable, but often remains stable thereafter. However, an increase in serum creatinine that exceeds 30% of the baseline value portends possible irreversible nephrotoxicity. In such instances the administered dose should be attenuated by 1 mg/kg/day and temporarily discontinued if the serum creatinine remains elevated. Provided the serum creatinine level returns to within 15% of the established baseline level, cyclosporine can be safely restarted at the attenuated dose (11). Hypertension is reported to occur in approximately 20% percent of patients but can be managed with either attenuation in the dose of cyclosporine or addition of antihypertensive drug therapy.

Other common side effects of cyclosporine include tremor, paresthesia, hypertrichosis, hyperkalemia, hypomagnesemia, and hyperuricemia. Liver enzyme abnormalities, particularly a rise in serum alkaline phosphatase, occur not uncommonly, but are seldom of clinical significance. While cyclosporine use in recipients of organ transplants has been associated with an increased risk of skin cancer and lymphoma, this association has not been confirmed among smaller cohorts of patients with RA treated with cyclosporine.

DAPSONE

Originally employed in the treatment of leprosy, dapsone is a sulfone with significant inhibitory effects on the function of neutrophils. Although there are few controlled trials examining its efficacy, it is most commonly used in the management of cutaneous leukocytoclastic vasculitis, urticarial vasculitis, bullous or ulcerative cutaneous lupus, and orogenital ulcers associated with Behcet's syndrome.

Use of dapsone requires attention to dose-dependent effects of the drug on erythrocytes and the potential for drug-induced agranulocytosis. Reversible agranulocytosis affecting as many as one of every 250 individuals may occur during the first 2 months of treatment. Some degree of methemoglobinemia and hemolysis is seen in almost all patients receiving doses of 100 mg daily or higher. Although individual variation exists, the adverse effects of dapsone on red cell membranes are usually well tolerated and often stabilize or resolve after 6 weeks. However, patients deficient in glucose-6-phosphate dehydrogenase are particularly susceptible to hemolysis that may be severe and life threatening, and it is advisable to prescreen patients for evidence of this deficiency prior to instituting treatment with dapsone.

The drug is best tolerated starting with a 25 mg daily dose, advancing to the target therapeutic dose of 100 mg daily over the course of several weeks. Blood counts should be monitored weekly until the target dose has been achieved for a month and then monthly thereafter. Should a significant fall in hematocrit and hemoglobin levels occur, the drug should be withheld and reintroduced at a lower dose. Liver function tests should be assessed within the first several weeks of treatment, following any dose increments, and periodically every 3 months thereafter. A rare hypersensitivity syndrome characterized by fever, exfoliative rash, jaundice, and hemolysis may occur with dapsone use; patients with this complication should not be retreated.

THALIDOMIDE

Following its withdrawal in 1961 because of its well-publicized and dramatic teratogenic effects, thalidomide was reintroduced specifically for the management of erythema nodosum leprosum, presently its only approved indication. Thalidomide has inhibitory effects on the production of tumor necrosis factor α (TNF-α) and has been reported to be of efficacy in the treatment of severe mucocutaneous ulcers associated with Behcet's syndrome, as well as severe cutaneous lesions associated with lupus, sarcoidosis, and pyoderma gangrenosum. It has also been reported to be of benefit in the management of graft-versus-host disease.

In addition to the known teratogenic effects, peripheral neuropathy is a frequent complication of thalidomide use, and aside from the teratogenic effects, it is the major limiting factor in its long-term use. Nerve damage from thalidomide is usually manifest by symmetric, painful paresthesias that often persist despite discontinuation of the drug. Since nerve conduction abnormalities may be noted prior to the onset of neuropathy symptoms, periodic electrophysiologic testing of peripheral nerves has been advocated for patients receiving thalidomide over extended time intervals, with discontinuation of the drug if neuropathy occurs.

COMMON PITFALLS TO AVOID WHEN USING TNF INHIBITORS

1. Infections especially with reactivated mycobacteria or hepatitis B

2. Infusion reactions with infliximab

Tumor Necrosis Factor α Antagonists

ETANERCEPT

Etanercept is a genetically engineered chimeric molecule comprising two of the human p75 soluble receptors for TNF-α adjoined to the Fc portion of a human IgG. By binding TNF, etanercept precludes ligation of TNF receptors on effector cells participating in immune and inflammatory responses promoted by this cytokine. Administered as a subcutaneous injection twice weekly, etanercept is predominantly used for the management of rheumatoid arthritis and juvenile idiopathic arthritis. Etanercept is also approved for and used in the management of other rheumatic diseases including psoriatic arthritis and ankylosing spondylitis; it has also been used with success in managing manifestations of Behcet's syndrome.

Since etanercept is a fully humanized molecule, it is usually well tolerated and its use does not require routine laboratory monitoring. Injection site reactions consisting of mild erythema and swelling lasting 1 to 3 days occur in more than a third of patients, but they are well tolerated and do not preclude continuation of therapy.

ANTI-TNF-α MONOCLONAL ANTIBODIES (INFLIXIMAB, ADALIMUMAB, GOLIMUMAB)

Originally approved for use in patients with severe complications of Crohn's disease, anti-TNF-α antibodies are approved for and most commonly used in the management of rheumatoid arthritis, psoriatic arthritis, and ankylosing spondylitis. They may also be useful in the management of severe manifestations of Behcet's syndrome.

Infliximab is a chimeric monoclonal antibody consisting of a murine domain in the variable region with binding specificity for human TNF-α; the remainder of the antibody is of human origin. Administered by intravenous infusion, infliximab binds and neutralizes secreted TNF-α. Binding of infliximab to cells expressing surface TNF-α may also result in antibody-mediated cytotoxicity. Infliximab is usually well tolerated and routine laboratory monitoring for toxicity is not required. Human antichimeric antibody responses to murine components of the antibody develop in up to 40% of patients given infliximab. Infusion reactions with pruritus, urticaria, and/or chills occur in a small minority of patients and respond favorably to halting of the infusion and administration of antihistamines. Retreatment of patients who have experienced an infusion reaction is not recommended. Although not required for initial efficacy, cotreatment with low-dose weekly methotrexate has been shown to decrease (but not abrogate) human antichimeric antibody responses and may extend the duration of infliximab efficacy.

Fully humanized antibodies to TNF-α are administered as subcutaneous injections at 1- to 2-week (**adalimumab**) or 4-week (**golimumab**) intervals. The development of neutralizing antibodies is rare, and although injection site reactions may occur, they are often transient and usually do not require cessation of therapy.

CERTOLIZUMAB

Certolizumab is a pegylated construct of F(ab') components of monoclonal reagents having specificity for TNF-α covalently bound to polyethylene glycol. Its efficacy in neutralizing TNF-α is comparable to that of anti-TNF-α antibodies, but the absence of the Fc-associated complement fixing domains may render it less likely to engender injection site reactions occasionally seen with etanercept, adalimumab, or golimumab.

SURVEILLANCE FOR INFECTION, MALIGNANCY, AND AUTOIMMUNE DISEASE

Since TNF-α likely plays a role in host defense, patients who are taking any of the TNF-α inhibitors should be cautioned about the occurrence of infection and all of these reagents should be used with caution in patients predisposed to serious bacterial infections. It is generally advisable to withhold anti-TNF-α in the setting of acute bacterial infection, resuming treatment once the infection has resolved with appropriate antimicrobial therapy. Reported reactivation of tuberculosis in patients given anti-TNF-α reagents emphasizes the need for caution and careful prescreening and surveillance when administering TNF-α neutralizing antibodies to patients with risk factors for or known prior history of tuberculosis (12). Disseminated fungal infections have also been reported, and careful monitoring for this complication is prudent.

In patients with active hepatitis C, treatment with anti-TNF-α reagents has not increased viral loads, unfavorably altered the course of disease, or impaired responses to antiviral therapy. However, exacerbation of hepatitis B viral (HBV) infection has been reported in the context of therapy with anti-TNF-α reagents, and this class of biologic therapy is best avoided in the context of active HBV disease; as such, screening for HBV is recommended before starting anti-TNF-α reagents. Patients with human immunodeficiency virus (HIV) disease who develop severe psoriasis may be treated with anti-TNF-α reagents; although doing so does not appear to adversely affect responses to antiretroviral therapy, extra vigilance for bacterial, fungal, and mycobacterial infection is required in patients receiving anti-TNF-α therapy who are immunocompromised from HIV.

Emergence of lymphomas has been reported in patients receiving anti-TNF-α therapy; however, the prevalence of lymphoid malignancies has not been shown to be higher in cohorts of patients with RA who have received anti-TNF-α reagents relative to those who have not. Given the role of TNF-α in host defense against malignancy, discontinuation of treatment is nonetheless advised in the context of the development of lymphoma and other malignant neoplasms.

Administration of anti-TNF-α monoclonal reagents is associated with the development of antinuclear antibodies in a minority of patients. Clinical manifestations of lupus have been reported to occur following administration of infliximab, and anti-TNF-α antibodies are not recommended for use in patients with systemic lupus erythematosus. Up to 15% of patients taking etanercept are reported to develop new positive antinuclear antibodies, antibodies to double-stranded DNA, or both. Although no patients in premarket controlled clinical trials who developed such antibodies developed clinical manifestations of systemic lupus erythematosus, a number of postmarket case reports have documented the occurrence of demyelinating syndromes following initiation of treatment with etanercept. Although laboratory monitoring for emergence of autoantibodies is not necessary, anti-TNF-α therapy should be discontinued should autoimmune disease manifestations not normally associated with rheumatoid arthritis or spondyloarthropathies emerge.

IL-1β Antagonists

Biologics targeting IL-1β include **anakinra** (recombinant human IL-1 receptor antagonist), **canakinumab** (an anti-IL-1β monoclonal antibody), and **rilonocept** (an IL-1β receptor/accessory protein construct fused to immunoglobulin Fc). Anakinra is approved for the treatment of rheumatoid arthritis and is commonly used in the management of systemic-onset juvenile idiopathic arthritis and adult Still's disease. Canakinumab and rilonocept are approved for use in managing patients with cryopyrin-associated autoinflammatory syndromes; IL-1β antagonists are also being studied for potential use in managing and suppressing flares of gout.

IL-1β antagonists are generally very well tolerated, and their use does not require laboratory monitoring other than periodic monitoring of blood counts to monitor for leucopenia that may develop in a very small minority of patients. Injection site reactions with anakinra are common, particularly during the initial weeks of therapy, but do not require cessation of treatment and often diminish in their frequency and severity with continued treatment.

IL-6 Antagonists

Tocilizumab, a humanized monoclonal reagent with specificity for the IL-6 receptor, is approved for use in patients with rheumatoid arthritis who have failed to respond to treatment with anti-TNF-α reagents. IL-6 has multiple effects on multiple cells of the immune system as well as hepatocytes. Elevations in serum cholesterol commonly occur following initiation of treatment with tocilizumab, and monitoring of serum cholesterol is recommended during the initial months of treatment. Dose-limiting elevations in liver transaminases may also occur in the context of treatment with tocilizumab, and monitoring of AST and ALT levels at 3- to 4-month intervals is recommended. Since IL-6 promotes thrombopoiesis as well as granulopoiesis, periodic monitoring at 3-month intervals for leucopenia and thrombocytopenia is also recommended for patients receiving tocilizumab.

Biologics Targeting T-Cell Activation

Abatacept is a human recombinant construct of CTLA4 and immunoglobulin Fc that binds to ligands on antigen-presenting cells required for sending costimulatory signals to T cells through CD28. The net effect of abatacept treatment is a decrease in activation of T cells by antigen-presenting cells. Abatacept is approved for use in patients with rheumatoid arthritis who have failed to respond to conventional nonbiologic DMARD therapy. Patients receiving abatacept do not require specific laboratory monitoring, and overall infection rates are not reported to be higher in patients with rheumatoid arthritis receiving abatacept. However, vigilance for infections with pathogens in which intact T-cell function may be required for resolution is appropriate. Titers of antibodies in response to primary immunization are attenuated in patients receiving abatacept relative to those not receiving abatacept. Although the clinical significance of this attenuation is unclear, it is recommended that patients in need of primary immunization receive such immunizations prior to initiating treatment with abatacept.

Ustekinumab is a human genome–derived monoclonal reagent with specificity for the p40 subunit shared by IL-12 and IL-23. Blocking IL-12 attenuates the maturation and activation of the Th1 lineage of T cells, while blocking IL-23 attenuates the maturation and survival of T17 cells, a subset of T cells implicated in the pathogenesis of a number of autoimmune disorders, including inflammatory bowel disease, psoriasis or psoriatic arthritis, and RA. Higher-than-expected rates of infection or malignancy have not been observed in controlled studies of ustekinumab; however, given the inhibitory effects on T-cell maturation and activation, vigilance for tuberculosis and fungal infections is nonetheless recommended.

Biologics Targeting B Lymphocytes

Rituximab is a chimeric antibody, with the murine component of the antigen-binding domain having specificity for CD20 expressed on B lymphocytes, with the net effect of treatment depleting CD20$^+$ B cells. Rituximab is approved for treatment of rheumatoid arthritis not responding to conventional DMARD therapy. Rituximab has also been used in the management of other autoantibody-mediated disorders including SLE, although clinical trials in SLE with rituximab have failed to achieve primary efficacy endpoints and it is not yet approved for this indication. B-lymphocyte depletion with rituximab is well tolerated by the vast majority of patients without significant increases in observed infection risk. However, cases of progressive multifocal leukoencephalopathy (PML) because of polyoma (JC) virus replication in the CNS have been reported in patients receiving rituximab in combination with other concomitant immunosuppressive therapy. As such, monitoring and vigilance for neurologic dysfunction is prudent in patients treated with rituximab. Although plasma cells do not express CD20, levels of IgG as well as IgA and IgM may decrease over time with repeated use of rituximab, and periodic assessment of immunoglobulin levels is recommended for patients receiving multiple courses of treatment.

SECTION 6 Diagnosis and Therapy

Belimumab is a human genome–derived monoclonal antibody with specificity for B-lymphocyte stimulator (BlyS), also referred to as B-cell–activating factor (BAFF), approved for the treatment of systemic lupus erythematosus. B-lymphocyte stimulator (BAFF) is required for the survival and proliferation of B lymphocytes into antibody-secreting plasmablasts. Belimumab treatment results in decreases in titers of autoantibodies but does not impair the survival of mature plasma cells and is not associated with significant hypoglobulinemia or decreases in antibody titers generated in response to previous immunization. However, hypoglobulinemia may potentially occur if belimumab is used in combination with other immunosuppressive therapies (such as azathioprine or mycophenolate), and levels of immunoglobulins should be periodically assessed in such patients.

References

1. Saag KG, Emkey R, Schnitzer TJ, et al. Alendronate for the prevention and treatment of glucocorticoid-induced osteoporosis. *N Engl J Med* 1998;339(5):292–299.
2. Fries JF. The epidemiology of NSAID gastropathy: The ARAMIS experience. *J Clin Rheumatol* 1998; 4(Suppl):S11.
3. Silverstein FE, Graham DY, Senior JR, et al. Misoprostol reduces serious gastrointestinal complications in patients with rheumatoid arthritis receiving nonsteroidal anti-inflammatory drugs. *Ann Int Med* 1995; 123:241.
4. Morgan SL, Baggott JE, Vaughn WH, et al. The effect of folic acid supplementation on the toxicity of low-dose methotrexate in patients with rheumatoid arthritis. *Arthritis Rheum* 1990;33:9.
5. Kremer JM, Alarcon GS, Lightfoot RW, Jr, et al. Methotrexate for rheumatoid arthritis: Suggested guidelines for monitoring liver toxicity. *Arthritis Rheum* 1994;37:316.
6. Pavy S, Constantin A, Pham T, et al. Methotrexate therapy for rheumatoid arthritis: Clinical practice guidelines based on published evidence and expert opinion. *Joint Bone Spine* 2006;73(4):388–395.
7. Easterbrook M. Detection and prevention of maculopathy associated with antimalarial agents. *Int Ophthalmol Clin* 1999;39(2):49–57.
8. Blyth C, Lane C. Hydroxychloroquine retinopathy: Is screening necessary? *BMJ* 1998;316(7133):716–717.
9. Talar-Williams C, Hijazi YM, Walther MM et al. Cyclophosphamide-induced cystitis and bladder cancer in patients with Wegener's granulomatosis. *Ann Intern Med* 1996;124:477.
10. McLeod HL, Lin JS, Scott EP, et al. Thiopurine methyltransferase activity in American white subjects and black subjects. *Clin Pharmacol Ther* 1994;55:15.
11. Panayi GS, Tugwell P. The use of cyclosporin A microemulsion in rheumatoid arthritis. Conclusions of an international review. *Br J Rheumatol* 1997;36:808.
12. Tuberculosis associated with blocking agents against tumor necrosis factor-alpha—California, 2002–2003. *MMWR Morb Mortal Wkly Rep* 2004;53(30):683.

Index

Page numbers followed by f indicate figures; those followed by t indicate tables.

Abatacept, 295
Abdomen, 105
Acetabular dysplasia, 57
Acetaminophen, 26
Acetylsalicylic acid (aspirin), 148
Achilles tendinitis, 39–40
Achilles tendinopathy, 70–71
Acromegalic arthropathy, 227
Acromegaly, 227
Acro-osteolysis, 115
Acute cutaneous lupus, 103, 105
Acute monoarthritis, 5
Acute transient synovitis, 55
Adalimumab, 293
Adhesive capsulitis, 225–226, 225t
Adventitious bursa, 38
Alendronate, 209
Alkaptonuria (ochronosis), 232
Allopurinol, 192
Alphaviruses, 260–262
Amaurosis fugax, 143
American College of Rheumatology (ACR), 85,
    86t, 89, 90t, 106t, 145, 145t
American–European Consensus Group,
    80, 81t
5-aminosalicylic acid, 286
Amyloidosis, 233, 233f
Anakinra, 193, 294
Analgesia, 34
  pharmacologic, 53
Analgesics, 179
Anaplasma phagocytophilum, 252
Anemia of chronic inflammation, 104
Ankle joint, 277
  stability, 72f

Ankle sprain, 43, 71–73, 71f, 72f
Ankylosing spondylitis, 3, 7, 96, 101
Anterior cruciate ligament, 51
Anterior right hip ligaments, 57f
Anterior talofibular ligaments (ATFL), 71, 71f
Anterior tarsal tunnel syndrome, 42
Antimalarials, 285–286
Antineutrophil cytoplasm antibody
    (ANCA), 134
Antinuclear antibodies (ANA), 126, 160
Antiphospholipid antibody, 108
Antirheumatic therapy
  antimalarials, 285–286
  B lymphocytes, biologics targeting, 295–296
  colchicine, 283
  corticosteroids, 280–281
  cytotoxic and antiproliferative drugs
    azathioprine, 290
    chlorambucil, 289–290
    cyclophosphamide, 288–289
    cyclosporine, 291
    dapsone, 291–292
    6-mercaptopurine, 290
    mycophenolate mofetil, 291
    tacrolimus, 291
    thalidomide, 292
  disease-modifying antirheumatic drugs
    (DMARDs), 283–284
  gold salts, 287
  IL-6 antagonists, 294–295
  IL-1β antagonists, 294
  leflunomide, 286–287
  methotrexate, 284–285, 285t
  nonsteroidal anti-inflammatory drugs
    (NSAIDs), 281–283, 282t

297

Antirheumatic therapy (*Continued*)
  sulfasalazine, 286
  T-cell activation, biologics targeting, 295
  tetracyclines, 287–288
  tumor necrosis factor (TNF)-α antagonists
    anti-TNF-α monoclonal antibodies, 293
    certolizumab, 293
    etanercept, 292–293
    surveillance for infection, 293–294
Anti-Scl70, 115
Antispasmodics, 180
Anti-TNF-α monoclonal antibodies, 293
Anxiolytics, 165
Apley grind test, 50, 50f
Arc sign, painful, 68f
Arthralgias, 6, 151, 231
Arthritis, HCV-related, 259
Arthritis–dermatitis syndrome, 3
Arthritis mutilans, 82, 82f
Arthrocentesis, 53, 274
  complications, 276
  equipment, 275, 275t
  techniques for, 275–276
    ankle joint, 277
    elbow, 278, 279f
    knee, 276–277, 277f
    metacarpophalangeal joint, 277, 277f
    metatarsophalangeal joint, 277, 278f
    shoulder, 277–278
    subacromial bursa, 278, 278f
    wrist, 278–279, 279f
Arthropathies, 224f. *See also* Gout and
    crystal–induced arthropathies
  amyloidosis, 233, 233f
  crystal-induced, 3
  with endocrine diseases
    acromegaly, 227
    adhesive capsulitis, 225–226, 225t
    charcot neuroarthropathy, 224–225, 224f
    diabetes mellitus, 223
    hyperparathyroidism and hypovitaminosis
      D, 227, 227f
    hyperthyroidism, 226–227
    hypothyroidism, 226, 227t
  with hematologic disorders

    hemophilia, 231
    sickle cell disease, 230, 230f
  with hereditary disorders
    alkaptonuria (ochronosis), 232
    of connective tissues, 232
    hemochromatosis, 231–232, 231f
    Wilson's disease, 232
  with malignancies
    carcinomatous polyarthritis, 228–229
    complex regional pain syndrome (CRPS), 229
    hypertrophic osteoarthropathy (HOA), 228, 228f
    multicentric reticulohistiocytosis (MR), 229,
      229f
    RS3PE, 229–230
  sarcoidosis, 234
Arthropathies, crystalline, 87–88
Articular complaints, patients with
  comorbidities, 6
  patient's background
    age, 3–4
    ethnic predilection, 4
    gender, 4
  symptomatology
    inflammatory changes, presence of, 5–6
    patterns of joint involvement, 4–5
    signs and symptoms, 6
Aspirin, low-dose, 113
Asymmetric oligoarthritis, 88
Atherosclerosis, 147
Atlas, anatomy of, 12, 13f
Atypical connective tissue disease (ACTD),
      150, 151t
Auranofin, 287
Aurothioglucose, 287
Autoimmune hemolytic anemia, 104
Autoimmune thyroiditis, chronic, 226
Avascular necrosis, 62f, 63f
Axis, anatomy of, 12, 13f
Azathioprine, 107, 290

Bacteremia, 274
Bacterial arthritis, 239–241, 239f
  in children, 244–245
  clinical course, 244
  clinical presentation, 241

examination, 241–242, 242t

in immunocompromised patients, 245

prosthetic joint infections, 245

studies, 242–243, 243t

treatment, 244

B-cell–activating factor (BAFF), 296

Behçet's disease, 4, 134

Belimumab, 108, 296

Benign hypermobility syndrome, 232

Bicipital tendinitis, 33

Bisphosphonates, 209–212, 210t, 211f

and teriparatide, 214

Black-legged tick, 249f, 252

Bladder toxicity, 289

Bleeding diathesis, 274

B lymphocyte(s), 295–296

B-lymphocyte stimulator (BAFF), 296

β_2-microglobulin amyloidosis, 233

Bohan and Peter criteria, 121t

Bone mineral density (BMD), 200, 201, 201f,
205, 205f

Bone scan, 19, 39

Bone scintigraphy, 221

Bone spurs, 175

Bone turnover, biochemical markers of,
204, 204t

Bony joint enlargement, 175f

Bony swelling, 231

Borrelia burgdorferi (Lyme disease), 159

Bosentan, 113

Bouchard's nodes, 175

Boutonniere deformity, 82, 82f

Braces, 45–46

Brown tumors hyperparathyroid, 227f

Buckling of knee, 49

Bunionette, 39

Bursectomy, 64

Cachexia, 143

Calcaneofibular ligament (CFL), 71, 71f

Calcific tendinitis, 35

Calcitonin, 209

Calcium, 207

and vitamin D, 207–208, 208t, 213–214

Calcium channel blockers, 113

Calcium pyrophosphate crystal deposition
(CPPD), 88

Calcium pyrophosphate dihydrate deposition
disease, 194, 195t

Calluses, 38, 43

Cancer-associated myositis, 122k

Capsaicin, 179

Carcinomatous polyarthritis, 228–229

Carpal tunnel syndrome, 115

Cauda equina syndrome, 26

Ceftriaxone, 255

Celiac sprue, 220

Centers for Disease Control and Prevention
(CDC), 247, 250f

Certolizumab, 293

Cervical collars, 19

Cervical radiculopathy, 19, 20

Cervical spine, 84–85

Cervical spondylosis, 18

Chapel Hill Consensus Conference (CHCC), 133

Charcot neuroarthropathy, 224–225, 224f

Chest, 105

Chlorambucil, 289–290

Chloroquine, 285

Chondroitin sulfate, 180

Chondromalacia patellae, 68–69

Chronic fatigue syndrome (CFS), 159

Chronic gout, 187

Churg–Strauss syndrome, 136

Clinical Disease Activity Index (CDAI), 89

Cocked-up toes, 39

Codman pendulum exercises, 34, 34f

Colchicine, 190, 283

Collateral ligaments, 51

Comorbidities, 55

Complete blood count (CBC), 284

Complex regional pain syndrome (CRPS), 229

Computed tomography, 19, 44, 52, 61

Connective tissue disease (CTD). See under
Overlap syndromes

Cooling of tissues, 46

Corticosteroids, 107, 129, 280–281

Corticotropin, 191

Cranial arteritis, 142–143

Crepitus, 40

Crescent sign, 221f
CREST syndrome, 113
Cricoarytenoid joint, 85
Crohn's disease, 97
Cryoglobulinemia, mixed, 259
Crystal deposition disease, 5
Crystal-induced arthropathies, 3. *See also* Gout
    and crystal-induced arthropathies
Crystalline arthropathies, 87–88
Cutaneous fibrosis, 115
Cutaneous lupus, 103–104
Cutaneous small-vessel vasculitis, 135
Cyclophosphamide, 288–289
  high dose, 108
Cyclosporine, 186, 291
Cytotoxic and antiproliferative drugs

Dapsone, 291–292
Decompressive laminectomy, 27
Deep peroneal nerve entrapment, 42
Deer tick, 249f, 252
Definitive diagnosis, 87
Degenerative disc disease, 21
Degenerative joint disease. *See* Osteoarthritis
    (OA)
Denosumab, 212
Depocorticosteroids, 180
Depression, 27
Dermatomes of cervical spine, 16f
Dermatomyositis (DM), 118, 119, 120f, 121t, 153.
    See also Inflammatory myopathies
Diabetes mellitus, 223
Diabetes myonecrosis, 8
Diagnostic test, 271–273, 272t
Diagnostic ultrasonography, 44
Diet and alcohol, 185
Diffuse scleroderma, 113
Dime ticks transmission, 249f
Disease Activity Score (DAS), 89
Disease-modifying antirheumatic drugs
    (DMARD), 283–284
  biologic, 90, 92
  synthetic, 90, 91t
Distal interphalangeal joint (DIP), 80, 82
Distraction test, 17

DMARD. *See* Disease-modifying antirheumatic
    drugs (DMARD)
Donut lesion, 221
Doxycycline, 255, 287
Drawer test, anterior, 72
Dual-energy x-ray absorptiometry (DXA),
    204, 205f
Dynamic sonography, 62

Elbow, 81, 278, 279f
Electrodiagnostic studies, 42, 43
Electromyography, 18, 126
Ely's test, 60
Encephalopathy, chronic, 254
Endocrine diseases. *See under* Arthropathies
Enteropathic arthritis, 97–98, 101
Enthesitis, 40
Enthesopathies, 96
Enzyme-linked immunosorbent assay (ELISA), 255
Epiphyseal ischemic necrosis, 230
Epiphysis, 56f
Erythema migrans (EM), 250, 252, 253f
Erythrocyte sedimentation rate (ESR), 140, 144
Estrogen, 208
Etanercept, 292–293
European League Against Rheumatism (EULAR),
    85, 86t
Exercise biking, 27
Exercises, 177, 207
  quadriceps-strengthening, 53
Extra-articular manifestations of RA (ExRA), 79,
    79t
Extracorporeal shockwave therapy (ESWT), 71
Extremities, 105

FABER maneuver, 59, 60f
Facial nerve palsy treatment, 255
Familial hypocalciuric hypercalcemia (FHH),
    218
Familial Mediterranean fever, 4
Febuxostat, 192
Feet and ankles, 83–84, 84f
Fibromyalgia (FM), 146, 158–159
  clinical course, 165
  clinical presentation, 159–160, 161t

examination, 162

   studies, 162, 163t

   treatment, 162, 163–165

Fibromyalgia impact questionnaire, 164

Fingers, 82, 82f

Flat feet, 38

Flavivirus, 258

Foot orthoses, 44

Footwear, 177

Forefoot varus and valgus deformities, 37

Frank arthritis, 262

FRAX WHO fracture risk assessment tool,
   206f

Freiberg disease, 39

Fructose, 185

Fungal infections, 293

Gabapentin, 26, 27

Gait abnormalities, 59

Gene expression analysis, 124

Giant cell arteritis (GCA), 132, 133–134, 140, 141f

   aortitis and peripheral arterial occlusion, 143

   clinical course, 148

   clinical presentation, 141–142, 142t

   cranial arteritis, 142–143

   polymyalgia rheumatica, 143

   studies, 144–145, 145t

     differential diagnoses, 145–147, 145t, 146t

   treatment, 147–148, 148t

   wasting and cachexia, 143

Glenohumeral arthritis, 30

Glucocorticoid, 280

Glucocorticoid-induced osteoporosis (GIOP),
   213–215, 214f

Glucocorticoid tapering, 148t

Glucosamine sulfate, 180

Gold salts, 287

Gonococcal arthritis, 240, 241

Gottron's papules, 119, 120f

Gout, 5

  and pseudogout, 3

Gout and crystal-induced arthropathies

   calcium pyrophosphate dihydrate deposition
     disease, 194, 195t

   clinical course, 197

   clinical presentation, 183–184, 185t, 194, 195

     diet and alcohol, 185

     genetics, 184–185

     medications and toxins, 185–186

   examination, 186–187, 186f

   studies, 187–188, 188t, 196, 196t, 197

     differential diagnosis, 188–189, 189t

   treatment, 197

     gout flares, management of, 189–191, 190t

     therapeutic approaches, 193–194

     urate-lowering therapy for hyperuricemia,
       191–193, 192f

Gout flares, management of, 189–191,
   190t

Haemophilus influenzae, 3, 244

Hallux limitus, 39

Hallux rigidus, 38–39

Hallux valgus, 38

Hammer toes, 39, 84

Hard corns, 43

Hashimoto's thyroiditis, 226

HCV. *See* Hepatitis C

Head, 105

Headache, 142

Heart, 105

Heart block, 251

Heating pads, 26

Heliotrope rash, 119, 120f

Hematologic disorders. *See under*
   Arthropathies

Hemochromatosis, 231–232, 231f

Hemophilia, 231

Henoch-Schonlein purpura, 135

Henoch-Schönlein purpura, 4

Hepatitis B (HBV), 260, 261f

Hepatitis C, 258–260. *See also under*
   Viral arthritis

Hepatosplenomegaly, 105

Hereditary disorders associated with
   arthropathies. *See under* Arthropathies

Herniated lumbar discs, 25

Highly active antiretroviral therapy (HAART),
   263

Hindfoot (calcaneal) varus, 43, 44

Hip, 84
    fractures, 201
    pain
        in adults, 56, 57–59, 58f
        clinical presentation, 55–56, 56f, 57f
        examination, 59–60, 59f, 60f
        studies, 60–63, 61f, 62f, 63f
        treatment and clinical course, 64
    protectors, 207
Hip bursae, 58f
HLA-B27, 100
Hoarseness, 85
Human immunodeficiency virus (HIV), 263
Human leukocyte antigens (HLA), 78
Hyalgan (hyaluronate sodium), 180
Hydroxychloroquine, 285
Hyperparathyroidism and hypovitaminosis D,
        227, 227f
Hyperthyroidism, 219, 226–227
Hypertrophic osteoarthropathy (HOA),
        228, 228f
Hyperuricemia, 184, 185t, 186f
Hypesthesia, 42
Hypocomplementemia, 169
Hypoglobulinemia, 296
Hypophosphatasia, 217
Hypophosphatemia, 217
Hyposplenism, 230
Hypothyroidism, 87, 226, 227t
Hypovitaminosis D, 227, 227f

Idiopathic inflammatory myopathy (IIM).
        See Inflammatory myopathies
IL-6 antagonists, 294–295
IL-1β antagonists, 294
Iliotibial band syndromes, 69–70
Immunosuppressive drugs, 107–108, 121, 122t
Impingement sign, 67f
Inclusion body myositis (IBM), 118, 121
Infarcts, acute, 230
Infectious Disease Society of America (IDSA),
        251
Inflammation, 5–6
Inflammatory arthritis, 259–260
Inflammatory bowel disease (IBD), 95, 97–98

Inflammatory myopathies
    biopsy findings in, 127f
    clinical chemistry, 125
    clinical course, 130–131
    clinical presentation, 118–119, 120f
        diagnostic criteria, 121, 121t, 122t
        differential diagnosis, 119
    electromyography, 126
    imaging studies, 128
    immunology, 126
    muscle biopsy, 126–128, 127f
    pathogenesis, 123, 124–125
    physical examination, 122–123, 124t
    treatment, 128–129
        rehabilitation, 129
        therapeutic approaches, 129–130
Infliximab, 293
Inguinal mass, 63f
Insertional tendinitis, 70
Interleukin 1β, 193
International Classification of Functioning,
        Disability, and Health (ICF), 11
International Myositis Assessment and Clinical
        Studies Group (IMACS), 129
International Society of Nephrology (ISN),
        104
Intraarticular corticosteroids, 180
Intra-articular therapy for OA, 180

Jaccoud's arthropathy, 82, 152
Jarisch–Herxheimer reaction, 256
Joint disease, 231
Joint effusions, 51
Joint involvement and diagnosis,
        4–5, 5t
Joint pain, 223

Knee, 84, 84f, 276–277, 277f
    braces, 177
    effusions, 254
    mechanical disorders of
        anatomical components of knee, 49f
        clinical course, 53
        clinical presentation, 48–49
        physical examination, 49–52

studies, 52
treatment, 52–53
Kyphoplasty, 212

Lachman test, 51
Large-vessel vasculitis. *See under* Vasculitis
Leflunomide, 107, 286–287
Legg-Calve-Perthes' disease,
    55, 56f
Ligament laxity, 45
Limited scleroderma, 113
Linear extensor erythema, 120f
Linear scleroderma, 113
Liver function tests, 286
Lofgren syndrome, 6
Low back pain
    clinical course, 27
    clinical presentation, 23–25, 24f
    examination, 25
    studies, 25–26
    treatment, 26–27
Lumber stenosis. *See* Low back pain
Lupus nephritis, 104
Lyme disease, 247–250, 247f, 248f,
    249f, 250f
    clinical course, 256
    coinfection, 252
    early disseminated disease, 250–251, 255–256
    early localized disease, 250, 250f
    late-stage disease, 251, 256
    physical examination
        cardiac symptoms, 253
        musculoskeletal, 254
        neurologic abnormalities, 253–254
        skin, 252–253, 253f
    in pregnancy, 252
    reinfection with *B. burgdorferi,* 252
    studies, 254
    treatment, 255
Lymphomas, 294

Magnetic resonance imaging (MRI), 12, 40, 52,
    61, 62f, 67, 221f, 231, 233f
Magnetic resonance imaging angiography
    (MRA), 144

Male osteoporosis, 215–216
Malignancies with arthropathies. *See under*
    Arthropathies
Marfan syndrome, 57
McMurray test, 50, 50f
Mechanic's hands, 120f, 123, 153
Medial retinacular laxity, 52
Medium-vessel vasculitis, 134
Meningitis treatment, 255
Meniscal tears, 52
    chronic, 49
6-mercaptopurine, 290
Metacarpal phalangeal joint (MCP), 80, 277,
    277f
Metacarpophalangeal joint, 82, 82f
Metatarsalgia, 39
Metatarsal stress fracture, 39, 40f
Metatarsophalangeal joint, 277, 278f
Methotrexate, 90, 107, 284–285, 285t
    oral, 130
Methylsulfonylmethane (MSM), 180
Midfoot disease, 84
Migratory arthritis, 3
Milwaukee shoulder, 197f
Minocycline, 287
Mixed connective tissue disease (MCTD),
    154–155, 154t
Monoarticular involvement, 5
Monosodium urate (MSU), 183
Morning stiffness, 15, 95, 158
Morton neuroma, 42
MRI. *See* Magnetic resonance imaging (MRI)
Mucosal ulcers, 96
Multicenter Arthroscopy of the Hip Outcomes
    Research Network, 59
Multicentric reticulohistiocytosis (MR), 229, 229f
Muscle disorders, 7–8, 8t
Muscle inflammation, 153
Musculoskeletal lupus, 104
Mycophenolate mofetil, 108, 291
Myopathy, 7

Nail-fold microscopy, 111, 111f
Narcotic analgesics, 34
Nasal ulcers, 105

National Arthritis Data Workgroup, 183
National Osteoporosis Foundation (NOF), 206
Neck pain
 clinical course, 20–22
 clinical presentation, 11–15, 14f
 physical examination, 15–17, 16f, 17t
 studies, 17–19
 treatment, 19–20
Neurologic lupus, 104
Neurologic symptoms and signs, 17t
Neuropathy, cause of, 43
Nighttime pain, 143
Nocturnal pain, 31
Nonsteroidal anti-inflammatory drugs (NSAID), 26, 101, 281–283, 282t. *See also under* Systemic lupus erythematosus (SLE)
NSAID. *See* Nonsteroidal anti-inflammatory drugs
Numbness of foot, 41

OA. *See* Osteoarthritis (OA)
Ober's maneuver, 59, 60f
Oligoarticular involvement, 5
Ophthalmoscope, 112
Oral analgesics, 27
Oral bisphosphonates, 210
Oral hygiene, 92
Oral ulcers, 105
Orthotics, 44
Orthovisc (hyaluronan), 180
Osgood–Schlatter disease, 220
Osteoarthritis (OA), 3, 174t
 clinical course, 181
 clinical presentation, 174
 diagnostic studies, 175
 epidemiology, 173
 examination, 175, 175f
 pathogenesis of, 174
 preventive therapy, 176
 symptomatic therapy of
  adjuvant agents, 180
  intra-articular therapy, 180
  medication-based, 178–179, 178t
  physical measures, 176–178, 176t

 psychosocial measures, 178
 surgical intervention, 181
 systemic oral agents, 179–180
 topical agents, 179
Osteoarthritis *versus* rheumatoid arthritis, 80f
Osteochondrosis, 39
Osteogenesis imperfecta, 219
Osteomalacia, 216–217
Osteonecrosis, 220–222, 220t, 221f. *See* Osteopenic bone diseases
Osteonecrosis of jaw (ONJ), 211, 211f
Osteopenic bone diseases, 200–201, 200f, 200t, 201f
 clinical presentation, 201–203, 202t
 examination, 203
 glucocorticoid-induced osteoporosis
  history and physical examination, 213
  prevention and treatment, 213–215, 214f
 hyperthyroidism, 219
 imaging, 204–206, 205f, 206f
 laboratory evaluation
  bone turnover markers, 204, 204t
  routine laboratory testing, 203, 203t
 male osteoporosis, 215–216
 metabolic bone manifestations, 219–220
 nonpharmacologic prevention, 207
 osteogenesis imperfecta, 219
 osteomalacia, 216–217
 osteonecrosis, 220–222, 220t, 221f
 pharmacologic prevention
  bisphosphonates, 209–212, 210t, 211f
  calcitonin, 209
  calcium and vitamin D, 207–208, 208t
  denosumab, 212
  estrogen, 208
  selective estrogen receptor modulators (SERMs), 208–209
  teriparatide, 212
 prevention and therapy, 206–213
 primary hyperparathyroidism, 218–219
 secondary hyperparathyroidism, 219
 surgical approaches, 212–213
Osteophytes, 32, 35, 38, 175
Osteotomies, 181
Ottawa Ankle Rules, 72

Overlap syndromes, 150–151, 151t, 152t
connective tissue disease (CTD)
mixed, 154–155, 154t
unclassified/undifferentiated, 155–157, 155t, 156f
rhupus, 151–153, 152f
sclerodermatomyositis or scleromyositis, 153
Oxalate crystal, 197

Painful feet
clinical course, 46
examination, 43
mechanical problems
achilles tendinitis, 39–40
achilles tendon rupture, 40
bunionette, 39
forefoot varus and valgus deformities, 37
Freiberg disease, 39
hallux rigidus, 38–39
hallux valgus, 38
hammer toes, 39
metatarsalgia, 39
metatarsal stress fracture, 39, 40f
peroneal tendon dislocation and peroneal tendinitis, 41
pes cavus, 38, 38f
pes planus, 38, 38f
plantar fasciitis, 41
posterior tibial tendinitis and rupture, 41
retrocalcaneal bursa, 40–41
sesamoid injuries, 39
subcutaneous achilles bursitis, 41
neurological problems, 41
anterior tarsal tunnel syndrome, 42
morton neuroma, 42
superficial peroneal nerve entrapment, 42–43
sural nerve entrapment, 43
tarsal tunnel syndrome, 42
studies, 43–44
treatment
braces, 45–46
modalities, 46

orthoses, 44–45
shoe modification, 45
steroid injections, 46
therapeutic exercise, 46
Palindromic rheumatism, 88–89
Palpation, 41, 43
Paresthesias, 42
Parvovirus B19, 257–258, 258f
Patellar laxity, 52
Patellofemoral disease, 51
Patellofemoral pain syndrome (PFPS), 68–69
Patrick's maneuver, 60, 99, 99f
Pedal edema, 105
Percutaneous vertebroplasty, 212
Peripheral arterial occlusion, 143
Peripheral neuropathy, 41
Peroneal tendon dislocation, 41
Pes cavus, 38, 38f
Pes planus, 38, 38f
Photosensitive diffuse erythroderma, 120f
Pistol grip deformity, 57
Plantar fasciitis, 41
Plaster casting, 224
Polyarthritis, 5, 89
Polyethylene glycol (PEG)–linked uricase (pegloticase), 193
Polymyalgia rheumatica (PMR), 4, 89–92, 140, 143, 146t, 148t. *See also* Giant cell arteritis (GCA)
Polymyositis, 118, 121t. *See also* Inflammatory myopathies
Popliteal cysts, 49, 84
Posterior longitudinal ligament, 12
Posterior talofibular ligaments (PTFL), 71, 71f
Posterior tibial tendinitis and rupture, 41
Prazosin, 113
Prednisone, 107
Pregnancy and rheumatic diseases
clinical course, 168–169
examination, 167
studies and treatment, 167–168
Pretest probability, 269, 270
Primary hyperparathyroidism, 218–219
Prophylactic therapy, 108
Prosthetic joint infections, 245

Prosthetic joints, 274

Proximal interphalangeal joints (PIP), 39, 80

Proximal muscle weakness, 8

Pseudogout, 5, 88, 194

Pseudorheumatoid arthritis, 195

Psoriatic arthritis, 3, 97, 101

Pulmonary disease, 115

Pulmonary fibrosis, 130

Pulmonary function tests, 117

Pulmonary hypertension, 105

Pulse therapy, 107

Pump-bumps, 41

Pyomyositis, 8

Pyrimidines, 286

Quadriceps-strengthening exercises, 53

RA. *See* Rheumatoid arthritis

Radiographs, 52, 60, 61f, 77f, 83f

Radionuclide scans, 243

Radionuclide scintigraphy, 61

Raloxifene, 209

Range-of-motion exercises, 34, 46

Raynaud's phenomenon (RP)
    clinical course, 113
    clinical presentation, 111–112
    studies, 112
    treatment, 112–113

Reactive arthritis, 3, 97, 101

Recombinant parathyroid hormone, 212

Referred pain, 55

Reflux esophagitis, 130

Reiter's syndrome, 3

Remitting, seronegative, symmetrical synovitis with pitting edema (RS3PE), 88–89, 229–230

Renal insufficiency, 284

Renal urate excretion, 184

Retrocalcaneal bursa, 40–41

Rheumatic diseases
    articular complaints, patients with
        clinical presentation, 3–6, 4t, 5t
        physical findings, 6–7

muscle disorders, patients with
    clinical presentation, 7
    physical findings, 7–8, 8t

Rheumatic disorders, diagnostic tests for, 269–273, 270f, 271f, 272t

Rheumatoid arthritis (RA), 4
    classification criteria of, 85, 86t, 87t
    clinical course, 92
    clinical presentation, 78–79, 79t
    crystalline arthropathies, 87–88
    diagnosis of, 85
    epidemiology, 77–78
        gender and hormonal influences, 78
        genetic and environmental risk factors, 78
    examination
        cervical spine, 84
        cricoarytenoid joint, 85
        elbow, 83
        feet and ankles, 83–84, 84f
        fingers, 82, 82f
        hips, 84
        knees, 84, 84f
        metacarpophalangeal (MCP) joints, 82, 82f
        shoulders, 83
        wrists, 82–83, 83f
    extra-articular manifestations of RA, 79, 79t
    medications, 89–90
        biologic DMARDs, 90, 92
        corticosteroids, 90
        NSAIDs, 90
        synthetic DMARDs, 90, 91t
    palindromic rheumatism, 88–89
    polymyalgia rheumatica (PMR), 89–90
    remitting, seronegative, symmetric synovitis with pitting edema (RS3PE), 88
    Sjögren's syndrome, 79
        diagnosis of, 80, 81t
        treatment of, 92
    SLE, 88
    spondyloarthropathies, 88
    treatment, 89, 90t
    viral arthritis, 89

Rheumatologists, 160

Rhupus, 151–153, 152f

Rituximab, 108, 295

Rose Bengal tests, 80

Rotator cuff, 31

Rotator cuff tendinitis, 66–68, 67f. *See also under* Sports–related injuries

Routine Assessment of Patient Index Data 3 (RAPID-3), 89

RS3PE. *See* Remitting, seronegative, symmetrical synovitis with pitting edema (RS3PE)

Rubella and rubella vaccine, 262–263

Rupture of achilles tendon, 40

Sacroiliac joints, 98

Sacroiliitis, 99
  testing, 98f, 99f

S-adenosylmethionine (SAM-e), 180

Sarcoidosis, 4, 234

Saturnine gout, 3

Schöber's test, 100f

Sclerodactyly, 114

Scleroderma sine scleroderma, 14

Sclerodermatomyositis, 153

Scleromyositis, 153

Secondary hyperparathyroidism, 219

Selective estrogen receptor modulators (SERMs), 208–209

Septic arthritis, 189, 239f

Serologic testing, 254

Seronegative spondyloarthropathies, 3, 4
  ankylosing spondylitis, 96
  clinical course, 101
  clinical presentation, 95–96
  enteropathic arthritis, 97–98
  examination, 98–99, 98f, 99f, 100f
  psoriatic arthritis, 97
  reactive arthritis, 97
  studies, 99–100
  treatment, 100–101

Serositis, 105

Serum urate, 187

Sesamoid injuries, 39

Sesamoiditis, 39

Shawl sign, 123

Shoe modifications, 45

Short tau inversion repeat (STIR), 128

Shoulder, 83, 277–278
  pain
    clinical course, 35
    clinical presentation, 30–31, 31f
    physical examination, 31–33, 32f
    studies, 33
    treatment, 34–35, 34f

Sickle cell disease, 230, 230f

Single-photon-emission computerized tomography, 165

Sjögren's syndrome, 108–109. *See under* Rheumatoid arthritis (RA)

Skin, 105
  lesions, 96
  rash, 252, 253f

SLE. *See* Systemic lupus erythematosus (SLE)

Sleep disturbances, 160
  with pain, 225

Slipped capital femoral epiphysis (SCFE), 55, 56

Small-vessel vasculitis. *See under* Vasculitis

Smoking, risk of, 78

Snapping hip syndrome, 58

Soft corns, 43

Spinal fracture, 205

Spine anatomy, 25, 26f

Spondyloarthropathies, 88

Spondylosis, 21

Sports-related injuries
  achilles tendinopathy, 70–71
  ankle sprain, 71–73, 71f, 72f
  iliotibial band syndromes, 69–70
  patellofemoral pain syndrome (PFPS), 68–69
  of rotator cuff
    clinical course, 68
    clinical presentation, 66, 67f
    examination, 66–67, 67f, 68f
    studies, 67–68
    treatment, 68

Spurling's test, 17

Standardized incidence ratio (SIR), 123

Staphylococcus aureus, 240

Staphylococcus aureus, 134

Sternocleidomastoids, 15

Steroid injections, 46

Steroid myopathy, 281

Stiffness, 95
Stinchfield test, 60
Straight leg raise against resistance test, 60
Straight leg-raising test, 25, 25f
Subacromial bursa, 278, 278f
Subacute cutaneous lupus erythematosus
    (SCLE), 104
Subcutaneous achilles bursitis, 41
Sulfasalazine, 286
Superficial peroneal nerve entrapment, 42–43
Supervised rehabilitation, 53
Supportive devices, 177
Sural nerve entrapment, 43
Swan neck, 82f
Swelling, 83
Symptomatic therapy of OA. *See under*
    Osteoarthritis (OA)
Symptom severity (SS), 162
Synovial fluid, 226
Synvisc (HYLAN GF 20), 180
Systemic lupus erythematosus (SLE), 4, 88, 271
  clinical course, 106
  constitutional, 105
  cutaneous lupus, 103–104
  epidemiology
  examination, 105–106
  hematologic lupus, 104
  laboratory assessment of, 106
  lupus nephritis, 104
  musculoskeletal lupus, 104
  neurologic lupus, 104
  NSAIDs
    antiphospholipid antibody, 108
    biologics, 108
    cardiovascular risk factors, 109
    immunosuppressive drugs, 107–108
    prednisone/corticosteroids, 107
    Sjögren's syndrome, 108–109
  organ manifestations, 103
  pathogenesis, 103
  serositis, 104
  treatment, 106–107
Systemic sclerosis (SSc), 4, 113–114. *See also*
    Raynaud's phenomenon (RP)
  clinical course, 116–117

clinical presentation,
    114–115
  studies, 115–116
  treatment, 116
Systemic vasculitis, 4, 86

Tacrolimus, 291
Tailor's bunion, 39
Takayasu's arteritis, 4, 134
Tarsal tunnel syndrome, 42
T-cell activation, 295
Telangiectasias, 114
Tenderness
  to palpation, 58
  on passive abduction, 33
Tenosynovitis, 3
Teriparatide, 212
Testosterone, 216
Tetracyclines, 287–288
Thalidomide, 292
Theileria microti, 252
Thenar atrophy, 83f, 84
Thermal modalities, 177
Thermoplastic materials, 44
Thiazide diuretics, 192
Thiopurine methyltransferase (TPMT), 290
  testing, 107
Thomas heel, 45
Thomas test, 60
Thompson test, 40, 70, 70f
Thrombocytopenia, 104
Tibiotalar joint, 277
Tinel sign, 42, 43
Tocilizumab, 294
Togaviridae, 260, 262
Tophi, 187
Tourniquet test, 42
Trabecular bone, 213
Tramadol, 179
Trapezius muscle, 30, 31f
Treatment algorithm for glucocorticoid-
    associated bone disease, 214–215, 214f
Trendelenburg sign, 59f
Tricyclic antidepressants (TCA), 26, 164
Trochanteric bursitis, 64

Trochanteric pain syndrome, 58
T-score, 204, 205f
Tumor necrosis factor-α, 292–294. *See also under*
　　Antirheumatic therapy

Ulcerative colitis, 97
Ulcers, 105
Ulnar deviation, 82, 82f
Unclassified/undifferentiated connective tissue
　　disease, 155–157, 155t, 156f
Urate-lowering therapy for hyperuricemia,
　　191–193, 192f
Urate oxidase (uricase), 193
Uric acid, 3, 184
Uricosuric drugs, 193
Ustekinumab, 295

Vaccinations for influenza, 106
Vacuolar myopathy, 283
Valgus deformities, forefoot varus and, 37
Vasculitis
　　clinical course, 137–138, 138t
　　clinical history, 135
　　clinical presentation, 132–133, 132f,
　　　133t
　　epidemiology, 133
　　examination, 135–136
　　large-vessel
　　　giant cell arteritis, 133–134
　　　Takayasu's arteritis, 134
　　medium- to small-vessel, 134
　　medium-vessel, 134
　　small-vessel
　　　cutaneous, 135
　　　Henoch–Schonlein purpura, 135

studies, 136–137
　　treatment, 137
Vasculopathy, 114
Vertebra, anatomy of, 13f
Vertebral fracture analysis (VFA), 205
Viral arthritis, 89
　　alphaviruses, 260–262
　　hepatitis B (HBV), 260, 261f
　　hepatitis C (HCV), 258
　　　coexisting inflammatory arthritis,
　　　　259–260
　　　HCV-related arthritis, 259
　　　mixed cryoglobulinemia, 259
　　human immunodeficiency virus (HIV), 263
　　parvovirus B19, 257–258, 258f
　　rubella and rubella vaccine, 262–263
Viral infections, 6
Viremia, 258
Viscosupplements, 180
Vitamin D, 207–208, 208t

Wasting and cachexia, 143
Weak hip abductors, 58f
Wegener's granulomatosis (WG), 134
Weight loss, 176
Whiplash injuries, 21
Widespread Pain Index (WPI), 163
Wilson's disease, 232
Wrist, 82–83, 83f, 278–279, 279f

X-rays, 18, 56, 62f, 224f

Zig-zag deformity, 81
Zoledronic acid, 210
Z-scores, 204, 205f